AF748848

THE LIBRARY

WESTMINSTER
MEDICAL SCHOOL.

HISTORY OF THE BRITISH MEDICAL ASSOCIATION

Volume II 1932-1981

THE LIBRARY
WESTMINSTER
MEDICAL SCHOOL.

HISTORY OF THE BRITISH MEDICAL ASSOCIATION

Volume II 1932-1981

by

ELSTON GREY-TURNER
C.B.E., M.C., T.D., M.D., M.R.C.S., L.R.C.P.
(Secretary, B.M.A., 1976-79)

and

F. M. SUTHERLAND
M.A., F.L.A.
(Librarian, B.M.A., 1961-81)

THE LIBRARY
WESTMINSTER
MEDICAL SCHOOL.

Published by the
BRITISH MEDICAL ASSOCIATION
TAVISTOCK SQUARE, LONDON WC1H 9JP
1982

© British Medical Association 1982.
ISBN 0 7279 0091 9

Made and printed in Britain by
Thomas Reed Printers Limited, Sunderland

Acknowledgments

The first volume of the *History of the British Medical Association* covered the period 1832-1932. When the BMA was considering suitable ways of celebrating the 150th birthday of the Association, which falls in 1982, it was decided that the history should be brought up to date with a second volume. With great reluctance, we accepted the invitation to undertake this daunting task.

We are deeply grateful for the help of many people. Much help was received from members of the BMA staff, especially Dr Stephen Lock and Mr A J Smith (the Editor and the Publishing Director of the *British Medical Journal*), Dr John Havard (Secretary), Dr Gordon Macpherson (Deputy Editor), Mr D J Wright (Librarian), and Miss Hilary Rhodes, who prepared the successive typescripts with her usual scrupulous efficiency.

Among many others who helped us with information or comment, and to whom we are grateful are: Mr C A Barker, Dame Josephine Barnes, Dr Hugh Clegg, Dr Dale Falconer, Sir Ronald Gibson, Dr J C Graham, Dr David Gullick, Mr H L Hacker, Lord Hill of Luton, Mr L T Morton, Sir Harry Platt, Major-General D H G Rice (Secretary of the Central Chancery of the Orders of Knighthood), Colonel A V Tennuci (Curator of the RAMC Historical Museum), Dr John Thwaites, and Mrs Heather Windle.

We are only too conscious that, despite all our researches and despite the help of so many others, this volume falls far short of perfection. We apologise in advance to those readers who detect errors either of omission or commission, and we hope that they will bring them to our attention (FMS for Chapters 1, 7, 8 and Appendix B; EG-T for the remainder). There may be an opportunity to "put the record straight" — perhaps in the bicentenary volume which will no doubt be published in 2032.

Finally, we are profoundly grateful to our wives for their

infinite patience and forbearance when they discovered that our retirement from the staff of the BMA, at any rate up to the present, has been an illusion.

ELSTON GREY-TURNER
F M SUTHERLAND
31 December 1981

Contents

List of illustrations

Chapter 1

The Association in 1932

> The future is only the past again, entered through another gate. — Sir Arthur Pinero, *The Second Mrs Tanqueray*, Act IV.

Early on the morning of Sunday, 24 July 1932, a group of about 400 doctors arrived at Paddington Station to board a special train for Worcester. When they reached their destination at about midday they were joined by many fellow members of the medical profession, who had travelled from different parts of Great Britain and her Empire.

After a formal welcome from the Mayor of Worcester, the party went in procession through the streets of the city from the Guildhall to the cathedral, where they took part in a special service — one feature of which was the unveiling of a memorial stained-glass window. This window portrayed the figure of the beloved physician, St Luke, together with a representation of the parable of the Good Samaritan, and bore the inscription:

> The British Medical Association on the celebration of their Centenary gave this painted window as a memorial of their Founder, Sir Charles Hastings, Physician in this City.

The event which had given birth to the BMA, and which was commemorated 100 years later by this pilgrimage of its members, was a meeting which took place on 19 July 1832 in the boardroom of Worcester Infirmary. Over 50 "medical gentlemen" from the surrounding region, including the Regius Professor of Physic from Oxford, had responded to an invitation from Dr Charles Hastings, physician to the infirmary, to discuss his proposal to establish a medical association "both friendly and scientific." Its name was to be the Provincial Medical and Surgical Association, and its principal objectives were to be the advancement of medical science and the maintenance of the honour and respectability of the profession, or, as the *Lancet* described it, the Association was to be "a congenial union of scientific research and professional honour."

The proposal was enthusiastically received, the Association was formally established, and the meeting adjourned to the nearby Guildhall Coffee House for an excellent dinner at 7/6d a head, and for lively conversation that was full of optimism for the prospects of the new society. Even the most imaginative of those present, however, could hardly have foreseen the developments that would transform this little gathering of 1832 into the assembly of over 4000 doctors who came together for the centenary meeting of the BMA in London in 1932, and who represented the British medical profession on a worldwide basis.

The evolution of the Provincial Medical and Surgical Association from a small local society into one of national and international importance took place relatively quickly, because the rapid growth of medical knowledge in the nineteenth century and the need for properly trained and identified doctors to practise that knowledge called for just such an organisation.

It began as a local society because Charles Hastings and his friends wished to counterbalance what they saw as the dominance of medical practice by London and by the Royal Colleges of Physicians and Surgeons. Under the terms of the constitution drawn up for the Provincial Medical and Surgical Association, members were to be recruited from provincial towns, the headquarters were to be in Worcester, and practitioners in London were to be excluded. The Association was to be a local and provincial one in the sense that it was to represent the whole country with the exception of its capital.

The professional and scientific aims of the Association, however, were so broad and so national in character that this restrictive policy could not be sustained for long, particularly if a reputation for success in achieving those aims was to be established in the medical world.

The irresistible pull towards London occurred at an early stage and in several different ways. In an age of primitive long-distance transport it was a fundamental weakness for any society to have its headquarters in a provincial centre such as Worcester. The attainment of many of the Association's aims depended on political means, and required close and effective contact with Parliament and Ministers in London. When the Association began to publish a regular weekly journal, the *Provincial Medical and Surgical Journal*, in 1840 it was found necessary to print it in London and to establish an editorial office there.

By 1853 the very successes of the Provincial Medical and Surgical Association in its early days created a demand for membership in the capital to the extent that a Metropolitan Counties Branch was formed, despite fierce opposition from Sir Charles Hastings and other provincial members. The name of the Association was changed to British Medical Association in 1856, and in 1857 its weekly journal became the *British Medical Journal*. Henceforth, the BMA was to be a national medical society. By 1932 it seemed to the provincial general practitioner that far too much power in the BMA rested with senior London consultants. Thus the wheel had turned full circle. These great men wore top hats and frock-coats at BMA House, and the clerical staff were instructed not to share the lift with them.

During the hundred years up to 1932 the internal structure of the BMA itself reflected its transformation from a minor society to a medical organisation of major importance. The group of 50 doctors who had inaugurated the Provincial Medical and Surgical Association had increased to 316 by the time of the first annual meeting at Bristol in 1833; when the centenary meeting of the BMA took place in London in 1932 the total membership of the BMA throughout the world had risen to the remarkable figure of 35 070.

Such a rise in membership naturally produced a substantial increase in financial resources. The Bristol meeting in 1833 received a report that the Association's income during the first year amounted to £261 5s 0d, with an expenditure of £214 15s 6d; the Annual Report of the BMA Council for 1932 records an income of £157 784 13s 9d and an expenditure of £157 675 13s 7d.

During its early years the Provincial Medical and Surgical Association had no permanent staff; its business was conducted by two Secretaries, Charles Hastings and James Sheppard, who operated on a part-time basis because both were busy physicians in Worcester. In 1872 the BMA appointed its first full-time General Secretary — not a medical man. By 1932 its affairs were in the hands of a Medical Secretary, a Financial Secretary, and the Editor of the *British Medical Journal*, who, between them, had at their disposal a staff of nearly 100.

With no permanent staff, the Provincial Medical and Surgical Association had needed no buildings of its own, and this remained the position while the headquarters were still at Worcester. From the 1850s onwards, editorial offices for the Association's journal were maintained in London, but it was not until 1878 that the first administrative offices were acquired there; these were at 161A Strand. Thereafter, the phenomenal growth of the BMA led to a move to 429 Strand in 1888, the reconstruction of that house and its adornment with the controversial Epstein statues in 1907-8, and, finally, the move in 1925 to the unfinished building in Tavistock Square, which had been designed by Sir Edwin Lutyens for the Theosophical Society. Sir Edwin was commissioned by the BMA to complete his work before it took possession, and in 1929 a new block was added by C Wontner Smith to the front of the building facing the square. The result—in 1932—was a handsome edifice and a home worthy of a society that had achieved national and international status as representative of the medical profession in the United Kingdom.

The BMA has always been a voluntary society; no doctor has ever been under any compulsion to join. In the light of this, the position of strength and influence which the Association had attained by 1932 can be explained only in terms of the attraction which its objectives had for the individual doctor, and of the success which it had achieved in furthering those objectives during the nineteenth and early twentieth centuries.

When, in 1832, the Provincial Medical and Surgical Association set out "to maintain the honour and respectability of the profession," a medical profession in the proper sense of the word did not exist. There was no uniform standard of medical education, and no formal qualification or licence was required to practise medicine. Bitter rivalry among different factions of practitioners raged alongside widespread incompetence and quackery, with the inevitable result that the doctor was held in poor esteem by the public at large.

When Sir Charles Hastings and his friends in Worcester sought to improve this unhappy state of affairs they were in tune with the spirit of a decade which was dominated by the Reform Act of 1832, but it took over 25 years of incessant lobbying on their part before Parliament passed the Medical Act 1858, in which their more important aims were embodied. The Act established the General Council of Medical Education and Registration, which was to set a minimum standard of education, and which would maintain a *Medical Register* of those doctors who achieved the necessary standard. This would enable the general public to distinguish between qualified and unqualified practitioners. Further improvements were brought about by the Medical Act 1886, which was also passed as a result of continual and unwearying pressure by the BMA. The creation of a true medical profession in the United Kingdom by these two Acts was the major achievement of the BMA in the nineteenth century, and it laid firm foundations for the future prestige of the Association.

These foundations were strengthened by the energetic way in which the Association promoted the cause of underprivileged sections of the profession. Foremost among these were those practitioners who were responsible for medical care under the provisions of the Poor Law Amendment Act 1834. So harsh were the terms of this Act that these local doctors suffered almost as much as the pauper patients for whom they were responsible. They were allowed to give treatment only if permission had been granted in the first place by the relieving officer, a layman. Fees paid to doctors were totally inadequate, and had to cover the cost of drugs as well as attendance on the patient. If the local doctor showed any spirit of resistance he could be supplanted by an inexperienced student brought straight from medical school.

The young Provincial Medical and Surgical Association took immediate steps to fight these abuses when, at the Oxford annual meeting in 1835, it formed a Poor Law Committee. The reports issued by this committee led to some improvement, but it took a long and persistent battle by the BMA in the later years of the century before the matter was finally resolved in 1909 by the Report of the Royal Commission on the Poor Law and Relief of Distress. The moral for the individual doctor, however, was clear —

if he was the victim of injustice from authority, there was a medical association which he could join, and from which he could expect powerful support.

Another downtrodden section of the medical profession, whose struggle was undertaken and won by the BMA during the nineteenth century, had been the doctors serving in the Army. In the period between Waterloo and the Crimean War the status of the regimental surgeon could hardly have been lower. He suffered the worst of all worlds as he had no military rank and enjoyed none of the benefits of civilian practice. The administration of the service itself was fragmented and inefficient, and the amount of money spent on supplies and equipment was niggardly in the extreme.

The years of peace after 1815 served to conceal this appalling state of affairs, but it was immediately highlighted when the Crimean War broke out in 1854. The part played by Florence Nightingale and by William Howard Russell's dispatches to *The Times* in publicising the horrors of the Crimea are well known; less well known, but no less effective in medical circles, were vivid reports from the Crimea published by the *Association Medical Journal* — the immediate predecessor of the *British Medical Journal.*

Some minor improvements in conditions followed the Crimean War, but it took another 40 years of constant pressure by the BMA before the resistance of the military authorities was overcome and the status of the army medical officer finally recognised with the formation in 1898 of the Royal Army Medical Corps.

The long and successful campaigns which the BMA waged on behalf of Poor Law medical officers and the Army Medical Service were only preliminary skirmishes in an ever-growing contest between the medical profession and Government. In 1911 came the first full-scale battle when Mr David Lloyd George, Chancellor of the Exchequer in the Liberal Government, introduced his National Insurance Bill.

With a membership of 25 000 out of about 40 000 doctors in the United Kingdom, and with a new, democratic constitution which had been adopted in 1902, the BMA was the one body equipped to represent the whole medical profession. It was not opposed to the principle of a comprehensive medical service for the poorer section of the population — indeed, it had already recognised the need for one by publishing a report on the subject in 1911. There were, however, aspects of the Lloyd George Bill which the Association considered to be inimical to the best interests of the profession, and which they were to oppose to the limit. We now know that the more advanced and radical ideas in the Bill came from Dr Christopher (later Viscount) Addison.

Every available weapon was used in the fight, including the new and effective one of a special representative meeting. In the end, the BMA was forced to concede defeat on the main points at issue. Even so, its leadership had learnt much about the process of hard bargaining with politicians, and, for individual doctors there had been a dramatic demonstration of the fact that only through a strong, united, and centralised body such as the BMA could they hope to resist the encroachments of political authority. These lessons had only recently been learnt in 1932, but proved valuable in times to come. Even then, however, negotiations consisted solely of exchanges of formal statements by the two sides; the cut-and-thrust of argument and debate did not develop until later.

By its efforts to establish and defend the medical profession, the BMA could justly claim in its centenary year that it had been true to one of the aims of Charles Hastings and the Provincial Medical and Surgical Association — the maintenance of the honour and respectability of the profession. In furthering its other aim of advancing medical science, the Association had also proved itself worthy of its founding fathers. It had never engaged in direct medical research, but had followed the sensible course of using the methods for which it was best equipped — pressure on political and public opinion, the expression of the collective experience and wisdom of its membership, the establishment of a library, and the publication of medical information.

Very early in the Association's history there had been an outstanding example of pressure on the Government in the interests of medical science. The registration of births and deaths in the United Kingdom at the beginning of the nineteenth century was rudimentary in the extreme. The importance of accurate medical statistics was clearly recognised by the Provincial Medical and Surgical Association, which immediately after its foundation sent recommendations on the subject to the House of Commons Committee on Parochial Registers. To a large extent these recommendations were embodied in the Births and Deaths Registration Act 1836.

Much later in its history — at the beginning of the twentieth century — the BMA exerted pressure on public opinion by its telling exposure of the patent medicine industry. Large profits were being made by the sale to a gullible public of remedies, most of which were worthless and many of which were potentially dangerous. Powerful vested interests supported the trade. Stamp duty on patent medicines contributed a substantial amount to the Exchequer and the national press received a large revenue from advertising.

To unmask this medical misrepresentation, the *British Medical Journal* began in 1906 to publish a series of articles that analysed individual remedies and supplied the true facts regarding their effects and their cost. To achieve a wider circulation, the articles were collected together in 1909 and published in book form under the title of *Secret Remedies — What they cost and what they contain*; in 1912 a further volume appeared, entitled *More Secret Remedies.* This was the start of a contest with the patent medicine industry, the press, and the Government that was not resolved satisfactorily until 40 years later. It did, however, help to establish the BMA's reputation as a champion of scientific medicine and as a defender of the interests of the individual patient. In due course the reputable pharmaceutical industry gave wonderful new weapons to the medical profession and conferred enormous benefits on mankind. The BMA and the Association of the British Pharmaceutical Industry (so named in 1948) became staunch allies.

As the BMA grew, the wide experience of its members was employed increasingly in the cause of medical advancement. The exploitation of this experience was achieved mainly through meetings of members, and through investigations into special topics by committees with a background of appropriate knowledge.

During the early days of the Provincial Medical and Surgical Association, discussions of scientific subjects were a feature of the Association's annual meetings, where they were interspersed with political and business debates. In 1865 the annual scientific meeting became a self-contained institution. Apart from the annual meeting, scientific meetings had always been an integral part of the programme for local BMA divisions.

In the latter part of the nineteenth century and in the period before 1932, a great many committees were appointed by the BMA to investigate and report on special subjects. From 1881 to 1889, the Collective Investigation Committee drew on the specialised knowledge of the membership to inquire into a whole range of diseases, publishing its findings first in its own journal, the *Collective Investigation Record*, and subsequently in the *British Medical Journal*. This project was somewhat too ambitious, however, and it became more usual to set up special committees to look into subjects of topical importance. In the years immediately before 1932, reports were published on *Tests for Drunkenness* (1927), *A National Maternity Scheme for England and Wales* (1929), *Psychoanalysis* (1929), *The Problem of the Out-Patient* (1931) and *Mental Deficiency* (1932). Reports such as these, backed by authoritative medical opinion, greatly enhanced the BMA's reputation.

By 1932, apart from adding to the store of medical knowledge, the Association was making a substantial contribution to the conservation and exploitation of that knowledge by means of its library. As early as the 1830s, there had been a strong move by members of the Provincial Medical and Surgical Association to establish a library, but the suggestion was not adopted because of communication difficulties between Worcester and other parts of the country. Only later in the century, when permanent offices were opened in London, did it become practical to reconsider the question, the prime mover in raising the matter again being Ernest Hart, Editor of the *British Medical Journal*. He proposed in 1887 that the BMA Council should form a library at its headquarters, 429 Strand. Hart himself was the first librarian, and, during the early years, with many other members he presented books to the library, which grew rapidly to become one of the largest medical libraries in the country. Its usefulness to members was somewhat limited until 1918, when the lending of books and journals was started, and in 1929 the introduction of an information service was a further improvement. During the year 1931-2, 16 699 volumes were lent to members, representing a rise of 13 000 since 1922, and providing solid evidence that the library was playing an important part, not only in storing medical knowledge but also in making it available to the practising doctor.

In the final event, however, it was in publishing — as represented by its periodical, the *British Medical Journal* — that the BMA was acknowledged to be a leader in the advancement of medical science in its centenary year of 1932. Not only was this opinion held by the profession — over half of whom were members of the Association, and received their copies of the *BMJ* every week — but also by Government and by the general public, which had come to regard the journal as a representative expression of current medical thought.

Transactions and periodical publications under different names were issued by the Association from 1832 onwards, but the rise of the *British Medical Journal* to its position of authority in 1932 was largely the work of two outstanding editors, Ernest Hart and Sir Dawson Williams. Hart, who had been on the staff of the *Lancet*, brought a journalistic professionalism and a zeal for reforming causes that led to numerous controversies, but added enormously to the reputation of the *BMJ* both at home and abroad. The membership of the BMA rose from 2000 in 1867, when Hart was appointed, to over 17 000 in 1898, the year of his death. His successor, Dawson Williams — friend of Dawson of Penn, Robert Jones, Berkeley Moynihan, and George Newman — was a scholar and brought to an already vigorous *BMJ* a standard of academic excellence that it had lacked under Hart. He became the first full-time Editor in 1902, and it was he who established the *BMJ* in the pre-eminent and influential position that it occupied in 1932 and has occupied ever since.

The year 1926, late in Dawson Williams's term of office, saw the introduction of two new journals: *Archives of Disease in Childhood* and the *Journal of Neurology and Psychopathology*. The publication by the BMA of journals devoted to specialist subjects marked a new and important contribution by the Association to medical science.

If the BMA of 1932 was a very different body from the

Provincial Medical and Surgical Association of 1832, the world in which it found itself was also a very different one from that of Charles Hastings and his colleagues.

1832 was a year of peace and of peaceful prospects. William IV was on the throne and 17 years had passed since the end of the Napoleonic Wars; apart from comparatively brief campaigns, such as those in the Crimea and during the Indian Mutiny, no other major military clash was to occur until the Boer War at the end of the century. Moreover, when it happened, war always took place overseas, was largely a matter for the professional soldiery, and had little impact on the population at large.

By contrast, 1932 was a year dominated by the shadow of military conflict. The carnage of the first world war had touched virtually every family in the land, and the horror that it inspired was still deeply felt. By the end of the 1920s the shaky foundations of peace laid by the Treaty of Versailles were already crumbling. The rise to power in Germany of the Nazi Party set the stage for another international conflagration. As war has always had a profound effect on the medical profession and on the advance of medical science, the progression towards military conflict in the period after 1932 was to overshadow all other BMA matters.

Other fundamental differences between 1832 and 1932 were the decline in British economic strength and the breakdown of a previously stable social order. In the 1830s, the changes brought about by the Industrial Revolution were already transforming the United Kingdom into a thriving manufacturing community. Large overseas possessions, which provided raw materials and markets for manufactured goods, were the basis for unprecedented prosperity and international political power. Society of the period was based on well-recognised social divisions, with power in the hands of a land-owning aristocracy and the commercial middle classes.

By the early years of the twentieth century, however, British economic strength was on the wane. Vigorous international competitors had appeared on the scene in the shape of Germany and the United States. Overseas markets were becoming less secure as increasing demands for independence were heard from the Colonies. Finally, the crippling cost of the first world war, followed by the worldwide recession of the late 1920s weakened the British economy and came to a head in the national financial crisis of 1931, which affected all classes of the community.

The stable social order of 1832 had collapsed through the effects of the industrial and agrarian revolutions, which had created a largely employed working-class population. During the course of the nineteenth century and early twentieth century the members of this work force obtained political power by acquiring the parliamentary vote, and economic influence by the formation and recognition of trade unions. It was the existence of this new class, with its political and economic strength in a nation which possessed diminishing economic resources, that made 1932 a vastly different year from 1832 so far as the medical profession was concerned. Inevitably, this new class made increasing demands that the limited provisions of the 1911 National Insurance Act be extended, and that full medical care be extended to all sections of the community — regardless of any inherent economic weakness in the nation. The shape of such a universal medical service, the quality of the care for the patient, and the implications for the medical profession were already matters of major importance to the BMA in 1932; they were clearly going to remain matters of major importance in the years ahead.

Charles Hastings and his friends had made use of Government to bring about the reforms which they felt were needed in medicine; the position in 1932 was the reverse, with the prospect of Government using the medical profession to provide a national health service. Such an intrusion by the state into the affairs of a highly individualistic profession would have been unthinkable in 1832, and could only pose new and serious problems for the BMA. It would certainly require a strong and stable membership from the medical profession as a whole, and skilled professional organisation within the Association itself.

The science of medicine had progressed by leaps and bounds during the first 100 years of the BMA's existence. To a large extent the dogmas and superstitions of previous ages had been abandoned, and medical research had become a matter of scientific observation and deduction. Fundamental discoveries, such as those of anaesthesia and radiology, had paved the way for a rapid expansion of medical knowledge and greater effectiveness in medical practice. By 1932, however, the process of scientific investigation had become so complex and so costly that research could no longer be the prerogative of the individual doctor, as it had been with Charles Hastings; it could be carried out only with the support of those state, academic, or commercial organisations that had sufficient funds at their disposal. It remained to be seen whether the BMA's traditional methods of research by meeting, committee, and publication would prove adequate to further the Association's aim of advancing medical science.

In 1932 the chemotherapeutic revolution had not yet broken out. Virology was in its infancy, so was cardiothoracic surgery. Transplant surgery was but a dream. The medical care of patients in the voluntary hospitals, without remuneration, was the dominant activity of the great majority of consultants. In the practice of surgery, especially in the provinces, Sunday was the principal day for private operations. The Poor Law hospitals had been "municipalised" in 1929, and were being upgraded. Some of the local authorities, such as the London County Council and the Middlesex County Council, ran fine hospital services. The voluntary hospitals were engaged in both specialist and general practice, their casualty departments being thronged with patients who could not afford to pay fees to a general practitioner. The general practitioner gave a large amount of free treatment and rarely pressed for his fees, and he usually commanded wide respect. Both the general practitioner and the specialist had no set hours; it was day and night, and a seven-day week.

The delegates to the centenary meeting of the BMA in London in 1932 exhibited the same buoyant optimism that their founding fathers had shown at Worcester a hundred years before. They had every justification for this, because they could look back on a century of considerable success in the face of formidable difficulties. As always, however, the future was uncertain, and it was the Prince of Wales, later to become King Edward VIII, in his speech at the centenary dinner at the Royal Albert Hall, who struck a wise note of caution. In proposing the toast of the BMA, he congratulated the Association on its past achievements, but went on to say:

> I would ask you to have in mind not alone the success it has achieved, but the bearing of such success upon the future, for success such as yours must carry with it, not only increased responsibilities, but expanding opportunities, and, if I may say so, the risks of both.

Chapter 2

The War

War is a game that is played with a smile. If you can't smile, grin. — Lt Col Winston Churchill, commanding 6th Bn Royal Scots Fusiliers, 1916.

The BMA celebrated its centenary in July 1932; six months later Adolf Hitler became Chancellor of Germany, and the writing was on the wall.

The BMA has never been lacking in patriotism and public spirit. On the very day that Great Britain and Ireland entered the first world war in August 1914, the Association placed its whole machinery at the disposal of the Government to help the war effort. Out of this offer arose the War Register of the medical profession, the Central Medical War Committee, which was entrusted with the task of selecting the doctors to be called up for military service, and the local medical war committees, all of which were organised by the BMA with the approval of the Government.

Between the wars the Government invited the BMA to co-operate in formulating proposals for the recruitment of medical practitioners in case of war. The BMA Council agreed to do so and in 1926 established a central emergency committee — which included the chairmen of the principal BMA committees — to prepare for any national emergency. Separate emergency committees were also appointed for Scotland and Northern Ireland.

For ten years these committees were merely precautionary: they were reappointed each year, but did not actually meet until 1936, by which time, although the nation turned a blind eye, the international outlook was deteriorating fast: Hitler had reoccupied the Rhineland, and Mussolini had seized Abyssinia. In that year the Secretary of the BMA was appointed to represent the Association on a subcommittee of the Committee of Imperial Defence which was considering the co-ordination of medical services in time of war; and the BMA made a statistical survey of the distribution of hospital beds and of the medical profession in its various sections throughout England and Wales.

In 1937 the Central Emergency Committee was augmented by representatives of the Ministry of Health, the Ministry of Pensions, the Air Raid Precautions Department of the Home Office and the medical branches of the three armed Forces. Representatives of the Royal Colleges of Physicians and Surgeons had already been added to the committee, and a representative of the Medical Women's Federation was now added too.

MOBILISATION OF THE PROFESSION

Local emergency plans were based on the local organisation of the BMA. With the approval of the Committee of Imperial Defence, steps were taken to establish in the area of each BMA division a register of established doctors who were willing to volunteer for service in the event of a national emergency. The objective was to classify doctors into (*1*) those willing to accept whole-time service at home or abroad, (*2*) those willing to accept part-time service at home, and (*3*) those willing to offer emergency service for the medical care of civilian casualties after air raids in (*a*) any part of the country, or (*b*) their own areas. At the same time, a model scheme for the protection of practices of absentee general practitioners was prepared and published. A similar scheme for consultants and specialists was approved by the BMA Council in June 1939. In 1937 the BMA placed at the disposal of the Air Raid Precautions Department of the Home Office the local machinery of the Association to help with the Government scheme for instructing medical, veterinary, and dental practitioners in antigas measures, and by the end of January 1938 over 10 000 doctors had been trained.

The Munich crisis in September 1938 gave the whole nation a severe jolt, and by the end of that month 93% of doctors had informed the BMA of their intentions of service. A central card register (the War Emergency Register) had previously been prepared on which all relevant details for each doctor were recorded.

On 22 April 1939 the BMA Council reported: "The international situation has caused the Council to give careful and detailed consideration to the emergency organisation of the profession. During the course of the Association's work in connection with the compilation of a register of medical personnel, especially at the time of the September crisis, the Central Emergency Committee has had brought home to it the supreme importance of the unified control of the medical measures for the protection of the civilian population and the need for efficient co-ordination of the different departments requiring medical personnel in time of emergency. It therefore asked the Minister for the Co-ordination of Defence to receive a deputation for the purpose of submitting to him certain resolutions passed by the Committee. The Central Emergency Committee urged the creation of a Government body which would, in time of emergency, control demands for medical personnel and co-ordinate civilian medical services with the medical services of the defence forces. It asked for full authority, in consultation with the appropriate Government organisations, to advise on *all* questions of medical personnel in time of emergency. This principle has now been accepted by the Government. The Central Emergency Committee, in order to enable it to deal with the important functions entrusted to it, has been entirely re-constituted so as to make it representative of all branches of the profession."

This development was of the highest importance. At the request of the BMA, the medical profession (alone in the entire population) was entrusted by the Government with responsibility for recruiting its members for military service and for deploying its personnel between the armed Forces and the civilian medical services in each area. The reconstituted Central Emergency Committee — from the end of 1939 it was called the Central Medical War Committee — was composed of 24 BMA representatives (including representatives of specialties) and nine representatives of the Royal Colleges, the Society of Medical Officers of Health, the Medical Women's Federation, the Medical Committee of the House of Commons, and the Medical Research Council. It also included advisers from the Defence departments, the Ministry of Pensions, the Home

Office, the Ministry of Health, and, later, an adviser from the Ministry of Labour and National Service. As already indicated, separate medical war committees were set up for Scotland and Northern Ireland, and every BMA division in England, Scotland, and Wales appointed a local medical war committee to provide local advice and administer the "Protection of Practices" schemes.

As in the first world war, there was a special local committee to deal with consultants and teachers on the staffs of the London hospitals. It was called the Committee of Reference, and, although it was appointed by the Royal Colleges, it was housed and staffed by the BMA. Special arrangements were also made for pathologists and research workers, the first being dealt with by a joint subcommittee of the Central Medical War Committee and the Medical Research Council, and the second by the Central Medical War Committee in consultation with the Royal Society.

At the request of the Central Medical War Committee, in 1941 Parliament set up a Medical Personnel (Priority) Committee to balance the competing numerical claims for doctors of the armed Forces, the civilian medical services, the Merchant Marine, the Colonial Medical Service, and other national needs. The Central Medical War Committee was of course represented on the Medical Priority Committee.

With some later modifications of titles and composition, this committee structure — which owed its creation almost entirely to the BMA — controlled the conscription of doctors throughout the second world war and in the period of compulsory National Service after the war. The cost was reimbursed only partially by HM Government. The Central Medical War Committee established an executive called the Services Committee, which met at least once a month from 1940 until 1960 and decided appeals from doctors for deferment of military service — often in order to complete some postgraduate training — and applications for entry to a particular service. The committee also decided applications from hard-pressed places or hospitals to retain a doctor, and from research units and Government departments for the services of individual doctors for particular work. Finally, the committee communicated with the Defence departments about the terms and conditions of service (including pay, allowances, and ranks) for doctors holding emergency commissions, and about the grading of some of them as specialists.

The Central Medical War Committee did its work efficiently, fairly, and to general satisfaction. This is one of the success stories in the history of the medical profession, and of the BMA in particular. Throughout the war and for some time afterwards the Chairman of the Central Medical War Committee was Mr (later Sir) Henry Souttar, who is the only person ever to have held the three highest offices in the BMA (President, Chairman of Representative Body, and Chairman of Council).*

A special problem which fell to the Central Medical War Committee was the employment of alien practitioners. Since 1933 there had been an influx of medical refugees from Germany, Austria, Czechoslovakia, and other countries who were anxious to "do their bit" in the war against the Axis powers. At first the problem was that their qualifications were not registrable in Britain, but about 300 doctors were allowed to undertake a course of study, obtain a British medical qualification, and settle in the United Kingdom. Others went overseas. After the outbreak of war security considerations became important and many were interned. In 1941 the Central Medical War Committee agreed to act as a clearing house in connection with the temporary registration of alien practitioners, both "enemy" aliens and "Allied" aliens, and the committee appointed a special Aliens Committee. Two matters of special interest were the establishment of the Polish Medical School at the University of Edinburgh, and the arrival, long before the United States entered the war, of volunteer American doctors. Among these, a whole unit — "The American Hospital in Britain" — arrived in England in September 1940, and performed orthopaedic and plastic surgery at Park Prewett Hospital, Basingstoke, and later at the Churchill Hospital in Oxford. In September 1941, Harvard University and the American Red Cross opened a hospital on the outskirts of Salisbury to deal with infectious diseases. At the end of the war Harvard University handed over this hospital as a free gift to the Ministry of Health: a generous memento of the fact that American doctors came voluntarily to Britain's aid in her hour of greatest need.

* Dr Solomon Wand has been Chairman of the Representative Body, Chairman of Council, and Treasurer, and is a Gold Medallist.

The BMA was also active in planning for a suitable organisation of civilian medical services in war. The Council reported on 24 June 1939: "Consideration has been given by the Central Emergency Committee to the subject of the methods of civilian hospital staffing in time of emergency and other cognate matters. The Committee has communicated to the Ministry its general proposals for the formation of a Civilian Hospital Emergency Medical Service composed of practitioners employed on a whole-time and on a part-time basis." The Government already had plans for an emergency hospital scheme. Thus was born the Emergency Medical Service, which — though this was unforeseen — laid the foundations for the nationalisation of the hospitals in 1948. Speaking in the House of Commons on 12 June 1945, the Minister of Health (Mr Henry Willink) said that: "Never before had the voluntary and municipal hospitals been welded together into an organic whole, working together under the regional and central direction of medical officers of the Government while preserving the internal autonomy of each hospital and the clinical freedom of the medical staff." The emergency hospital scheme was based on the 11 regions into which Great Britain had been divided for civil defence purposes. The London region was divided into ten sectors, each radiating from one of the large undergraduate teaching hospitals. The BMA spent much time ironing out the early difficulties in organising the EMS, and in negotiating the terms of service (including pay) of the doctors who staffed it.

One of the first wartime economy measures to affect the medical profession seriously was the rationing of petrol. The BMA took energetic action in the early weeks of the war to secure from the authorities recognition of the special position of doctors. The Board of Trade appointed divisional petroleum officers in each region. It was arranged that each of these should have a medical adviser and that medical practitioners would be placed in the highest category of priority for petrol supplies. It is interesting that in 1943 the Government agreed that doctors could use petrol granted for "professional purposes" in order to attend local meetings called to discuss the comprehensive medical service envisaged in the Beveridge Report (see Chapter 3).

In each area the scheme for the protection of practices of doctors who joined the Forces was administered by the local medical war committee. (A similar scheme was operated in 1950-3, during the Korean War and in the Suez emergency of 1956.) This was an arduous and unenviable task. In 1946 the BMA Council reported: "There were great difficulties in the practical administration of the scheme which could not have been foreseen when the plans were evolved before the war. . . . That large numbers of acting practitioners faithfully discharged their obligations to their absent colleagues is not open to doubt, but it must regretfully be admitted that there were others who did not loyally carry out their agreement to protect the practices of those of their colleagues on whole-time war service." Nevertheless, the detailed report concluded: "The Council has tried to give an objective picture of the working of its Protection of Practices Scheme . . . and believes that with all its inevitable faults it has played a part in the war of which the profession has good reason to be proud."

At first the needs of HM Forces for doctors could be met entirely by volunteers, but in April 1940 the Central Medical War Committee advised the Government that conscription should be applied to medical practitioners who were within the age limits of current proclamations, and that their conscription should be administered through the machinery of the Central Medical War Committee. The Government accepted this advice. In 1941 the Central Medical War Committee reviewed the establishments of all hospitals and laid down a sanctioned establishment for each hospital, which was not to be exceeded. As the war intensified, the needs of the Forces for doctors grew apace, and there were two occasions (in September 1942 and November 1943) when some young doctors had to be called up after only three months in their first house posts. Already the Medical Personnel (Priority) Committee had recommended the use of final-year students as housemen, albeit under supervision.

Back in 1940, the Central Medical War Committee had advised the Defence departments that women doctors could be employed with the armed Forces, either as civilian medical practitioners or as attached medical officers with military status. From then on the recruitment of women doctors was organised by the committee.

As the war progressed, the depleted civilian medical service came under increasing strain. The civilian doctors had to work very long hours, many general practitioners having to carry on single-handed a practice previously served by two or even three partners, and many retired doctors returned to harness in general practice and in hospital. But the reverse happened for a time on the east and south-east coasts when, after the fall of France, the civilian population was evacuated from certain towns in anticipation of a German invasion. The local doctors were temporarily deprived of their means of livelihood, and the Central Medical War Committee negotiated with the Ministry of Health that the doctors required for the remaining population would be employed as whole-time medical officers of the Emergency Medical Service.

The committee also negotiated terms of service for civilian doctors staffing first-aid posts under the Air Raid Precautions scheme. On the formation of the Home Guard in 1940, the BMA offered to find doctors to provide, free of charge, first-aid treatment for those members of the Home Guard who were wounded or injured on duty. Medical officers were later appointed to Home Guard units, and the nomination of doctors for this service was administered by the local medical war committees.

During the war the Central Medical War Committee had to adjudicate on some appeals for premature release of doctors from the Forces, and at the end of the war the BMA concerned itself with arrangements for demobilising doctors from the Services, and reabsorbing them into civilian practice.

In 1947 the BMA considered the application of the National Service Bill (which was to continue conscription in peacetime) to the medical profession, and expressed the opinion that young men intending to enter medicine should be given the option of performing their conscripted service either before starting their medical studies or after qualification — so that their course of undergraduate medical training should not be interrupted by the call-up.

In 1952 the Central Medical War Committee was renamed the Central Medical Recruitment Committee, and it continued to administer the call-up of doctors under the National Service Acts until conscription ended. It also undertook the task of "screening" the lists of doctors with a reserve commitment to HM Forces, in order to earmark those who should be exempted from recall in any national emergency because of the essential nature of their civilian medical work. This "screening" was a huge and delicate task.

Altogether, a great burden of important work, all voluntary, was shouldered by the central and local medical war committees on behalf of the nation. Their plans and machinery were adapted to meet the changing circumstances of war, and of return to peace (or "cold war"), but their objectives remained the satisfaction of Service requirements with the least possible disturbance of the medical service to the civilian population. Call-up for National Service ceased at the end of 1960, and in 1961 the BMA Council stated: "In 21 years of conscription, over 27 000 doctors were recruited for the Forces, and the recruitment committees dealt with an enormous number of applications for deferment. The Council considers that the recruitment committees succeeded in striking a very fair balance between the competing claims of the Forces and of the civil medical service, without losing sight of the aspirations of the young doctors themselves, and the Council desires to place on record its warm appreciation of the conscientious and efficient manner in which the Central Medical Recruitment Committee and the Scottish Central Medical Recruitment Committee discharged their onerous and invidious tasks."

TERMS AND CONDITIONS OF SERVICE FOR DOCTORS IN HM FORCES

We must now digress and discuss a subject which was important both in wartime and in peacetime. The BMA's function of negotiating suitable terms and conditions of service for doctors was exercised on behalf of Forces doctors very early in its history. As Ernest Muirhead Little wrote in his centenary *History of the British Medical Association,* "The Association stands in a position of peculiar responsibility to its members in the Services. By the nature of their employment they are subject to regulations and discipline, and are not allowed to combine in the way open to persons engaged in practically every other form of employment. It is therefore necessary that there should be some outside responsible body which is able to take a comprehensive view of the conditions of employment inside the Services as compared with those outside, and be able and willing when necessary to make representations to the Department concerned or to Parliament. . . ."

In 1933 the BMA was seriously concerned at inadequacies in the terms and conditions of service of Forces medical officers and, not having received any satisfactory response to its representations, the Council recommended: "That members of the profession be advised seriously to consider the disadvantages to which they are liable if they accept service as officers in the Royal Naval Medical Service, the Royal Army Medical Corps, or the Royal Air Force Medical Service under the existing terms and conditions." In July 1933 the Warren Fisher Committee (to which the BMA had given evidence) reported, mainly recommending accelerated promotion and accelerated increments of pay, but the BMA was not fully satisfied and continued to press for further improvements. Certain special concessions were won, and the BMA then decided to co-operate to the fullest extent in the recruitment of medical officers for the Forces.

As has already been stated, during the second world war the BMA kept a watchful eye on the pay and conditions of service of the many doctors serving in HM Forces. When peace returned the remuneration of doctors in the National Health Service (the bitter battles fought then are described in later chapters) established a yardstick against which the remuneration of all other employed doctors could be measured. Applying this yardstick to the pay of medical officers in the Forces, in March 1949 the BMA submitted a memorandum of detailed proposals and new rates to the Ministry of Defence. The calculation of comparable rates for general-duty medical officers was based on an estimate of the average annual remuneration of general practitioners (always a difficult thing to estimate) plus a supplement which, in the BMA's view, should be added to compensate for the disadvantages of a Service medical officer's career. Discussions with the Ministry of Defence were protracted, and eventually a meeting was held with the four Defence Ministers at the House of Commons and new rates of pay were introduced with effect from 1 September 1950. The new rates for general-duty medical officers represented an increase of 10% over previous remuneration and were

8-10% more than the remuneration for corresponding civilian general practitioners. The BMA was not satisfied with the rates for specialist medical officers, however, and said so.

Recruitment of regular medical officers continued to be unsatisfactory, and the BMA continued to make proposals to the Government for making a medical career in the Services more attractive. In 1954 the Government set up a committee under the chairmanship of Viscount Waverley to examine all aspects of the problem. The BMA submitted a powerful memorandum of evidence, drafted by a distinguished committee specially assembled by the Association. The Waverley Report appeared in 1956 and was regarded by the BMA as disappointing.

While compulsory National Service was in operation, of course, the Forces could rely on conscript doctors to fill their establishments, but the day of reckoning came at the end of 1960 when conscription ended. On 20 December 1961 a deputation from the BMA met the four Defence Ministers and urged that the Forces had no alternative but to offer pay and conditions that were favourable enough to compete successfully with the National Health Service.

The deputation also made suggestions for widening the scope of the professional work of doctors in the Forces. Another meeting with the four Defence Ministers took place in March 1962, and a month later the Minister of Defence, Mr Harold (later Viscount) Watkinson, said in Parliament: "In particular, the British Medical Association has advised me that we cannot hope to attract newly qualified young doctors in adequate numbers and of good quality unless we can offer them a substantial lead over the remuneration which they could expect to get as doctors in civilian life. The Government have accepted this advice."

A "new deal" for Forces doctors, which included a medical cadet scheme, was hammered out between the BMA and the Government, and in June 1962 the BMA Council gave its approval to the new terms and resolved to give wholehearted support to the Government's campaign for the voluntary recruitment of doctors to the Forces. A year later recruitment had improved dramatically.

Unfortunately, this happy situation was soured by the Government's "pay standstill" in 1966 (described in full in Chapter 5). The BMA withdrew its co-operation from the recruitment campaign and even refused to accept advertisements of medical vacancies in the armed Forces for publication in the *British Medical Journal* — an action which incurred both support and criticism in the correspondence columns of the *BMJ.* In 1968 the BMA submitted a detailed memorandum to the National Board for Prices and Incomes. As a result the board restored the analogue between the pay of Forces doctors and NHS general practitioners which had been so abruptly broken by the Government in 1966. Harmony was restored, and in 1969 advertisements for Forces vacancies were again accepted by the *BMJ.*

In 1970 a Review Body for the Armed Forces was established, and each year the BMA has carefully submitted evidence on behalf of medical officers, continuing its policy that they should be analogued with the National Health Service and should also receive compensation for the inescapable disturbance of a career in the Forces, either in an adequate "X factor" applicable to the Forces as a whole, or in the form of a "medical betterment factor." In 1975 the Review Body on Armed Forces Pay dismissed the BMA's case for a special medical betterment factor, but nevertheless awarded an increase of 38% to Forces doctors — proof, indeed, of the value of the BMA's championship of doctors in the armed Forces.

The BMA has frequently made representations to the authorities and various commissions of inquiry about the career structure and professional scope of the medical branches of the armed Forces, and is proud of the fact that the Royal Army Medical Corps owes its creation to representations made by the Association. In 1958 Sir Gordon Gordon-Taylor delivered an oration at BMA House to celebrate the diamond jubilee of the corps.

THE BMA IN WARTIME

After this long but important digression, we must complete the story of the BMA in wartime. On 27 September 1939 the BMA Council appointed an executive committee "to conduct the business of the Association" during the war, but the full Council continued to meet fairly regularly. There were, for example, four Council meetings in the blackest year of the war, 1940-1.

The annual meeting, which was to have been held in Birmingham in 1940, was cancelled, and an extraordinary general meeting was held at BMA House on 16 May 1940 (the same day that, at the height of the Battle of France, Churchill flew to Paris for his first crisis talks with the French leaders) for the purpose of passing a resolution conferring certain emergency powers on the Council for the duration of the war, in case the Representative Body should be unable to meet. This period was defined as "the period beginning with the 3rd day of September 1939 and ending on such date as His Majesty may by Order in Council declare to be the date on which the emergency which was the occasion of the passing of the Armed Forces (Conditions of Service) Act 1939 and other like Emergency Legislation came to an end." In fact, no annual representative meetings were held in 1940 and 1941.

Of the staff, 23 members were away serving with the Forces in April 1940. BMA House was blacked out every night and, because typewriters were unobtainable during the war, all the BMA House machines were taken down to the air-raid shelter in the basement every night before the staff went home and were brought up again next morning. A copy of the War Emergency Register was kept for safety at the Secretary's home in Harpenden, and was brought up to BMA House once a week to be updated. BMA House was frequently struck by incendiary bombs, which were quickly extinguished by the teams of firewatchers drawn from the staffs of the Association and of the tenant organisations. On 16 April 1941 the house was struck by a high explosive bomb and the south wing was destroyed. There were several near misses on other occasions. Parts of BMA House were occupied by the Royal Canadian Air Force and by the Royal Norwegian Navy, and, on one occasion, King Haakon of Norway visited the building.

As a precaution against the possibility that London might be completely destroyed or invaded by the enemy, early in the war the BMA took a lease of a house in Buxton, Derbyshire, to which the head office could be transferred if necessary. Members of Council and committees (and of course the staff) were frequently delayed on the trains to and from London, but everybody carried on and the motto was "business as usual," although a great deal of normal committee activity was suspended.

Throughout the war the *British Medical Journal* gave good service to the profession and to the country. Many a medical officer in the North African desert or the jungles of Burma gained news and comfort from the *BMJ*, however erratic and delayed its delivery might be. In the early months of the war the BMA provided a lending library for the British Expeditionary Force in France. The BMA was instrumental in forming a Medical War Relief Fund to help doctors who were in difficulty or distress because of damage by enemy action to their surgeries and equipment.

The Council report of April 1940 contains a small paragraph which illustrates the therapeutic revolution that was gathering momentum: "The Ministry of Health has agreed to the inclusion, as from February 1st 1940, of M and B 693 in the list of drugs and appliances for the supply of which a dispensing practitioner is entitled to claim special payment. The preparation is being referred to under the heading of 'sulphapyridine'."

In 1942 the Council publicly expressed its "heartfelt sympathy with the members of the Hong Kong and China, Malaya and Burma Branches, and with their families, in the tragedy which had befallen them." They had been overrun by the Japanese. In the same Council report there is a paragraph with an old-fashioned flavour, entitled "Reservation of Maidservants" (which concerned their exemption from conscription to the Forces).

The Association's membership increased by a quarter (from 40 000 to 50 000) during the war, possibly because medicopolitical battles were seen to be looming. A more likely explanation is that the BMA was seen by doctors as the body which was organising the profession's war effort. In at least one instance this surmise went far beyond the facts. On 5 November 1939 the *Sunday Pictorial* published an article entitled "The Banned Doctor" which opened with the words: "Because they do not belong to the British Medical Association, or have not rendered past services to the Association, 21 000 doctors, it is declared, may never get a chance of serving with the Forces." There was not a shred of truth in this, and the Association's solicitors extracted from the *Sunday Pictorial* a published apology and a sum of 100 guineas, which the BMA donated to the Lord Mayor's Fund for the British Red Cross Society.

In the second world war 542 members died on active

service, and four civilian members were killed by enemy action. Their names are inscribed in a Roll of Honour at BMA House. After the war the BMA Council gave much thought to providing a suitable war memorial. A fund was raised from the members, and a proportion was set aside to help with the education of the children of the fallen. In addition, a permanent memorial was built in the Court of Honour at BMA House. It takes the form of a central fountain based on the shape of the staff of Aesculapius, surrounded by four statues representing Sacrifice, Cure, Prevention, and Aspiration. The memorial bears the inscriptions "In Memoriam 1939-45" and "In Honour of the Medical Men and Women of the British Empire and Commonwealth of Nations who gave their Lives in the Second World War." The memorial was designed by Mr James Woodford RA, and was dedicated on 2 November 1954 by the Archbishop of Canterbury, assisted by the Moderator of the General Assembly of the Church of Scotland, a representative of the Free Church Federal Council, and the Vicar of St Pancras. The singing was led by the choir of the Queen's Chapel of the Savoy, and the music was played by the Band of the Royal Army Medical Corps. Many relatives of the dead were present at the intensely moving service.

Each year, at Remembrance time, the memorial is quietly decorated with a wreath of poppies.

Chapter 3

Into the National Health Service

> To reconcile individual freedom with collective responsibility is perhaps the leading problem of the world today. — Dr G C Anderson, Secretary of the BMA, 1932-43.

The most important event for the BMA in the 50 years covered by this volume was not the war or the therapeutic revolution, but the nationalisation of medicine in 1946-8. A long history led up to this, starting with the National Insurance Act of 1911 (the Lloyd George Act). The events of that time were fully described in the centenary history of the Association. Here we pick up the story just after the first world war.

THE DAWSON REPORT

Under the Minister of Health Act 1919, which created the first Ministry of Health, a Consultative Council on Medical and Allied Services was established. The Chairman was Lord Dawson of Penn, and it included three prominent representatives of the BMA: Dr (later Sir) Robert Bolam, Dr (later Sir) Guy Dain, and Dr J A Macdonald. This council published a report in 1920 on *The Future Provision of Medical and Allied Services.* The report made recommendations that were well ahead of its time: for example, that all the medical services in each area, curative and preventive, should be brought together in close co-ordination under a single health authority, on which the medical profession would be represented; and that each authority should have a local medical advisory council, elected by all the registered medical practitioners in the area. The report mentioned the growing cost of medical services but dodged that issue, saying merely: ". . . We do not mean that the services are to be free; we exclude for the moment the question how they are to be paid for."

THE ROYAL COMMISSION ON NATIONAL HEALTH INSURANCE

The BMA gave evidence to the Royal Commission on National Health Insurance, which reported in 1926. It found that national health insurance was already established as a permanent feature of the social system of Britain and should be continued, but that there should be no wider charge on the Exchequer in respect of it. The commission recommended that at that time inpatient treatment in hospitals, major operations in the home, maternity services, and dental services should not be included, and that, because of the large cost, there should be no extension in the provision of medical benefit for the dependants of insured persons. The commission recommended that insurance committees should be abolished and that their powers and duties should be transferred to committees of the local authorities. This recommendation was not implemented.

A GENERAL MEDICAL SERVICE FOR THE NATION

In 1929 the BMA published proposals for "A General Medical Service for the Nation." It is important to remember this because there are some who have alleged that the BMA has always been opposed to a national health service. The opposite is true. Long before governments and political parties* produced plans for the nationalisation of medicine the BMA had produced its own proposals for a national medical service.

In its annual report for 1938 the BMA Council said: "In 1930 the Representative Body approved a series of proposals for a General Medical Service for the Nation. These proposals were submitted to those public bodies and public men and women interested in the subject, with an intimation that the Association would be glad to receive comments, criticisms, and suggestions. ... The Council has

---

*Professor Harry Eckstein of Harvard wrote (in *The English Health Service*, Harvard University Press, 1964): "Of all the people and organisations articulately concerned with medical reform before the war the socialists were the last and, in some ways, the most half-hearted in the field."

thought it wise to review the proposals for a General Medical Service for the Nation in the light of recent developments and experience, and at the same time to co-ordinate with those general proposals the policies of the Association in regard to hospitals, to a National Maternity Service, and to open-choice public assistance medical services. The Council recommends this revised report, the culmination of many years' medico-political work, to the serious consideration of every member of the Association."

The revised report stated four main basic principles: (*1*) that the system of medical service should be directed to the achievement of positive health and the prevention of disease no less than to the relief of sickness; (*2*) that there should be provided for every individual the services of a general practitioner or a family doctor of his own choice; (*3*) that consultants and specialists, laboratory services, and all necessary auxiliary services, together with institutional provision when required, should be available for the individual patient, normally through the agency of the family doctor; (*4*) that the several parts of the complete medical service should be closely co-ordinated and developed by the application of a planned national health policy.

The report suggested that the National Health Insurance scheme should be extended to cover the families of the insured workers, and also to include hospital and specialist treatment. The hospitals of the country should be integrated on a regional basis, each region being based on a large hospital and medical school.

With regard to consultant and specialist services, the report said: "In a national health service there should be made available the services of consultants and specialists in all branches of medicine. . . . It would be necessary to establish lists of consultants and specialists who satisfy a certain standard of eligibility and who desire to render service under the scheme." This was logical enough: to establish in each region a "panel" of participating consultants and specialists. But this would have constituted the makings of a specialist register, against which the BMA set its face in later years.

What came later to be known as the "100% issue" was nowhere specifically mentioned, but the report clearly implied that the "wealthier classes" would not be covered by the proposed service. The report suggested two categories of pay-beds in hospitals: one category at fees within the capacity of the middle-class person to pay; and the other category available for "the wealthier classes, the institutional and professional charges varying with the economic standing of the patient." Thus we see the origin of the two categories of pay-beds which were provided at the inception of the National Health Service — those with a ceiling on professional charges, and those with no ceiling.

Like the Dawson Report before it, this report avoided the issue of the cost of the service: "... Different views have been expressed as to the best method of financing an extended service — and it is not within the province of the medical profession to express a view on this subject."

Surprisingly, the report seemed to envisage that the service would be managed mainly by the larger local authorities: "The Association considers ... that changes in local government, so far as the medical and public health services are concerned, are urgently necessary. . . . The objects to be aimed at in England and Wales should be: the creation of a system of complete and all-embracing units for local public health administration; the treatment of hospital services and related medical services as regional problems. ... The medical officer of health of the administrative area concerned would be the administrative head of those parts of the scheme under local administration."

The report emphasised the importance of prevention, drawing attention especially to "the evil of atmospheric pollution by smoke" and "the safety of such an important food as milk." It also emphasised the need to co-ordinate the maternity services, and to develop industrial medical services, fracture and rehabilitation services. It looked forward to the creation of specialised accident and emergency departments: "It is believed that segregation of cases into one department where they can be uniformly handled by a specially trained and experienced staff is highly desirable.... All the stages of treatment of each case need not only expert supervision but supervision by one expert."

Though this report is not as clear as it should be in several passages, and shows signs of "committee drafting" and compromise formulae, it is a most important document for which the BMA deserves credit. It shows that long before many other national bodies the BMA saw the need for an integrated national policy on health.

In the 1930s while "A General Medical Service for the Nation" was being revised, other events occurred. In March 1933 the Chairman of Council, Sir Henry Brackenbury, published an address on the essentials of a national medical service. The next month the BMA Council published a new model scheme for public medical services. These were local schemes promoted and managed by the medical profession, "For the provision of medical attendance and treatment for the dependants of insured persons and others of a like economic status." (The Council had first issued model rules for such schemes in 1909.) And in 1936 the Cathcart Report, published in Scotland, recommended an integrated medical service based as far as possible on the family doctor. But the next main landmark was the Medical Planning Commission.

THE MEDICAL PLANNING COMMISSION

With what Paul Vaughan* has called "incongruous sangfroid," the BMA set up a medical planning commission in the blackest year of the war, 1940. This courageous and forward-looking action was drily reported in the Council's annual report of May 1941: "In the belief that national post-war reconstruction will involve profound changes in medical practice, the Council, in co-operation with the English Royal Colleges and the Scottish Corporations, has set up a Medical Planning Commission to study wartime developments and their effects on the country's medical services both present and future."

Eventually, the Medical Planning Commission consisted of 73 members appointed by the BMA, the Royal Colleges in England and Scotland, the Society of Medical Officers of Health, the Faculty of Radiologists, the Medical Women's Federation, and the Parliamentary Medical Committee. There were observers from the Ministry of Health, the Department of Health for Scotland, and the Ministry of Home Affairs for Northern Ireland. The political left-wing was represented by Dr Haden Guest MP, Mr Somerville Hastings FRCS, and Dr D Stark Murray. Other notable

---

* *Doctors' Commons* by Paul Vaughan (Heinemann, 1959).

members were Dr G F Buchan (medical officer of health of Willesden), Dr Guy Dain, Sir Allen Daley (chief medical officer of the LCC), Sir Francis Fremantle FRCP, MP, and Professor R M F Picken. At the time of writing (1981) survivors of this commission are Dr Mason Bolam, Dr Frank Gray, Sir Harold Himsworth, Dr Doris Odlum, Sir Harry Platt, and Dr Solly Wand.

At the first meeting on 7 May 1941 Viscount Dawson of Penn proposed and Sir Alfred Webb-Johnson seconded that Mr H S Souttar (Chairman of Council of the BMA) be elected chairman of the commission, and this was agreed unanimously. Lord Dawson said that the most important question to settle was the regionalisation of hospitals and health services. He hoped that the commission would not attempt to issue a single report at a particular time, but would publish interim reports. The commission proceeded to set up five committees and a sixth, co-ordinating, committee, and the BMA asked its local divisions to form study groups to discuss the various problems relating to the future of medical practice: 190 such study groups were formed.

A "draft interim report" by the Medical Planning Commission was published in the *BMJ* on 20 June 1942. It covered 11 pages. The commission asked that the interim report "should be freely discussed by the profession, and that comments and criticisms should be made available to it."

The report opened with criticisms of the existing patchwork quilt of medical services. "There are too many central and local bodies concerned with one or another aspect of the country's health services, and too little collaboration between statutory bodies and between statutory and voluntary bodies." The report went on to discuss some principles. "Some maintain that the existing system can be so augmented and rearranged as to provide a comprehensive and wholly satisfactory medical service. Others argue that the ideals of medical service cannot be achieved without radical alterations in the basis of existing services, and suggest that a whole-time salaried service under Government control is essential. A third group favour a combination of private practice and a Government service."

The report discussed each of these possible lines of

development, and offered some tentative conclusions. "The majority view of the committees which have discussed this matter is against a whole-time salaried Government service . . . changes could be achieved without any violent break with the traditional basis of medical practice . . . National Health Insurance has proved a greater success than was anticipated either by its supporters or by its opponents. Today it is an integral part of the social structure. Its medical service contains features which have proved to be essentially sound, such as free choice of doctor, the minimum of interference by the State, and the central negotiation of terms and conditions of service."

The report advocated a central authority, which might be a Government department or a "corporate body formed under Government auspices." For local administration the report proposed the creation of regional authorities, elected for new areas with populations much larger than those of most of the existing major local authorities. The regional authority, which would have a statutory advisory medical committee and a chief medical officer, would administer the hospital, medical, and allied services, including the environmental and personal health services, as well as the health centres in which general practitioners would be encouraged to work. An alternative would be to establish appointed regional councils, representative of the local authorities in the region and of voluntary hospitals, and including nominees of the central authority and an adequate representation of the medical profession. It is of interest that 35 years later the BMA suggested to the Royal Commission on the National Health Service that the regional health authority should consist of one-third elected by the local authorities in the region, one-third elected by the staff of the authority (including of course medical staff), and one-third nominated by the "central authority," the Secretary of State.

The report of the Medical Planning Commission suggested that the remuneration of a principal in general practice should consist of three parts: (*a*) a basic salary with additions for special qualifications and length of service; (*b*) a capitation fee; and (*c*) any fees received in respect of services not covered by the capitation fee. For senior hospital staff, the report suggested payment by salary, and three types of contract: whole time; geographical whole time (described as "a whole-time salaried post with the right to undertake a certain amount of private practice within the hospital"); and part time, with freedom to undertake private practice either inside or outside the hospital.

The report emphasised the importance of the machinery of selection of the medical staff of hospitals, and recommended that "the selection of consultants and specialists . . . should be made on the advice of a medical appointments panel specifically appointed by the regional council or authority. The panel should include representatives of the university or universities in the region and, for certain senior appointments, assessors from outside the region."

The report also emphasised the importance of a medical staff committee in each hospital. "In the council hospitals . . . too much of the responsibility for internal administration is vested in the medical superintendent and too little is allowed to the other members of the medical staff."

The commission remarked that: "It would be an advantage to both the community and the practitioner if, when the medical student has passed his final examination, he could spend some time in practice under supervision before he embarked in practice on his own account. It is suggested that the student should be registered provisionally when he has passed his final examination, and that he should then be required to practise under supervision in some approved hospital or health service. The period of such practice should be one year. . . ."

The commission also said that: "The problem of industrial health . . . demands a special reference. At the present time [1942] the whole of the country's effort is directed to the development of adequate and efficient fighting and defence services. This effort largely depends on production by industry and the output of the individual worker. Conservation of health in industry, therefore, is one of the most immediate problems before the medical profession, and an urgent issue is to ensure that its contribution is made in the best possible way."

The question of how to finance a health service was obviously seen as less of a problem 40 years ago than it is today, and the Medical Planning Commission had very little to say about it. The report envisaged an extension of National Health Insurance to cover all domiciliary care, and regional contributory schemes to cover hospital care.

For persons "above contributory scheme limits there should be insurance provision of a provident character, with 'full cover' for those within specified limits and possibly only 'grant in aid' for those above these limits."

Finally, the report ended with a list of questions to be decided, of which one on the "100% issue" was especially important: "Should provision, whatever its character, be made by Government for the whole community or for a part of it only? If the latter, to which section of the community should it be limited?" The annual representative meeting in 1942 resolved — by 94 votes to 92 — that provision, of whatever character, should be made by the Government for the whole community.

Enough has been quoted above to show that the interim report of the Medical Planning Commission, a widely representative body of doctors set up by the BMA, propounded many of the fundamental features eventually embodied in the National Health Service: no whole-time State salaried service; remuneration of general practitioners by capitation fee but with some elements of salary; regionalisation of the hospital service; choice of whole-time or part-time contracts for consultants; and advisory appointments machinery for consultant posts. It also recommended the compulsory preregistration year, which was introduced by the Medical Act 1950; and raised a problem which is still with us 40 years later — how to integrate occupational medicine into the National Health Service.

Michael Foot — not a boundless admirer of the BMA — wrote*: "Yet the Medical Planning Commission's report did represent an imaginative breakthrough. It was the boldest document ever issued by the British Medical Association. Its principal draughtsman was Dr Charles Hill, at that time the BMA's Deputy Secretary."

THE BEVERIDGE REPORT

On 12 August 1941 Mr Churchill and President Roosevelt issued a joint declaration which came to be known as the Atlantic Charter. It opened with the words: "The President of the United States of America and the Prime Minister, Mr

*Volume 2 (1945-1960) of *Aneurin Bevan*, by Michael Foot (Davis-Poynter, 1973).

Churchill, representing His Majesty's Government in the United Kingdom, being met together, deem it right to make known certain common principles in the national policies of their respective countries on which they base their hopes for a better future for the world."

The declaration then spelled out eight principles, including these two: "Fifth, they desire to bring about the fullest collaboration between all nations in the economic field, with the object of securing for all improved labour standards, economic advancement, and social security. Sixth, after the final destruction of the Nazi tyranny they hope to see established a peace which will afford to all nations the means of dwelling in safety within their own boundaries, and which will afford assurance that all the men in all the lands may live out their lives in freedom from fear and want."

So "social security" and "freedom from want" became Allied war aims. The UK Government immediately established an Interdepartmental Committee on Social Insurance and Allied Services. The Chairman was Sir William Beveridge, who had been director of the London School of Economics from 1919 to 1937, almost the whole period between the wars. In December 1942 the Interdepartmental Committee presented its report, the "Beveridge Report," which at once caught the attention of the British public.

Its scheme was to insure the whole nation against unemployment, illness, injury, and retirement, the necessary finance being provided by contributions from individual citizens, employers, and the Government. Beveridge said that his scheme was based on certain assumptions, one of which — the famous Assumption B — was spelled out thus:

> That a comprehensive national health service will ensure that for every citizen there is available whatever medical treatment he requires, in whatever form he requires it, domiciliary or institutional, general, specialist, or consultant, and will ensure also the provision of dental, ophthalmic, and surgical appliances, nursing and midwifery, and rehabilitation after accidents.

Beveridge justified his Assumption B by saying: "It is a logical corollary to the payment of high benefits in disability that determined efforts should be made by the State to reduce the number of cases for which benefit is needed." The Beveridge Report said many other interesting things too: "The primary interest of the Ministry of Social Security is not in the details of the national health service or in its financial arrangements. It is in finding a health service which will diminish disease by prevention and cure, and will ensure the careful certification needed to control payment of benefit at the rates proposed in this Report." There was also a storm signal: "The possible scope of private general practice will be so restricted that it may not appear worthwhile to preserve it."

Statements such as these caused unease in the BMA, but the Beveridge Plan stirred the imagination of politicians. In a note circulated to the Cabinet on 14 February 1943 the Prime Minister (Mr Churchill) said: "This approach to social security . . . constitutes an essential part of any postwar scheme of national betterment. . . . We cannot, however, initiate the legislation now or commit ourselves to the expenditure involved. . . . We do not know what Government is going to be in power after the war, or what Prime Minister. We should get everything ready for them, and leave them a free hand to take up or reject a scheme which will be perfected in itself."

And so the mighty Government machine, although preoccupied with the supreme task of winning the war, began to plan a national health service. In fact, since the early months of the war, some senior officials of the Ministry of Health had been looking ahead to postwar health services.*

At the invitation of the Minister of Health (Mr Ernest Brown), representatives of the main bodies of the medical profession, including the British Medical Association, met him on 9 March 1943 to consider his suggestions on the procedure to be adopted for consultation in the months ahead. The Minister asked that a committee, representative of the medical profession as a whole, should be set up to consider with him and his officers the many important problems and difficulties.

---

*See *The Making of the National Health Service* by John E Pater, p 23 (King Edward's Hospital Fund for London, 1981).

THE REPRESENTATIVE COMMITTEE

The BMA took the initiative in setting up the Representative Committee which eventually consisted of 40 members, including 25 from the BMA, the six presidents of the Royal Colleges in England and Scotland, and nine representatives of the Society of Medical Officers of Health, the Medical Women's Federation, the Society of Apothecaries, and the Provincial Teaching Staffs Association.

At a joint meeting of the BMA Representative Body and the Panel Conference held on 31 March 1943, the action of the Executive Committee of the BMA Council in forming a representative committee without referring the matter to the peripheral organisation of the Association was sharply criticised by several speakers. But Sir Kaye Le Fleming said: "If the Executive or Council had said that it was not prepared to meet the Minister with a committee of this kind until the matter had been referred to the whole country, the Minister would have asked the Royal Colleges and some other bodies to do what he wanted. The occasion was urgent, and the action taken was in the best interests of the profession." After a vigorous debate, the motion "That the Government's invitation to enter into discussions without commitment be accepted" was carried with only two dissentients in a meeting of about 400 and the composition of the representative committee was approved by a large majority. These decisions were confirmed later the same day by separate meetings of the Representative Body and the Panel Conference.

The discussions between the Representative Committee and the Minister of Health made an unpromising start. The annual report of the BMA Council published on 10 July 1943 summarised the position thus: "During the course of the discussions the Ministry put forward certain tentative proposals for a comprehensive medical service based on . . . the employment of doctors as salaried officers, mainly whole-time, by a new type of local authority. The Representative Committee, considering that further discussion on the basis of such proposals would be unfruitful . . . made it clear that, although it was not empowered to commit the medical profession, it believed that such proposals would be contrary to the public interest and would be unacceptable to the great majority of the profession. It therefore asked for the withdrawal of the proposals . . . the Minister agreed to relegate the proposals to 'the discard' and consented to a re-examination of the whole position." A leading article in the *BMJ* commented drily: "This, we understand, is a term used in the game of poker. It is well to remember that cards in the discard are reshuffled and find their way back into subsequent games."

Discussions continued between the Representative Committee and the Ministry of Health. A special meeting of the Council was held on 28 July 1943 to take stock of the position, but first the Council decided unanimously to recommend to the annual meeting that Sir Beckwith Whitehouse be requested to continue in office as President for another year. Unhappily, Sir Beckwith died suddenly from a heart attack on the evening of the Council meeting. Eventually Lord Dawson of Penn was elected President (for the second time).

On 7 August 1943 the BMA Council reported that the discussions "ranged over a wide field of subjects, such as central and local administration, health centres, free choice of doctor, private practice, and methods of utilising the services of medical practitioners, including methods of remuneration. Though the Committee did not in any way commit the medical profession, it reached the conclusion that there should be an early statement by the profession of the fundamental principles that should form the basis of any future reorganisation of health services, whatever the contents of the White Paper."

The Council went on to state a series of principles in the form of 14 recommendations. Some of these were nebulous and idealistic, such as recommendation C: "That the efficiency of a country's medical services, both preventive and curative, depends upon the available medical and scientific knowledge, upon the character and extent of medical education, and upon the absence of any economic barriers that impede the utilisation of such services. Thus in order to improve the country's medical services, the facilities and resources for medical research should be greatly increased and methods devised for their adequate application; medical education, both undergraduate and postgraduate, should be maintained on a high standard and be adapted to modern needs; the facilities for post-graduate medical education should be greatly increased;

and wherever economic barriers prevent an individual taking advantage of medical services such barriers should be removed."

Other statements were more forthright: "It is not in the public interest that the State should convert the medical profession into a salaried branch of central or local government service."

Again: ". . . Every member of the community should be free to consult the doctor of his choice either officially, as when he consults the doctor he has selected under an official service, or privately. . . ."

The views of the BMA Council were summed up in recommendation M: "That . . . Assumption B [in the Beveridge Report] should be satisfied by an extension of National Health Insurance to include dependants of insured persons and others of like economic status and to cover consultant and specialist services and laboratory and hospital facilities as well as general practitioner service. Those persons with incomes above the existing limits could, if Parliament decides to make the service available to every member of the community, be permitted to become voluntary contributors to the extended service. . . ."

THE WHITE PAPER

The phase of non-committal discussion with the Minister ended with the publication of a Government White Paper on 17 February 1944. By then Mr Henry Willink had succeeded Mr Ernest Brown as Minister of Health, and Dr Guy Dain had succeeded Mr Henry Souttar as Chairman of Council. Moreover, on the first day of 1944, the Secretary of the BMA, Dr G C Anderson, had unexpectedly died. His successor was his deputy, Dr Charles Hill (now Lord Hill of Luton). The Council passed the following resolution: "That the Council records its sense of the overwhelming loss the Association has suffered by the death of its Secretary, George Anderson, and pays tribute to the outstanding and single-minded service he has given so devotedly to the British Medical Association, as indeed to all the members of his profession."

The White Paper illustrated the aptness of the *BMJ*'s comment about the discard in a game of poker. Mr Ernest Brown's plan for a salaried service controlled by the local authorities was revived. But first some unexceptionable general principles were stated: everybody in the country — irrespective of means, age, sex, or occupation — should have equal opportunity to benefit from the best and most up-to-date medical and allied services available; no compulsion into the new service, either for patient or for doctor; no interference with the making of private arrangements at private cost, *if anyone still prefers to do so* (our italics); the doctor not to be subject to outside clinical interference.

Central responsibility was to lie with the Minister of Health. At his side was to be a "new central and statutory organisation for voicing professional views," the Central Health Services Council (with a parallel council in Scotland). A special executive body was also to be set up, the Central Medical Board. This was to be mainly professional in composition, but was to be appointed by the Minister and act under his "general direction."

The local organisation was to be the county councils and county borough councils, and, for running the hospital service, new joint authorities of these councils. Each joint authority was to be advised by a local health services council. The Central Medical Board was to be the contractual employing authority of general practitioners, and the local insurance committees were to be abolished. The voluntary hospitals were to remain autonomous but could participate by entering into contract with a joint authority. Consultants would be salaried, either whole time or part time.

The White Paper placed considerable emphasis on health centres, and implied that general practitioners would be encouraged to work in them. The health centres would be owned, equipped, and maintained by the county and county borough councils. General practitioners in health centres would be paid by salary, and the county and county borough councils would be joint employers with the Central Medical Board.

Two other important functions would be discharged by the Central Medical Board. General practitioners wishing to enter the public service, or to move to new areas or new practices, would be required to obtain its consent; and the board would have power to require newly qualified doctors to work full time in the public service in their early years "if necessary." This last function did not appear extraordinary at a time when a large proportion of doctors had been conscripted into HM Forces.

Finally, the service was to be free to everyone (apart from possible charges for certain appliances). The White Paper admitted that "Any estimates of cost made at the moment can only be conjectural." It suggested tentatively that 27% of the cost would be met by the new social insurance scheme, and the remaining 73% would be shared equally by the taxpayer and the ratepayer.

The Council went to great trouble and expense to keep the profession fully informed. They issued a copy of the White Paper, together with an analysis of it and a questionnaire prepared by the British Institute of Public Opinion, to every member of the profession, including non-members of the BMA and doctors serving with the Forces overseas. It was even hoped to obtain the detailed views of medical prisoners-of-war, but it proved impossible to send the questionnaire because of censorship regulations. Prisoners-of-war were therefore sent the White Paper and the analysis, and were informed that if they cared to make a brief comment on the White Paper in one of their monthly letters or postcards, full weight would be given to any opinions expressed, along with the views of other doctors serving in the Forces. In the UK, BMA divisions were encouraged to arrange meetings of the whole profession (including Forces doctors stationed in their areas) to discuss the White Paper.

THE BMA'S REACTION

The *British Medical Journal* of 13 May 1944 opened with a report of the Council to the Representative Body consisting of a draft statement of BMA policy on the Government's White Paper on a National Health Service, together with the replies by the Minister of Health to 44 questions which had been submitted to him by the Representative Committee. The same issue also contained a leading article entitled "Before negotiations begin" and the Annual Report of Council for 1943-4, in which it was stated that a negotiating committee of 30 members was now to be set up; 16 to be appointed by the BMA (eight by the Council and eight by the Representative Body); three each to be appointed by the Royal College of Physicians and the Royal College of

Surgeons; two to be appointed by the Royal College of Obstetricians and Gynaecologists; one each to be appointed by the three royal Scottish medical corporations; two to be appointed by the Society of Medical Officers of Health; and one by the Medical Women's Federation. Soon afterwards a representative of the Society of Apothecaries was added. This Negotiating Committee remained in being until the National Health Service was eventually introduced in July 1948, Dr Guy Dain being its chairman throughout.

The special report of the Council on the White Paper contained some forthright passages: "The medical profession is in complete agreement with the Government's aim to ensure that every man, woman, and child should be able to obtain all the advice and treatment and care which they may need in matters of health, and that the country's full resources are brought to bear upon reducing ill health and promoting good health in all its citizens. The profession, particularly in the last quarter of a century, has again and again pressed upon the Government of the day developments and amplifications of health provision to this end. That pressure has been almost without avail.... A controversial issue has [now] been raised at a time when the energies of the profession, like those of the whole community, should be directed to one objective — the winning of the war. ... There is suspicion, not without basis, that these proposals found their first inspiration in a desire to control an independent profession in order to control medical certification and so the outgoings of a Social Security Fund. ... Until full details are known of the proposed administrative and professional arrangements and of the social security plan as a whole, and until more information is available as to the proposed machinery for safeguarding private practice among that section of the community which prefers it, the Association cannot commit itself to any acceptance of the 100% principle. . . . According to the White Paper, practitioners working in health centres would be remunerated by salary or similar alternative, the practitioners being in contract both with the Central Medical Board and with the authority owning the centre. The profession sees in this proposal the thin end of the wedge of a form of service to which it is overwhelmingly opposed — a State-salaried service under local authorities."

The *BMJ* leading article also had some pointed things to

say, not all directed at the White Paper: "Of the emotional cross-currents in the life of the profession today, the strongest is suspicion. . . . It is as well to remember that there are now 46 195 members of the BMA, and that there cannot be 46 195 separate plans for reorganising the medical profession. . . . It would be a mistake to think that the public is generally sympathetic to the medical profession as a whole." But the *BMJ* clearly pinpointed the *casus belli*: "Except for a vocal minority of doctors grouped round a party political flag, by far the greater part of the profession is rigidly opposed to a whole-time State salaried medical service, and it is upon this one issue that opposition must be unshakably offered in the coming months."

Almost all of the four days of the annual representative meeting 1944 were taken up with debating the White Paper. The Chairman (Dr Peter Macdonald of York) opened by saying that this was the most important ARM within his memory. Criticism of the White Paper was muted, perhaps because (as Mr Henry Souttar pointed out) a large part of the Government's proposals were based on the findings of the Medical Planning Commission, which had represented the whole profession and whose conclusions had been accepted by the Representative Body. The ARM 1944 resolved: "That the Central Medical Board, if formed, should not have any powers of direction," and "That the profession should not be controlled by the local authority as at present constituted." In addition, the meeting declared that there should be no whole-time salaried service for general practitioners, and that the profession would accept no clinical control. The meeting also passed an important resolution to the effect that any health service proposals should be the subject of a separate Bill, and should not be incorporated in a social security measure. The Representatives* were aware that the social insurance provisions emanating from the Beveridge Report enjoyed a good deal of popularity in the country, and that it would be easier to fight the health service provisions on their own.

After the ARM, the Negotiating Committee had frequent meetings with the Minister of Health, Mr Henry Willink. On 21 March 1945 the BMA Council received a

* Representative with a capital 'R' is a member of the Representative Body of the BMA.

confidential report from the Negotiating Committee and decided to call a special representative meeting in May 1945. The report of Council to this SRM was not published, but was sent under confidential cover to every member of the profession, both members and non-members of the Association. Some irritation was expressed in the House of Commons over the fact that doctors were privy to information that Mr Willink had not yet chosen to make available to Members of Parliament. The BMA Council's confidential document indicated that the Health Ministers had made substantial concessions to meet the BMA's criticisms of the White Paper. Ministers were prepared to drop the Central Medical Board's proposed powers of direction, or to omit the Central Medical Board altogether. Joint authorities would be abandoned, and there would be no question of any contract of employment in a health centre with the local authority.

On 3 and 4 May 1945 the special representative meeting was held. It authorised the Negotiating Committee to continue negotiations; requested the Minister to drop the proposal for a Central Medical Board; and voted against any "basic part salary" for general practitioners. On the 100% issue the meeting rejected an amendment that there should be an income limit for participation in a National Health Service, and passed the following resolution by a large majority: "That the Association, regarding the 100% issue as one for Parliament to decide, is willing to negotiate terms and conditions for such a 100% service, if such be decided upon, provided that ample safeguards are introduced to ensure that any member of the community, whatever his income, should be enabled to obtain his medical service, in part or in whole, privately, as for example by grant-in-aid provisions."

The *BMJ* commented: "There is no doubt that at the meeting last week the representatives appreciated the hard work the Negotiating Committee had put in, and, by their voting on some outstanding issues, believed the results of the negotiations to be such as to provide a sufficient framework for the proposed National Health Service. . . . On one issue that has perplexed many — the 100% issue — the meeting hardly needed to be reminded that 60% of those who answered the [1944] questionary were in favour of including the whole population in a comprehensive health service." So the principle of a universal service was accepted.

Incidentally, the 1944 questionnaire had also yielded some other interesting replies. Although 53% voted against the White Paper, 68% expressed themselves in favour of health centres and 62% were in favour of salaried service for general practitioners *in health centres.*

At the SRM, Dr Guy Dain scored a personal triumph. The meeting expressed its appreciation and gratitude to him for his outstanding services in the negotiations, and the *BMJ* commented: "Not often in representative meetings has the note of affection as well as of admiration been so conspicuous. Some of the great leaders of the past, like the late Sir Henry Brackenbury, inspired great respect and could sway decisions, but they hardly evoked the feeling which was evident in the singing of 'For he's a jolly good fellow' in Dr Dain's honour as the meeting ended."

ENTER ANEURIN BEVAN

The negotiations with the Coalition Government were thus nearing agreement when an event occurred which radically altered the position. This was the General Election of June 1945, the result of which was announced on 26 July 1945. To the world's astonishment the Labour Party was swept into power with a huge Parliamentary majority (180). Sir Winston Churchill wrote afterwards*: "... The verdict of the electors had been so overwhelmingly expressed that I did not wish to remain even for an hour responsible for their affairs. At seven o'clock therefore, having asked for an audience, I drove to the Palace, tendered my resignation to the King, and advised His Majesty to send for Mr Attlee."

Mr Attlee appointed Mr Aneurin Bevan as Minister of Health. He was a Welshman, had started life as a coal miner, and had been prominent in the councils of the South Wales Miners' Federation. Professor Harry Eckstein wrote†: "In 1945, he was still something of an unknown quantity, not having held any political position, senior or junior, until that time. He was known chiefly as a promising nuisance on the extreme left wing of the party." Another

* Winston Churchill *The Second World War*, Vol VI, p 583 (Cassell, 1954).

† *Pressure Group Politics: The Case of the British Medical Association* by Professor Harry Eckstein (George Allen and Unwin, 1960).

opinion is that of Lord Hill of Luton*: "We were to find in Aneurin Bevan a formidable negotiator. Charming and sympathetic at one moment, he could be hotly indignant at the next. In a flash he could spot a point or detect a flaw in an argument, without waiting, or wanting to wait, for a speaker to finish. He would purr or pounce according to his mood. Gaily argumentative in debate, he preferred giving it to taking it."

In April 1943 the Labour Party had published a statement in favour of a full-time, salaried, pensionable State medical service. Aneurin Bevan wanted the National Health Service to be his memorial. He at once pressed ahead with his Party's policy and, without negotiation with the medical profession, introduced a National Health Service Bill on 21 March 1946. Meanwhile, scenting trouble, the BMA Council had established two emergency funds, with a guarantee of £100 000 of BMA money to Fund A (which was to provide the sinews of war), and an appeal to the National Insurance Defence Trust and to the whole profession to guarantee substantial amounts to Fund B (which was to compensate individual doctors who might suffer financial hardship in the fight).

The Bill was accompanied by a White Paper (Cmnd 6761) giving a general description of the proposed health service. Some notable features were as follows.

> All the service, or any part of it, is to be available to everyone. . . . The health service is to be financed partly from the Exchequer, partly from local rates, partly from the . . . National Insurance contributions. . . . There will be some charges.
>
> The existing premises and equipment of voluntary and public hospitals are transferred to the Minister under the Bill. . . . Medical and dental schools are not to be transferred to the Minister or to the Board of Governors of the teaching hospital with which they are associated . . . the Minister is empowered to provide separate pay-bed rooms or blocks for which people can pay the whole cost privately and in which part-time specialists within the service can treat private patients.
>
> A main feature of the personal practitioner services is to be the development of health centres . . . remuneration should take the form of a combination of fixed part-salary and of capitation fees. . . . Actual rates of remuneration for doctors can be determined, in consultation with the profession, only

* *Both Sides of the Hill* by Charles Hill (Heinemann, 1964).

> after the report has been received of the Spens Committee — a special committee set up, by agreement with the profession's representatives and under the chairmanship of Sir Will Spens,* with a membership half medical and half non-medical, to make an independent report on the appropriate range of remuneration for doctors taking part in a publicly organised service of this kind. . . . The total amount of compensation [for loss of the right to buy and sell the goodwill of practices] to be made available under the Bill is a sum of £66 million. . . .

This last point was important. The sum of £66m was generally thought to be fair, and this probably coloured the views of some general practitioners towards the Bill. In a powerful speech at Wimbledon Town Hall on 24 March 1946 Dr Charles Hill said that nobody would be able to criticise these proposals on the ground of inadequate compensation for capital values. That might bring delight to some, he said, but it brought anxiety to others, for one thing was quite clear: "The proposal to abolish goodwill in practices must be examined as a principle rather than as a business proposition." (Applause.)

Dr Hill had stood unsuccessfully as an Independent for Cambridge University in the General Election. He was a brilliant orator, and ended the same speech at Wimbledon with these words: "My job is to express as vigorously as I can the views of the profession as a whole, and I shall go on doing that job in the next few months. But it is your job as a profession to make up your minds on these issues. We are on trial now. This is the most critical phase in the history of the profession. Let us not consider it as a matter of compensation or remuneration. Let us look at principles and determine where in fact the principles lie, and let us, at last, learn to stick together."

SEVEN PRINCIPLES

The *BMJ* of 30 March 1946 included the text of the White Paper, and also seven principles which were stated by the Negotiating Committee to crystallise the views of the medical profession as a whole on the subject of a National Health Service.

---

* Master of Corpus Christi College, Cambridge, and later Chairman of the National Insurance Advisory Committee.

> (*1*) The medical profession is, in the public interest, opposed to any form of service which leads directly or indirectly to the profession as a whole becoming full-time salaried servants of the State or local authorities.
>
> (*2*) The medical profession should remain free to exercise the art and science of medicine according to its traditions, standards, and knowledge, the individual doctor retaining full responsibility for the care of the patient, freedom of judgment, action, speech and publication, without interference in his professional work.
>
> (*3*) The citizen should be free to choose or change his or her family doctor, to choose, in consultation with his family doctor, the hospital at which he should be treated, and free to decide whether he avails himself of the public service or obtains independently the medical service he needs.
>
> (*4*) Doctors should, like other workers, be free to choose the form, place, and type of work they prefer without governmental or other direction.
>
> (*5*) Every registered medical practitioner should be entitled as a right to participate in the public service.
>
> (*6*) The hospital service should be planned over natural hospital areas centred on universities in order that these centres of education and research may influence the whole service.
>
> (*7*) There should be adequate representation of the medical profession on all administrative bodies associated with the new service in order that doctors may make their contribution to the efficiency of the service.

There followed a report by the BMA Council to a special representative meeting called for 1 and 2 May 1946. Here are some notable extracts from this five-page report.

> The Association criticises the proposed administrative arrangements as likely to divide the service into at least three compartments. ... In the Association's considered view, co-ordination should take place at the regional level. Regional boards should assume responsibility for the planning and administration of hospital and non-hospital medical services alike.... This regional integration is essential not only to efficient administration but in the interests of the public. ... The three proposals (*a*) to abolish buying and selling, (*b*) to institute basic salaries, (*c*) to control the distribution of doctors ... would take the profession much nearer the whole-time State-salaried service to which it is so strongly opposed."

And the Council strongly criticised the exclusion from the scheme of the industrial medical services.

No effort was spared by the BMA to keep the profession fully informed. A leading article in the *BMJ* of 20 April

1946 entitled "The Press, the Minister and the Bill" gave an excellent summary of the whole of the National Health Service argument up to date. The following paragraphs are worth quoting *in extenso.*

> It may therefore still serve some purpose if we state as plainly as is possible what the position of the BMA is at this moment. . . . First of all we have, in common with Mr Bevan and his predecessors, the aim of providing a comprehensive health service. . . . Second, we agree that all the resources of modern medicine should be at the disposal of everyone: we differ on the means of achieving this. Third, we approve of the Minister's plan for administering the hospital service on a regional basis, and of his proposals for national laboratory and transfusion services. What are the points of disagreement? There is disappointment that the Minister has not been able to integrate in his Ministry the various services still administered by other Government departments. The administrative separation of hospital, general practitioner, and clinic services makes, in the view of the BMA, proper co-ordination of the work of doctors taking part in them difficult. What is worse, there seems to be a sharp separation of the general practitioner from the hospitals. The failure to give details of the composition of the Regional Board, and the failure to make the Central Health Services Council a really effective body, are further measures on which the Minister is criticised.
>
> If the Bill is looked at as a whole and in relation to the future evolution of the medical profession, there are two features which the Council of the BMA finds not only disappointing but profoundly disturbing. The first is the proposal to disinherit the voluntary hospitals, and to deprive local communities of the part they should play in the development of local institutions. With the ownership of all hospitals vested in the Ministry of Health, given absolute power subject to Treasury direction, the hospitals of this country will in effect be run by the civil servants of the Ministry — for they are permanent, while the Minister is but a temporary figure. A State hospital service means in the long run that medical men working in it will be wholly or partly State employees working under Civil Service direction. State ownership of hospitals can mean nothing less.
>
> The future general practitioner will, it is proposed, practise in the public service in an area only with the permission of a Government committee, be paid in a substantial part by salary, and conduct his practice in and from a health centre owned and administered by local health authorities. This, it is not unreasonable to assume in view of the Labour Party's declared policy, is the first step to a whole-time salaried basis.
>
> Considering the hospital and the general practitioner

plans together, we cannot avoid the conclusion that they form the nucleus of a whole-time salaried State medical service.

This was the paramount fear of the BMA and of most doctors, and a public relations campaign was started on "B-day" (the day on which the Bill was published) to explain it to the press and public. *A Charter for Health* was published,* and a film illustrating the work of the family doctor was produced. Significantly, a joint committee was set up with the Royal College of Nursing, though the passage of time was to show that this alliance between the professions of medicine and nursing was not as close or as influential as had been hoped.

ENTER THE COLLEGES

On 16 April 1946 Lord Moran initiated a debate in the House of Lords on the Government's proposals. Lord Moran (formerly Sir Charles Wilson) had been Dean of St Mary's Hospital Medical School from 1920 to 1945 and was President of the Royal College of Physicians. He was also personal physician to Mr Winston Churchill, who had obtained a peerage for him in 1943.† He drew attention to the fact that one-third of the voluntary hospitals had fewer than 100 beds. He said that in many of them major surgery was performed by men without surgical training, and the duties of physicians were usurped by those who had not been trained as physicians. Every discussion among consultants and specialists who worked in the voluntary hospitals had been dominated by the fear that the hospitals would come under the control of local authorities. Because the present White Paper appeared to lift that menace from the profession, many consultants and specialists were reconciled to the passing of the voluntary system. It was difficult to say what the general practitioner thought of the proposals in the White Paper, but there was fairly general disquiet among practitioners for only one reason, and that was the dread that these proposals might lead to a whole-time service. He himself, after 25 years as dean of a

* *A Charter for Health*, by a committee of the British Medical Association under the chairmanship of Sir John Boyd Orr (George Allen and Unwin, 1946).

† Lord Moran lived to the age of 94, dying in 1977.

medical school, was unable to say what effect a whole-time service would have on the practice of medicine.

Lord Horder, a distinguished physician and a member of the BMA Council, said he was glad that Lord Moran had made it clear that he was speaking for himself. In the previous week the Royal College of Surgeons and the Royal College of Obstetricians and Gynaecologists had dissociated themselves definitely from approval of the transfer of ownership of the voluntary hospitals to the Government. The day before the debate this matter had come under discussion in the College of Physicians, but Lord Moran, in his speech to the House, had made no reference to the opinions of the college over which he presided.

Replying to the debate, Lord Moran said he was an unrepentant advocate of health centres. The reason why the motion had been brought forward was that meetings all over Britain were not having presented to them the considered views of people who had followed the subject on negotiating committees, but in many cases were given just slogans, and great harm was being done. It was imperative that somebody should try to rescue this question from slogans. Lord Horder had mentioned the Royal College of Physicians. Consequently, Lord Moran read the motion passed by that college, which was: "That the College approves the central direction and co-ordination of the general policy of hospitals provided the composition of regional boards is satisfactory."

The second reading debate on the Bill took place in the House of Commons on 30 April and 1 May 1946. Mr Aneurin Bevan adopted a conciliatory tone. "This Bill will universalise the best of advice and treatment. It will strengthen democracy by giving doctors full participation in the administration of their own profession." Doctors would not become civil servants. He was not in favour of a fully salaried service. He had made a further concession: the general practitioner — and the specialist — would still be able to obtain fees. Specialists in hospitals would be allowed to have fee-paying patients. Unless some fee-paying patients were permitted there would be "a rash of nursing homes" all over the country. Only in respect of the sale of goodwill was Mr Bevan provocative: "I have always regarded the sale and purchase of medical practice as an evil in itself. It is tantamount to the sale and purchase of patients."

Mr Ungoed-Thomas (Labour) referred to "the BMA bureaucracy, which so largely misrepresents the interests and the views of the doctors." Sir Wavell Wakefield (Conservative), representing St Marylebone with many consultants and specialists among his constituents, said it was tragic that a measure in the preparation of which the doctors had given their help in the past two decades should be opposed by an almost united medical profession. The reason for this was that doctors felt deeply that the public would be worse served instead of better. The Bill would alter fundamentally the relationship between doctor and patient, and do away with the voluntary principle in our great hospitals.

Mr Reid (Unionist) observed that "the Minister is out for a full-time salaried service as soon as he feels he can impose that upon the country," and Mr Bevan interjected "There is all the difference in the world between plucking fruit when it is ripe, and plucking it when it is green." Mr Reid went on to ask whether the Labour Party's pamphlet *A National Service for Health*, published in April 1943, still held good. In this was written: "In the Labour Party's opinion it is necessary that the medical profession should be organised as a national full-time salaried pensionable service."

Mr Arthur Greenwood, the Lord Privy Seal, wound up for the Government and supplied the answer: "What was published by my party in 1943 . . . we of course stand by. We have never repealed any of our policy, and we shall continue to march on in the light of that policy." So there was ample foundation for the BMA's intense suspicion that the medical profession might be dragooned into a whole-time State-salaried service.

The Lord Privy Seal also made an interesting statement about negotiating machinery: "It is my right honourable friend's intention before prescribing any terms of service or rates of remuneration to use the familiar machinery of discussion and negotiation with employees. Where suitable machinery exists and is in operation it will be used with such adaptations as may be necessary in the new circumstances. What my right honourable friend has in mind where there is no machinery is to set up some machinery of the Whitley Council type behind which there may be provision for agreed reference to arbitration." The NHS Whitley machinery still, 35 years later, has no provision for agreed reference to arbitration.

THE OTHER PARLIAMENT

Starting one day later (on 1 May 1946) the "parliament" of the medical profession, the Representative Body of the BMA, met not far away (in Bloomsbury) in special session to debate the National Health Service Bill. Dr J G Hunter of Sydney, Secretary of the Australian Federal Council of the BMA, was present and said that the members of the profession in Australia were with their British colleagues unanimously in the fight for professional freedom.

The fact that the second reading debate in the House of Commons had started the previous day was held to be important. Dr W N Leak of mid-Cheshire said that it was right that they should express their deep resentment at the way the second reading had been timed. It showed that the Government did not care about the opinion of the profession. Dr Leak moved an amendment to alter the agenda of the meeting "to give Parliament at once some idea of the general reaction of the medical profession to the Bill."

This amendment won a good deal of support, but not the two-thirds majority which it required. The contrary view was that the Representative Body of the BMA should not be hustled into making "a snap diagnosis before anything had been done in the way of inspection, palpation, percussion, and auscultation." (Mr Lawrence Abel of St Marylebone.)

The meeting went on to approve unanimously the seven principles elaborated by the Negotiating Committee and resolved, also unanimously, that "The profession, while anxious and willing to co-operate with the Government in evolving a complete Health Service, is opposed on grounds of public interest to certain important features of the Government's proposals which render the Bill, in its present form, not only unacceptable to the profession but also constitute strong reasons for advising the public against its acceptance."

The meeting voted that "the principle of regional organisation should apply to all health services," and also urged the "immediate publication of the exact constitution of the Regional Hospital Board." An amendment to approve State ownership of hospitals provided that the constitution of the regional boards was acceptable to the profession was lost by a large majority, the meeting preferring the Council's view that "it is unnecessary and undesirable for the Minister to proceed to assume actual ownership of hospitals. . . ."

The Representative Body resolved by huge majorities: "That this meeting regards as essential to the freedom of patients and the profession the right to buy and sell practices as at present," and "That there shall be no control over doctors in regard to the choice of area in which they shall practise." The meeting also voted by an overwhelming majority: "That the remuneration of general practitioners under any National Health Service should take the form of an adequate capitation fee without a fixed part salary and without a tapering scale of payment."

On the second day (2 May 1946), Dr P Inwald (City of London) moved: "That this meeting regards the National Health Service Bill as an important step towards the provision of a comprehensive service available to the whole community, and therefore approves its general framework." He said that his division (which included not only the City of London but six metropolitan boroughs as well) had sent in resolutions year after year supporting a comprehensive health service. They had done this because they thought, as in 1911, that an evolutionary period in the medical service was beginning and that this was the next step. In his division they had a number of socialists, and those who put forward this amendment did belong to the Labour Party and supported the Government; they were not thinking of the Government, however, but of the profession and the people. Their ideal was that no man in a civilised society should suffer or die because of preventable disease or lack of efficient medical attention.

Despite this courageous and persuasive advocacy, and after considerable debate, the amendment by the City Division was overwhelmingly defeated. The meeting went on to resolve: "That while agreeing on the need for improvement in and co-ordination of existing medical services, this meeting disapproves of the methods proposed in the National Health Service Bill to achieve these ends."

Many points of detail were then debated, and the Council

was requested to consider holding a referendum or plebiscite of the whole profession to determine its collective opinion on the Bill. A far-sighted motion was passed "That the medical profession, while anxious to co-operate in any approved National Health Service, is fully aware that the inception of the service as planned by the Minister will entail a vast amount of new work. The profession warns the Minister and the public that the medical manpower and hospital facilities that will be immediately available will fall far short of requirements, with the inevitable result of an overworked and consequently inefficient service." Finally, at the end of the two-day special representative meeting, a vote of confidence was passed in the Council "in its efforts to negotiate with the Minister over the present Bill."

In the same month as the special representative meeting and the second reading debate in the House of Commons, another important event occurred: the publication of the Report of the Interdepartmental Committee on Remuneration of General Practitioners — the first Spens Report. The second Spens Report, on Remuneration of Consultants and Specialists, was published in 1948. The two Spens reports were to prove of great importance. The terms of reference for the first inquiry were:

> To consider, after obtaining whatever information and evidence it thinks fit, what ought to be the range of total professional income of a registered medical practitioner in any publicly organised service of general medical practice, to consider this with due regard to what have been the normal financial expectations of general medical practice in the past, and to the desirability of maintaining in the future the proper social and economic status of general medical practice and its power to attract a suitable type of recruit to the profession, and to make recommendations.

The Spens committee on general practitioners had been set up by the Coalition Government in February 1945, the Chairman being Sir Will Spens; it included four general practitioners chosen by the BMA, and four lay members (in addition to the chairman). One of the joint secretaries was Dr A V (Peggy) Kelynack of the BMA staff. In June 1946 the BMA Council stated that the report had been well received by general practitioners throughout the country and particularly by the Insurance Acts Committee of the Association. The Council recommended that the Representative Body should welcome and approve the report. Its implementation was destined to cause years of controversy.

Another event, disconcerting to those who feared that the Government's plan was to put shackles on the medical profession, was an attempt by the Willesden Borough Council to compel all its employees (including its medical officers) to be members of trade unions — in other words, to impose a closed shop. This was a problem that was to recur from time to time in succeeding years. In a long and cogent article in the *BMJ* of 18 January 1947 analysing some constitutional and medical issues raised by the National Health Service Act, Mr Reginald T Payne FRCS wrote: "An organisation where union membership is a primary condition of employment, and that union is linked to one political party, rapidly approaches the one-party State."

The National Health Service Bill became law on 6 November 1946. The BMA immediately conducted a plebiscite of the whole profession to determine whether or not the doctors should agree to enter into discussions with the Minister on the necessary regulations. Voting papers were sent to all doctors in the United Kingdom and in HM Forces and strict precautions were taken at the headquarters of the BMA to ensure that the secrecy of individual voting was preserved. In Great Britain 37% of doctors voted yes; 55% voted no; and 8% did not reply.

A majority of 55% against co-operation in the National Health Service was indecisive, but it was sufficient to warn the Minister that his cherished scheme was in danger. The presidents of the three London Royal Colleges (Lord Moran, Sir Alfred Webb-Johnson, and Mr William Gilliatt) decided to write to the Minister. Their letter (dated 2 January 1947) began: "The opposition of a substantial part of the medical profession to any renewal of discussions with the Government regarding the National Health Service is causing us concern. We fear that it may lead to an impasse, and we wish to do what we can to prevent such an impasse arising." The presidents went on to ask for clarification and assurances on several contentious matters such as the basic salary for general practitioners, the liberty of movement of general practitioners, and the continuation of private practice by specialists. Mr Bevan replied on 6 January 1947 and appealed for negotiations. "I agree with you that an impasse between the Government and the medical profession would be a grave misfortune. . . . I can certainly assure you that, if discussions take place, I shall endeavour to meet any views of the profession which do not conflict with the principles of the Act." In a general and conciliatory way, he went on to deal with the specific points mentioned by the presidents, and had this to say on the continuation of private practice by specialists: "In the case of a consultant on a hospital staff . . . he will be able to treat his private patients in the private beds of his own or other hospitals, subject to availability, and I recognise with you the need for both public and private accommodation, as indeed I have made clear in Parliament on a number of occasions."

The presidents incurred widespread criticism for writing their letter. In 1948 Mr Reginald T Payne FRCS wrote: "The action of the Presidents of the three Royal Colleges in January 1947 was a risky one and it failed in its object. It damaged the prestige of the Colleges, endangered relations between consultants and general practitioners, encouraged the Minister, and misled the press." But a different view has been expressed by Dr A M Cooke*: "Someone authoritative had to make some move and the letter certainly removed more bad feeling than it created."

The BMA Council convened a special representative meeting on 28 January 1947 to consider the following recommendation from the Council: "That the Association, having considered the final results of the plebiscite and the Minister's letter of 6 January to the Presidents of the Royal Colleges, and desiring to secure for the people the best possible health service, is willing that discussions be entered into with the Minister to that end, provided that such discussions are comprehensive in their scope, and that the possibility that they may lead to further legislation is not excluded; and that after the conclusion of these discussions a second plebiscite of the profession be taken on the issue of entering the Service." In presenting the recommendation, the Chairman of Council (Dr Guy Dain) said: "If the Minister refuses to negotiate we have done no harm in making the offer, and we have had the opportunity of putting ourselves right with the public."

Dr W D Steel (Worcester and Bromsgrove) said that the plebiscite showed a bare majority, not strong enough to

* *A History of the Royal College of Physicians of London*, Vol III (Clarendon Press, 1972).

justify the use of brute force. Tactful diplomacy was necessary, and the Council's recommendation exactly filled that prescription. Lord Horder (St Marylebone) said it was weak to refer to the correspondence between the Minister and the Royal Colleges, in view of the fact that such correspondence did not alter the main issue. It was vital that the Minister from the first should be aware of the necessity for some fresh legislation. After considerable debate the Council's motion was passed by 252 to 17, but several speakers had demanded a promise from the Minister of amending legislation. There was also some criticism of the membership of the Negotiating Committee. Dr R W Cockshut (of Hendon) said that it was of vital importance that when this matter was put to the Minister it should be put by people who believed in the principles established by the profession. The Royal Colleges did not believe in these principles. In the end, however, the meeting decided to leave the composition of the Negotiating Committee unaltered, accepting the view of the Chairman of Council that "a certain price had to be paid for the great advantages of having in the Negotiating Committee all the elements of medical life in this country."

NEGOTIATIONS RESUMED

On 31 January 1947 the Permanent Secretary of the Ministry of Health (Sir William Douglas) wrote to the BMA: "The Minister wishes me to say that he has considered the terms of the resolution [of the special representative meeting] and will be glad if the Negotiating Committee will resume discussions with him, in the light of that resolution, at their early convenience." So Mr Bevan at last agreed to begin real negotiations: one of the BMA's main complaints was that until then he had refused to negotiate in any real sense of the word.

In May 1947 the second Spens committee — on the remuneration of consultants and specialists — was appointed. It consisted of Sir Will Spens (chairman) with five medical representatives (Professor D Murray Lyon, Lord Moran, Sir Harry Platt, Dr S Cochrane Shanks, and Mr J R H Turton) and five lay representatives. One of the two joint secretaries was Dr D P Stevenson of the BMA staff.

The greater part of 1947 was occupied by discussions

between the Negotiating Committee (and its six subcommittees) and officials of the Ministry of Health. The discussions culminated in meetings with the Minister himself on 2 and 3 December 1947. The Negotiating Committee urged the Minister to make changes in the scheme to meet the points raised by the committee, where necessary by amendment of the Act itself.

On 20 December 1947 the Negotiating Committee published an account of the results of the negotiations in the past year. Altogether 27 pages of that issue of the *BMJ* were devoted to arguments about the National Health Service. It is not necessary to reproduce here all the detailed objections to the Act. Suffice it to give the following extracts from the first leader in the *BMJ* of that week: "Yet a crisis of confidence has been precipitated, and it cannot be denied that Mr Bevan himself has helped to precipitate it. . . . He has made, it is true, concessions to the consultants and specialists, in particular by his offer to set aside in State hospitals a limited number of beds in which consultants and specialists may treat patients with no restriction on the fees to be charged. . . . Mr Bevan refuses to remove the ambiguity and anomalies of Section 35* of the Act in spite of the fact that his interpretation of the wording in particular of Subsection 4 of this section is challenged by two of the most prominent legal advisers in this country, Sir Cyril Radcliffe KC and Mr J H Stamp. . . . Mr Bevan claims that his Act does not conflict with any of the profession's principles. We believe, on the contrary, that the Act is the first step towards a whole-time salaried State medical service, and the refusal of Mr Bevan to amend the Act strengthens this belief."

On 27 December 1947 the BMA Council announced that a second plebiscite of the whole profession was to be held, and on 8 January 1948 a special representative meeting expressed the opinion that "the National Health Service Act 1946 in its present form is so grossly at variance with the essential principles of our profession that it should be rejected absolutely by all practitioners."

The plebiscite form invited the voter to state, firstly, whether he or she approved or disapproved of the National

---

* This was the section that prohibited the sale of medical practices. It contained 12 subsections, and included in subsection 4 some tortuous provisions affecting partnership agreements.

Health Service Act 1946 in its present form; and, secondly, whether he or she was or was not in favour of accepting service under the Act in its present form. The preamble stipulated that if the votes of consultants and specialists, general practitioners, and whole-time voluntary hospital staffs showed a majority against accepting service under the Acts, and this majority included "approximately 13 000 general practitioners (out of a present total general practitioner strength of 20 500)," the Association would advise the profession not to enter the Service.

The result of the second plebiscite was unmistakable: 84% of the profession voted, and of these no less than 90% disapproved of the Act in its present form. Every section of the profession, and all age groups, showed large majorities against the Act. Even the doctors already in whole-time Government service voted heavily against the Act — striking evidence of the profession's confidence in the secrecy of the ballot, which was audited by a leading firm of chartered accountants. Of those concerned, 86% (including 17 000 general practitioners) voted against accepting service under the Act in its present form.

Several important meetings were held after the announcement of the results of the plebiscite. On 10 March 1948 a conference of representatives of Scottish divisions and local medical and panel committees was held in Edinburgh. On 16 March a special conference of representatives of local medical and panel committees was held at BMA House, London, and on 17 March another special representative meeting was held.

At the special panel conference an important question was raised. Dr P Y Lyle of Southport moved that the conference would welcome a definite assurance that there was in existence an alternative plan for the medical services of the nation should the profession be advised not to accept service under the Act. Dr E A Gregg said that a committee had been set up, with Dr Frank Gray as chairman, which had gone into the whole question of the conduct of practice in the event of a dispute of this kind with the Government, and the report of that committee had been circulated to all panel committees. It appeared that panel committees did not wish to have a stereotyped standard method applied all over the country, and that this was a matter which should be determined in each locality. Dr Lyle was disappointed with this reply and pressed his motion to a division, in which it was carried by 99 votes to 56. Later, Dr Gregg remarked: "Our alternative is the National Health Service scheme with the changes in it for which we have asked." This revealed a serious weakness. There appeared to be no clear-cut plan as to how doctors were to carry on practices, and earn their incomes, if they refused to join the National Health Service.

The special representative meeting on 17 March 1948 opened with an expression of gratitude (carried with "prolonged acclamation") to Dr Dain and the Council for their untiring efforts in addressing meetings of divisions and making known the important matters at stake; and also to Dr Hill and the headquarters staff for the efficient manner in which they had kept in touch with members in all branches of the profession. A further motion was carried expressing appreciation of the work of the Editor (Dr Hugh Clegg) and staff of the *British Medical Journal*, both in keeping the profession informed of the progress of events and in "moulding opinion by means of a valuable series of leading articles."

Lord Horder then moved: "That in view of the continued misleading statements made by the Minister of Health and supported by some sections of the press, this meeting wished to place on record its opinion that the British Medical Association is thoroughly representative of the medical profession and that the Council and the BMA representatives on the Negotiating Committee could not be elected more fairly or freely." He said that the Minister had accused the BMA of being engaged in a "squalid political conspiracy" and that the Rt Hon Hugh Dalton had spoken of the Negotiating Committee as a handful of elderly doctors dictating to the profession. Lord Horder continued: "We believe that the Association has got the confidence of the public in a fuller measure today than ever before. This is reflected in the fact that, of 68 350 doctors registered in the British Isles in January of this year, 58 000 are members of the Association. But I would not put the profession's confidence today at the height at which I believe it to exist merely on numerical strength. I believe it to be due to the realisation that the Association's policy . . . commands the adherence of the whole profession." Lord Horder's motion was carried unanimously.

The Chairman of Council, Dr Guy Dain, then presented

a masterly review of the position,* and moved: "That the Representative Body, reaffirming the whole-hearted desire of the medical profession for a comprehensive health service available to everyone, urges that in the public interest such changes should be made in the National Health Service Acts of 1946 and 1947 [the second of these was the Scottish Act] as are necessary to maintain the integrity of medicine and to prevent doctors being turned into State servants, with harmful consequences to patient and doctor alike. The Representative Body therefore expresses the hope that the Government will make it possible for the profession to co-operate by making such changes, and states its view that it is not in the best interests of the public or of medicine for members of the profession to enter the Service until such changes are made." The motion was carried unanimously. The BMA's objective was now plain for all to see: amendment of the Act.

Later, the representative meeting unanimously resolved to establish an independence fund (to take the place of the guarantee funds established two years previously) in order to finance the profession's activities during the present dispute with the Government, with an initial donation of £400 000 from the National Insurance Defence Trust.

Some idea of the passions aroused at this time may be gleaned from what a correspondent wrote to the *BMJ* on 10 April 1948: "As soon as the appeal [for the independence fund] arrived yesterday morning I filled in the form and enclosed a cheque for £100. I could not do otherwise when I remembered Nuremberg. . . . It is because of fear of this degradation if we surrender our liberty to the State under the authority of Ministers as devoid of culture as those who held sway in the Germany of the recent past that I hasten to support the Independence Fund." Even so, only 6000 doctors contributed to the independence fund.

There was another outburst of passion at the end of the SRM, when a motion was passed instructing the Council, the profession having expressed its emphatic view through the plebiscite, not to be influenced by any "quislings" — however exalted they might be. A few days later the Royal College of Physicians of Edinburgh submitted several resolutions to the Prime Minister urging the resumption of

---

* *British Medical Journal*, Suppl, 27 March 1948, pp 50, 51.

negotiations. And on the 22 March 1948 the Comitia of the Royal College of Physicians of London, still under the presidency of Lord Moran, passed two resolutions and sent them to the Minister of Health.

> (*1*) The College affirms its desire for unity and recognises that the comprehensive health service cannot be successful without the willing co-operation of all branches of the profession. The College believes that this can be furthered if the Minister of Health makes clear in an amending Act that a whole-time service shall not be brought in by Regulation; so that if any future Government desires to introduce such a service, a fresh Act of Parliament would be required. The College reaffirms its opposition to a whole-time medical service.
>
> (*2*) A principal cause of the present discontent with the National Health Service is the power possessed by the Minister of Health to change its character by Regulations. The College therefore suggests than an amending Bill should be introduced to make Regulations affecting the National Health Service subject to special procedure.

These resolutions were supported by the Royal College of Obstetricians and Gynaecologists, and somewhat less firmly by the Royal College of Surgeons, whose President (Sir Alfred Webb-Johnson) said that "the legislation suggested ... would not by itself be sufficient to secure the willing co-operation of all branches of the profession." The same point was made by Dr Guy Dain in a letter to *The Times* of 7 April. But at least the main objective of the BMA — some amendment of the Act — was publicly supported by the Royal Colleges.

Meanwhile, despite the BMA's dislike of the Act as it stood, the BMA Council was giving detailed consideration to the question of suitable representation of consultants and specialists vis-à-vis the new regional hospital boards. The Council had before it the example of the local medical and panel committees which had been set up under the National Insurance Act of 1911 to represent general practitioners vis-à-vis the insurance committees, and which were copied into the National Health Service Act of 1946. The Council decided to set up similar machinery for consultants and specialists. In each region the BMA would take steps to secure the election by consultants and specialists (including those who were not members of the BMA) of a regional consultants and specialists committee;

and at the centre the Council decided to replace two of its existing standing committees (the Consultants and Specialists Committee, and the Hospitals Committee) by a new Central Consultants and Specialists Committee, consisting mainly of representatives elected to it by the regional committees. This was an extremely important new committee which posed an obvious challenge to the claim that the Royal Colleges spoke for the hospital branch of the profession.

BEVAN HOLDS OUT AN OLIVE BRANCH

At the special representative meeting on 17 March 1948 Dr Dain said: "We are ready to enter into any discussions directed to making it possible for the medical profession to co-operate with the Government. If the Government can show us other ways, new ways, of preserving our independence we are willing to listen." In the House of Commons on 7 April Mr Aneurin Bevan made a statement in which he undertook to make clear by statute that a whole-time service would not be brought in by regulation, but would require further legislation to make it possible, Mr Bevan also suggested important modifications of his previous proposal for a universal basic salary. In reply to questions, Mr Bevan affirmed his wish to discuss these matters with representatives of the medical profession. The next day (8 April) the National Health Service Executive Committee of the BMA Council issued a statement welcoming the observations made by the Minister, noting that they presented a changed approach, and inviting him to receive a deputation to consider a series of written questions. The executive committee's statement was put out through the news media without any prior consultation with the Council. This was unfortunate, because many doctors had not read Mr Bevan's latest remarks in Parliament and were surprised, to say the least, when they read in the newspapers that the deadlock between the Minister and the doctors had been resolved. As a result, many doctors gained an impression that their leaders, having taken their followers to the brink, had now begun to waver. Accusations were made subsequently that these events had caused a crisis of confidence, which had influenced the voting in the third plebiscite. As stated on 17 April 1948 in an editorial in the *BMJ*, the plain fact was, however, that: "Mr Bevan has made a gesture of conciliation, and has taken steps to meet two of the principal objections of the medical profession to the present Act."

The BMA's 14 questions and the replies of the Minister of Health and the Secretary of State for Scotland were published in the same issue of the *BMJ*. In the next issue there was a statement by the BMA Council, which included the following passages: "We now have the new proposals. In order that the profession may, in the most democratic way, determine its views and intentions on the new situation created by these statements, the Council submits the issue afresh to the profession in plebiscite form. ... We have succeeded on some points, such as the bar on the introduction of a whole-time salaried service by regulation, and the universal basic salary. We have failed on others, such as the ownership of goodwill and the right of appeal.... Bearing in mind that what we have secured falls short of what we sought, the Council's view is that, while progress has been made to that end, the freedoms of the profession are not sufficiently safeguarded. Whatever your views, please vote in order that the plebiscite may faithfully represent the views of the profession and guide those whose heavy responsibility it is to act on its behalf. Meetings of the profession will be held in your area between April 21 and April 26. Please do your best to attend your local meeting."

So the decision was made to hold a third plebiscite of the whole profession. The plebiscite form again made it clear that if in the aggregate vote the replies (from general practitioners, consultants and specialists, and whole-time voluntary hospital staffs) showed a majority against accepting service under the Acts, and this majority included at least 13 000 general practitioners (out of a total general-practitioner strength of 20 500), the BMA would continue to advise the profession not to enter the Service.

The first leader in the *BMJ* of 24 April 1948 said: "We must therefore take note of the fact that public opinion, as expressed by those who represent their constituents in Parliament and by responsible daily and weekly newspapers, considers that Mr Bevan has made a conciliatory move towards a solution of present difficulties. It is recognised that this move has been made as the direct result of the enormous vote of no confidence in the present Act given in the plebiscite earlier this year. The Government had to take this into account and has in consequence modified its policy. Doctors must now ask themselves whether the modifications go far enough to remove their underlying fears of the Act in its unmodified form." A correspondent in the same issue of the *BMJ* supplied his own personal answer: "Our net gains, then, from these "conciliatory" assurances would seem to be *nil*, and we are likely to lose from their possible weakening effect on some in our ranks."

This is exactly what happened. The April plebiscite form was sent to 54 667 doctors, of whom 40 462 (74%) voted. In section A, 25 842 (64%) expressed disapproval of the National Health Service Acts, notwithstanding the modifications now proposed by the Government, and 14 620 (36%) expressed approval. In section B (the vital question about taking service under the Acts), 13 891 (52%) were not in favour of accepting service under the Acts, and 12 799 (48%) were in favour of accepting service. But the majority against accepting service included only 9588 general practitioners, a figure far short of the 13 000 which had been clearly stipulated as necessary to make the Act unworkable. The great and natural fear of many general practitioners was that enough of their colleagues might join the Service on the appointed day to make it workable, and so would take away the bulk of the patients.

On 5 May 1948 the BMA Council met to consider the results of the plebiscite. Be it noted that the National Health Service (with much other related social legislation, none of which had caused any controversy, strange to say) was due to come into operation only two months later, on 5 July 1948. At the end of a long, difficult, and tiring day's discussion, the Council decided to recommend to the Representative Body that the profession should "co-operate in the new service on the understanding that the Minister will continue negotiations on outstanding matters, including terms and conditions of service for consultants and specialists, general practitioners, public health officers, and others." The Council also resolved to accept the Minister of Health's invitation to enter immediately into discussions on the details of the promised Amending Bill, and on other outstanding matters.

A leading article in the *British Medical Journal* entitled

"What we have gained," said some things for which the Editor was later bitterly criticised. The article said: "We have only to contrast the scheme put forward by a Liberal Minister of Health [Mr Ernest Brown] with the present scheme to see what great changes have been made as a result of the intermittent negotiations that have been going on for the past five years." It went on to detail ten gains which the BMA had secured by its tenacity. The article continued: "It would seem that some of our correspondents do not have a 'whole-hearted desire,' or, indeed, any desire at all, for a comprehensive medical service available to the whole community. This is a tenable position, but it is not the policy of the British Medical Association. . . . Mr Bevan, in the light of his own statements and of the policy of his own Party, has by his promise of an Amending Bill and other concessions in written answers to questions gone a considerable way to meeting the demands of the medical profession. He has offered a compromise, and compromises are the traditional English way of settling disputes. For the medical profession to reject the compromise and to be intransigent would cost it the support of public opinion. . . . During the past months the medical profession has shown its strength and has shown, too, that it can use it with wisdom."

DECISION TO CO-OPERATE

The momentous special representative meeting called by the Council to consider the results of the third plebiscite and the consequent recommendation of the Council to co-operate in the new health service was held in the Great Hall, BMA House, London, on Friday, 28 May 1948. Dr J B Miller of Bishopbriggs presided, supported by Sir Hugh Lett Bt, President of the Association, Dr H Guy Dain, Chairman of Council, Dr J W Bone, Treasurer, and the chief officials of the Association. The atmosphere was charged with excitement, and heated debates continued all day. Very early in the day a motion by Newcastle upon Tyne was carried: "That the Council's action in calling for a third plebiscite so quickly after the second one was premature, and indicated approval of the new conditions which had been offered, and prejudiced the voting. The meeting considers that such a step should only have been taken on the decision of a special representative meeting."

There then followed a long debate on the Council's recommendation A (to co-operate in the new service). Dr Guy Dain confessed: "I was never so disappointed in my life as I was when the figures of the April plebiscite came in." Lord Horder said that in St Marylebone they thought that the men and women who were signing on daily to join the National Health Service were signing on for economic reasons and for motives of fear, especially the fear that they might lose their compensation [for the loss of the right to sell their practices]. Dr S Wand said that the army was so satisfied with the achievements of the generalship that it had started to go home. That was the present position whether they liked it or not. Throughout the country the press and important bodies of professional men had congratulated the BMA on the magnificent fight it had put up for freedom and the victory it had won. Dr A C E Breach (Bromley) spoke of this "tragic meeting." The smell of appeasement was concentrated here. Dr Wand had said that their army was "going home." The truth was that the army thought its leaders had gone home.

In reply to the debate, Dr Dain said that the statement that they accepted defeat was nonsense. They had gained the greatest victory against the Government, which had been compelled to accept an Amending Act before the main Act came into force.

This was indeed an unusual achievement. The Council's recommendation, as follows, was carried by a large majority:

> That, despite the insufficiency of the safeguards to the profession's freedom and the misgivings of a substantial section of the profession, the Representative Body, anxious as ever that in the public interest a comprehensive health service should be made available to the community, is prepared to advise the profession to co-operate in the new Service on the understanding that the Minister will continue negotiations on outstanding matters, including terms and conditions of service for consultants and specialists, general practitioners, public health officers, and others.

A motion by Guildford of no confidence in the Council, and calling for its resignation, was then lost by an overwhelming majority. There followed a motion by Burnley complaining of the disastrous effect on the plebiscite of the *BMJ* leaders of 17 and 24 April and calling for the discharge of the Editor. After a brisk debate this also was lost by a large majority.

Finally, an important motion by Dr A G Manley of Richmond (based on a recommendation from the Council) was carried: "That the public be adequately informed that, for reasons outside the control of the profession, the inception of the new Service cannot be followed for some time to come by all the improvements promised by the Government in the medical services of the country, because of the shortage of personnel, medical and nursing, and of the difficulty of providing the necessary premises and equipment, and although the medical profession will make every endeavour to work the scheme, it cannot hold itself responsible for the Government's promises."

So ended a momentous day. That night a young assistant secretary of the Association (EG-T) wrote in his diary: "Today was the day of the vital representative meeting of the BMA. All day the Great Hall at BMA House was packed and the debate raged, before a full visitors' gallery and press bench. In the morning the 'rebels' — so-called because they disapproved of the Council's recommendation to co-operate now in the Health Service — were in bellicose mood. They attempted to alter the agenda so that the votes of censure on the Council would be heard first, and if they had succeeded in this I think the day might have gone differently. As it was, a motion of censure on the Council for holding the [third] plebiscite was proposed by Dr Mona MacNaughton in a powerful speech and carried. This blew off a good deal of the rebel steam. The Council's famous recommendation A, to co-operate in the Service, was debated at great length. Lord Horder made a long but not very telling speech against it — he was generally regarded as the leader of the 'revolt.' The vote was finally taken after tea and the Council's recommendation was adopted by a substantial majority. After that the Guildford motion, calling for the resignation of the Council, and the Burnley motion, calling for the discharge of the Editor, were both heavily defeated."

THE END OF THE STORY

Immediately after the SRM the Negotiating Committee and its subcommittees were reconvened and recommenced urgent negotiations with the Health Ministers and their officials. The *BMJ* of 5 June 1948 printed an explanatory statement from the Ministry of Health about the remuneration of general practitioners taking part in the National Health Service, and also a statement for patients "of the changes that will take place on July 5 under the National Health Service as compared with the present position under the National Health Insurance Scheme."

The same issue of the *BMJ* published several letters bitterly critical of the line just taken by the BMA, and this bitter criticism was to continue for years. Two examples will suffice:

> Outmanoeuvred, outwitted, and stampeded, the Council rushed that plebiscite upon us without our having sufficient time to consider and discuss the full implications of the Minister's tardy modifications to certain details of the Act which we could not accept.
>
> We are mostly an inarticulate profession and leave letter writing to the other man. However, that does not mean to say that we do not feel deeply how badly we have been let down by our Council.

But outside observers saw things differently. The *Economist* commented: "Undoubtedly the doctors have won a big victory, for Mr Bevan does not easily climb down to the extent that he has done."

In a detailed analysis of the long negotiations between the Government and doctors (*BMJ* supplement, 29 January 1949, p 46) Dr R W Cockshut of Hendon wrote: "When, therefore, Mr Bevan in the House of Commons in April 1948 promised on behalf of the Government to introduce legislation to make it impossible to institute a salaried service under the present Act, and retreated from his proposal for a universal basic salary, the position changed radically. Here was a triumph for the BMA. Looking back at the Minister's cocksureness, at the astounding debate, at the insults and bullying, it was truly remarkable. . . . There is still no certainty about what the diehards wanted to fight for. The time has come when somebody should say quite clearly whether appeal to the courts and buying and selling were issues in which the Representative Body should have led the great rebellion, and those who claim that the profession has been let down should be more explicit and let us know just what should have been done."

After a lapse of a third of a century, we may wonder why a National Health Service scheme which incorporated much of what had been advocated by the BMA itself in *A General Medical Service for the Nation* (1938) and the report of the Medical Planning Commission (1942) should have aroused such determined hostility from the Association in 1948. This hostility was not so illogical as it might seem. The planning reports had not been deeply studied by the rank and file of the profession. But when Mr Aneurin Bevan's Bill appeared, they did not like the feel of it. Most doctors sensed that it presented a threat to their independence of action in the practice of their profession. This did not mean that they had withdrawn their support for a general medical service for the nation — only that they did not approve of the sort of service that Bevan intended to impose on them. When he promised to amend his Act, enough doctors agreed to co-operate to make it work.

Many people at the time were puzzled by the sudden volte-face in the BMA's attitude. The fact is that there was an emotional, even political, undercurrent to the dispute. In July 1945, when the great war-leader Churchill was (in his own words) "immediately dismissed by the British electorate from all further conduct of their affairs," many in the middle classes were uneasy. Their misgivings were increased by the utterances of some of the Labour leaders. The Attorney-General (Sir Hartley Shawcross) was reported to have declared: "We are the masters now." The Secretary of State for War (Mr Emanuel Shinwell) said that he did not care a "tinker's cuss" for the middle classes. And Mr Bevan himself (albeit at a later date) said that as far as he was concerned the Tory Party were "lower than vermin." This kind of attitude provoked resentment and belligerence in professional people. So long as the Minister of Health exhibited a high-handed, truculent attitude towards the medical profession the doctors were united against him. The pretexts of the dispute were technical and were not understood by the general public, who were not much interested in an abstract concept of "professional freedom" and could not fathom why general practitioners should object so strongly to receiving a salary. The second plebiscite forced Mr Bevan to make important concessions to the BMA. As soon as he showed that he had learnt that he could not ride roughshod over the BMA and the medical profession, the attitude of the doctors changed.

In the House of Commons on 7 April 1948 the only Communist MP, Mr Willie Gallacher, asked the Minister of Health: "While agreeing that it is very desirable that the National Health Service should start off in a healthy manner, would it be permissible for the Government or the Minister to advise the workers to show the same solidarity and tenacity as the doctors?"

Aneurin Bevan did not reply. The BMA had won its spurs as the standard-bearer of the middle classes.

Chapter 4

Decolonisation

> These are ties which, though light as air, are as strong as links of iron. — Edmund Burke, 1775. Quoted on the back of the presidential chair at BMA House.

In 1932 the BMA had 57 overseas branches (that is, branches outside the United Kingdom). They were in Australia (six branches), New Zealand (one branch), South Africa (11 branches), Southern Rhodesia (two branches), the Indian subcontinent (11 branches), the Irish Free State (three branches), and one in each of the 23 colonies and dependencies of: Jamaica (the oldest overseas branch, founded in 1877), the Leeward Islands, St Lucia, Barbados, Trinidad and Tobago, Grenada, British Guiana, Bermuda, Gibraltar, Malta, Egypt, Mesopotamia, Kenya, Uganda, Tanganyika, Zanzibar, Northern Rhodesia, Nyasaland, Sierra Leone, Burma, Hong Kong, Malaya, and Fiji. The BMA branches in Canada had been dissolved in 1926 after the British and Canadian Medical Associations had entered into an affiliation agreement — which was to set the pattern for many others to follow.

Since 1932 the BMA has formed new overseas branches in British Honduras, St Vincent, Cyprus, the Sudan, Aden, the Seychelles, Mauritius, Lesotho, the Gambia, and ten other areas in which the new branches have subsequently been dissolved. The branches in all the "great Dominions" have also been dissolved and replaced by affiliation agreements, as described below. The BMA now (in 1981) has 15 overseas branches.

Before the second world war, a considerable section of the annual report of Council was devoted each year to overseas affairs. At that time the British Empire still existed and the BMA ruled its own overseas empire, albeit benevolently and on a loose rein. At the centenary meeting in 1932 a conference of representatives of the overseas branches was held, together with members of the Council, to discuss matters of common interest. This was the first overseas conference which, for several years, became a regular feature of the annual meeting, reaching a peak of importance in the 1950s.

Examples of the kind of activity undertaken by the overseas branches are shown in the following extracts from the 1933 Annual Report of Council.

> The Malaya Branch held a number of meetings, and its annual meeting was held in Singapore, in January 1933. The matters discussed included the remuneration of estate medical officers and the proposed formation of a group of these practitioners within the Branch; retrenchment of officers in the Malayan Medical Service; publication of articles in lay press; fees in estate and Government hospitals; the outpatient problem; blood transfusion service; the best method of organisation of the Branch; fees for medical examination for life insurance; medical education in Malaya; the *British Pharmacopoeia* 1932; history of the Singapore General Hospital; and the present state of medical knowledge of the anopheline mosquito in Malaya. A golf competition and annual dinner were also held.
>
> The Gibraltar Branch held five general and three council meetings; also a social function. At its clinical meetings cases and specimens were displayed and discussed. Smallpox was one of the subjects dealt with, and *x*-ray films of abdominal diseases were shown. The collection of books for the Branch library (recently formed) is progressing. The Branch entertained the medical officers of the Mediterranean and Atlantic Fleets on two occasions.

These examples clearly illustrate the functions of overseas branches of the BMA: to promote scientific discussion and exchange of information; to represent the profession on terms and conditions of service; and to provide some social events for the local doctors and their families.

In 1934 the Council expressed great concern at the proposal by the 1930-1 Indian Round Table Conference to abolish the civil branch of the Indian Medical Service. In forthright terms, the Council stated: "The Indian Medical Service is acknowledged to be one of the finest medical services in the world. In the past it has attracted to it medical men of the highest professional attainment, whose work in India and elsewhere has been of outstanding importance in the fields of medicine, surgery, public health, education, and research. There is every justification for asserting that the work of members of the service has been, and still is, of incalculable value to the welfare of the peoples of India." The Council went on to describe in detail the work of the IMS (both military and civil), and to examine the best ways of recruiting doctors to the service, concluding that "the successful recruitment of the Indian Medical Service would not be maintained if the civil branch of the service were discontinued as proposed by the Services Subcommittee of the Round Table Conference." It is interesting to note, however, that the Bombay Branch of the BMA formally dissented from the views expressed by the Council, and its dissenting memorandum was forwarded by the Council to the Joint Select Committee of Parliament which was considering proposals by the Imperial Government for Indian constitutional reform.

The BMA has always been prepared to adopt new and flexible constitutional arrangements to meet changing times. As long ago as 1921, the Articles and Bylaws were amended to allow overseas groups of branches or individual branches to become locally incorporated and self-governing. In 1934 the Federal Committee of the BMA in Australia became incorporated, with the title of Federal Council of the BMA in Australia. Thus was born a powerful new member of the world family of medical associations, but it is interesting to record that the Australian branches of the BMA did not choose to form themselves into an independent Australian Medical Association (affiliated to the BMA) until 1 January 1962. The six BMA branches were then formally dissolved and the BMA Council commented: "Although this is a matter for regret, it is also one for rejoicing and congratulation."

The annual meeting in 1935 was held in Melbourne (Australia), and a package tour round the world (by sea, of course) was arranged for those attending from the United Kingdom. There had previously been four annual meetings outside the UK, three of them in Canada (Montreal, 1897; Toronto, 1906; and Winnipeg, 1930), and one in the Irish Free State (Dublin, 1933). Several more annual meetings were held overseas:

1952 Dublin (Republic of Ireland)
1955 Toronto (Canada)
1961 Auckland (New Zealand)
1966 Karachi (Pakistan)
1968 Sydney (Australia)
1973 Vancouver (Canada)

All these meetings were highly successful, and on each occasion chief officers and officials of the Association took the opportunity to visit overseas branches and affiliated associations on the outward and return journeys. The meetings were held jointly with the relevant national association, and it was the custom for the two associations to share the same president.

In 1976 the annual meeting was a tripartite affair, being a joint meeting in Dublin of the British, Canadian, and Irish Medical Associations. Mr Barry O'Donnell FRCS, FRCSI of Dublin was installed as President of all three associations. In fact, at that time the Irish Medical Association was still an incorporated, self-governing group of branches of the BMA. A special agreement between the BMA and the IMA signed in 1936 remained in force until 31 December 1977, when the Irish Medical Association finally separated from the BMA, but became allied to it by another special agreement. On the occasion of the Dublin Meeting in 1976 the British and Canadian Medical Associations presented a ceremonial mace to the Irish Medical Association.

The joint meetings overseas did much to cement the ties between the BMA and the overseas branches and affiliated associations. In addition, special visits took place from time to time. At a meeting of the Dominions Committee on Empire Day 1937, consideration was given to the desirability of sending a member of the medical secretariat on what was referred to as a "colonial tour" in order to establish contacts, investigate difficulties on the spot, and increase the likely effectiveness of action by the Association. In 1939 the Secretary of the Association visited the West Indian branches, in connection with comprehensive evidence which the BMA presented to the Royal Commission on the West Indies, but the war prevented further realisation of this plan. Then, in 1949, the secretary of the Colonies and Dependencies Committee (as it had then become) was sent on a tour of the BMA branches in East Africa. This was followed by a tour of the Caribbean branches in 1950, a tour of the Mediterranean and Middle Eastern branches in 1951, a tour of the West African branches in 1955, and a tour of the Far Eastern, Central African, and East African branches in 1959. These tours were immensely instructive and valuable to the secretaries of the Overseas Committee who undertook them, and also demonstrated to the overseas branches and members that the BMA was anxious to take a real interest in their affairs. In addition, visits to overseas branches were made from time to time by chief officers, members of Council and chairmen of the Overseas Committee. In 1962, for example, the President of the BMA (Sir Douglas Robb of Auckland, New Zealand) visited Sydney, Melbourne, Adelaide, Singapore, Kuala Lumpur, Penang, Bangkok, Hong Kong, Jorhat, Calcutta, Madras, Bombay, Delhi, Agra, Karachi, Beirut, Jerusalem, Nicosia, London, Belfast, New York, Toronto, and Papeete.

In 1948 the BMA Council established the Empire Medical Advisory Bureau, which was to become a department at BMA House where overseas doctors would be welcomed on their arrival in Britain, and where they could obtain general information and advice on postgraduate work, accommodation, and contacts they might make with their British colleagues. The foundation of this special department (to be followed shortly by the International Medical Visitors Bureau, for foreign doctors) was an altruistic action by the BMA which was outstandingly successful. In terms of hard cash it has cost the BMA between a quarter and half a million pounds in the past 33 years, and the BMA has not always received due credit from HM Government and other bodies for its public-spirited effort. One of the first actions of the bureau was to compile a "Summary of Regulations for Postgraduate Diplomas and of Courses of Instruction in Postgraduate Medicine" which was of immense value and was published annually by the BMA for many years. Another was to arrange regular receptions for Commonwealth and foreign medical visitors at BMA House, to enable them to meet leading members of the BMA and other representatives of British medicine. These friendly receptions for overseas doctors continued for many years. Much of the success of the Commonwealth and International Bureaux was due to the genial personality and fatherly wisdom of the first medical director, Brigadier H A Sandiford, who retired in 1957.

We must now return to our earlier narrative. In 1939 the Australian Federal Government passed a National Health Insurance Act and a royal commission was set up to take evidence from interested parties. The BMA made a special additional grant of £1000 to the Federal Council in Australia to help it present the views of the medical profession. In 1942 South Africa followed suit and a National Health Services Commission was appointed to conduct an inquiry into the provision of a service "in conformity with the modern conception of health" which would ensure adequate medical, dental, nursing, and hospital attendance for all sections of the people of the Union. The report of the commission was published in 1945 and, unlike some other reports, was received with great satisfaction by the medical profession.

At this time the Medical Association of South Africa was an incorporated group of branches of the BMA, but before the war a desire for complete independence had been expressed by some of the BMA members in South Africa and in 1945 the Federal Council of the Medical Association of South Africa consulted their members by referendum. A substantial majority voted for separation of the MASA from the BMA, but with an affiliation agreement. The BMA Council in London immediately acquiesced in this desire, and the BMA branches in South Africa were formally dissolved on 31 December 1945. Soon afterwards the BMA and the MASA entered into an affiliation agreement, and cordial relations continued between them. It is worth remarking that the Medical Association of South Africa has never countenanced any racial discrimination among its own members, and has strenuously fought against it (with a great deal of success) wherever it has been imposed in the terms and conditions of service of doctors in South Africa.

Plans were made for the annual meeting of the BMA to be held in South Africa in 1941 but the war led to postponement. The plan was revived after the war and a joint meeting with the Medical Association of South Africa was due to be held in Johannesburg in July 1951. Dr A W S Sichel of Cape Town, President of the MASA, was nominated for election as President of the BMA. Dr Sichel was indeed elected and inducted as President of the BMA, but the joint meeting in South Africa was cancelled by the BMA because doubts arose whether those BMA members who happened to be coloured would all be admitted by the South African Government to attend the meeting. The cancellation was a grievous disappointment to the Medical Association of South Africa, which had made elaborate and hospitable arrangements to receive all visiting BMA members, regardless of race.

When India achieved independence in 1947, negotiations between the BMA and the Indian Medical Association were undertaken and were harmoniously concluded in 1952. The BMA branches in India were dissolved, and an affiliation agreement was made between the British and Indian Medical Associations. (In due course affiliation agreements were also made with the Pakistan and Ceylon Medical Associations.) One branch of the BMA in India was preserved at its own special request, and with the concurrence of the Indian Medical Association. This was the Assam Branch, which still had a high proportion of British members (mainly doctors working on the tea estates). In due course conditions changed, however, and the time came for the Assam Branch to request dissolution. This was done on 27 April 1966. So ended the BMA's long and honourable presence in the Indian subcontinent.

In 1966-7 the BMA branches in New Zealand, Nigeria, Rhodesia, and Sierra Leone were dissolved and replaced by independent medical associations, all of them affiliated with the BMA. The affiliation agreements which were made all over the world followed the same pattern. They provided for reciprocal membership for members of one association in the territory of the other, for the regular exchange of journals and other official documents, and for the exchange of delegates at the respective annual meetings.

Affiliation also means mutual assistance when the occasion arises. In 1961 the Government of Saskatchewan passed a Medical Care Insurance Act, despite objections by the medical profession. The starting date of the medical care plan (in 1962) was postponed because of the doctors' opposition, and the Government of Saskatchewan started to recruit British doctors to work the Act. At the request of the Canadian Medical Association, the BMA placed Saskatchewan in the "Important Notice" in the *British Medical Journal.* Within a few weeks (as a result of mediation by

Lord Taylor FRCP, from Britain) the Saskatchewan Government undertook to amend the Act and the dispute was settled. In 1965, when the Government of Mr Ian Smith made its unilateral declaration of independence in Rhodesia, the British Government imposed sanctions and stopped all movement of goods and persons to Rhodesia. The BMA, with which the Rhodesian Medical Association was affiliated, was unhappy with this policy so far as medicine was concerned. The BMA Council stated publicly its "firm conviction that the political situation should not be allowed to deny to the peoples of Rhodesia the benefit of life-saving drugs and new medical knowledge and information." Believing that medicine is international, and that only in times of outright war should medical links be severed, the BMA made representations to the Foreign and Commonwealth Office to obtain permission for British doctors to go out to fill medical vacancies in Rhodesia, and some success attended these efforts.

While moves towards the formation of independent associations from the pre-existing BMA branches had been taking place in the self-governing Dominions, and towards the creation of new linkages through affiliation and the formation of new international medical associations, the BMA continued to take a great interest in the affairs of its branches in the colonies, and to help with their problems. The war had put a stop to most of the activities of the smaller overseas branches: as peacetime conditions gradually returned, these branches were systematically revived, and several new branches were formed. In these respects the visits by chairmen and secretaries of the Overseas Committee were invaluable: the visitor met the local BMA members (both in the capital and upcountry), met the Governor, the chief officials, and political leaders, and made representations to them about any grievances or problems that had been reported by the BMA members.

In 1949 the BMA in London submitted detailed proposals to the Colonial Office for substantial improvements and rationalisation of the terms of service of Colonial Medical Officers. In drawing up its proposals on pay, the BMA attempted to do two things (*1*) to arrive at a fair colonial equivalent of the Spens recommendations for the remuneration of the profession in the National Health Service ("Spens" having become the yardstick for judging

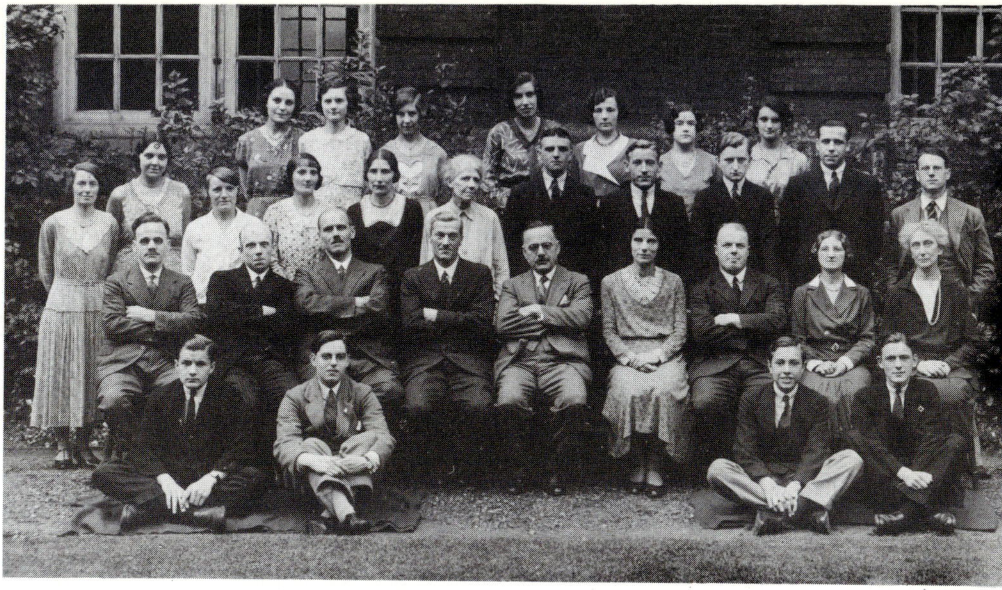

1932 THE MEDICAL SECRETARY, DR ALFRED COX, AND HIS CLERKS. MR GEORGE PERKINS IS STANDING IMMEDIATELY BEHIND DR COX.

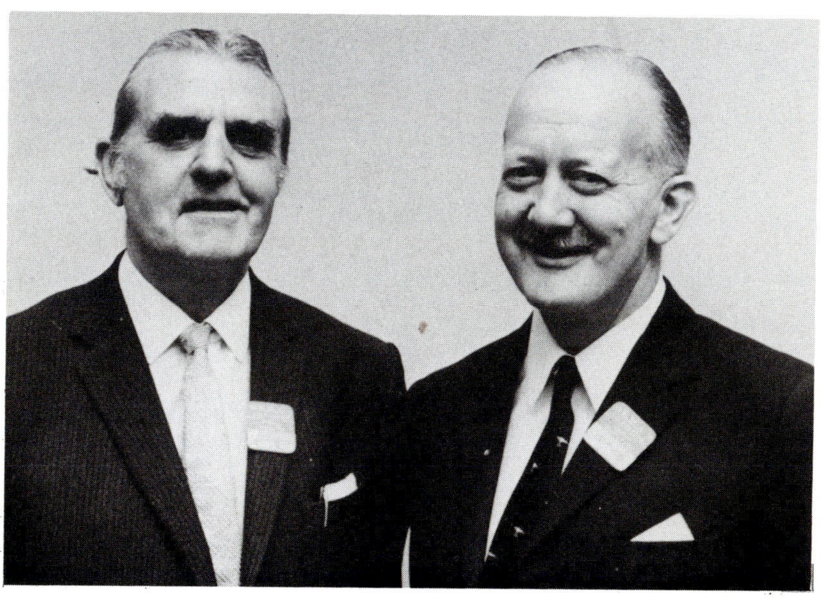

1973 MR GEORGE PERKINS AND MR JOHN HUISH, ON THEIR RETIREMENT.

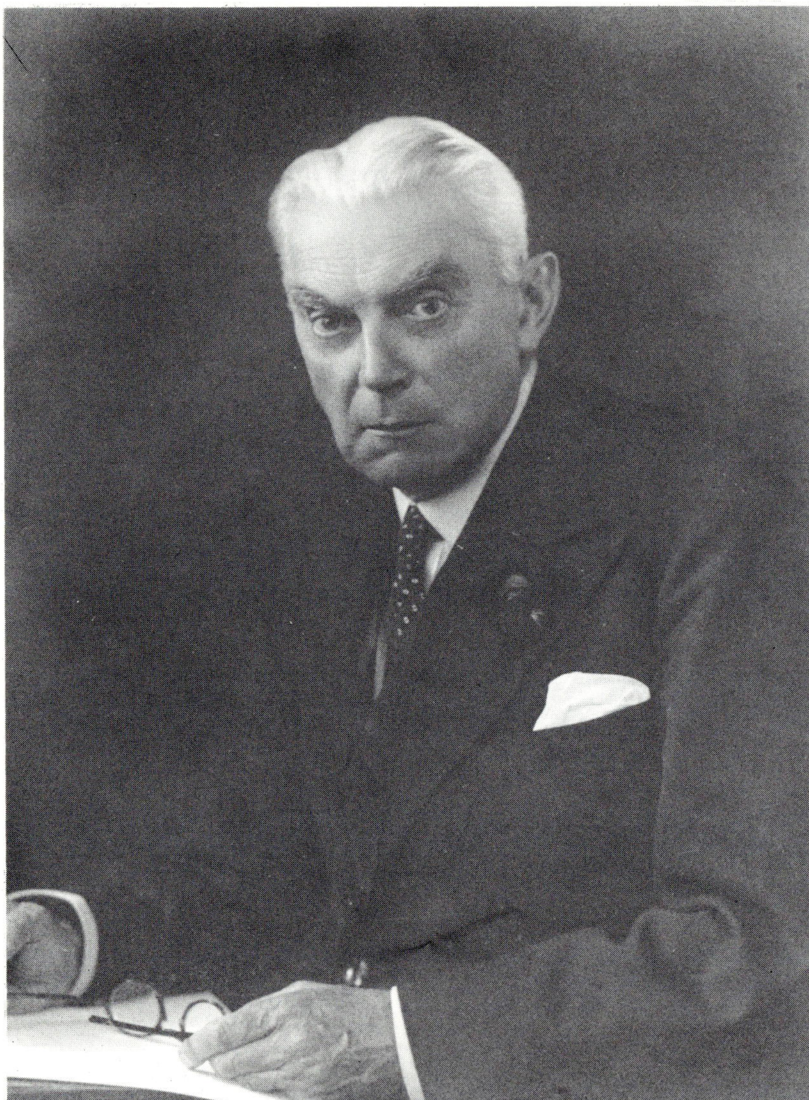

Sir Kaye Le Fleming
Chairman of Representative Body 1931–4.
Chairman of Council 1934–9.

the remuneration of BMA members in any publicly organised medical service), and (*2*) to draw up a single uniform scale applicable to all colonial territories. With regard to this second objective, it became apparent in the negotiations with the Colonial Office that because of the wide variation throughout the colonies in such matters as taxation levels, cost of living, and conditions of work, a scale of salaries which might be a fair equivalent of Spens in one colony would be far from equivalent in another. Consequently, the attempt to produce a single uniform scale of figures was abandoned in favour of "the achievement of a broad equality of real reward" (words used in the annual report of Council for 1949-50). A thorough examination was made of the various advantages and disadvantages of a Colonial Medical Officer's career and an attempt was made to assess their value in terms of money. The conclusion was reached that the (recently improved) salary scales in the Far Eastern and West African colonies were satisfactory, but that considerable amelioration was required in the East African and Central African colonies. Proposals were agreed with the Colonial Office for correcting the deficiencies. The painstaking analysis of the various factors which had been made in a joint working party of the BMA and the Colonial Office was noticed by *The Times* in a complimentary leading article.

A conference of the Caribbean branches of the BMA was held in 1951, presided over by Dr Guy Dain of the BMA Council and attended also by Dr H B W Morgan, the representative of the Caribbean branches on the BMA Council. Some resolutions passed by the Caribbean conference were remitted to the Colonial Office for consideration, and a Caribbean Council of the BMA was established in anticipation of the federation of the British West Indies which was then envisaged. The BMA Caribbean Council continued to hold meetings for the next 20 years.

In 1953 Mr (later Sir) Ian Fraser of Belfast (a member of Council) visited the Gold Coast and on his return representations were made to the Colonial Office about the feeling of insecurity which existed among British doctors as to the future of the Gold Coast medical service, with a consequent reluctance to take up vacancies as they occurred. The suggestion was made that a civil service (including a medical branch) might be organised on a Commonwealth basis.

In that same year (1953), appointments under the Government of Cyprus were "blacklisted" in the *British Medical Journal,* after two years of fruitless negotiations about the remuneration of Government specialists. A salaries commissioner was appointed and the Cyprus Branch submitted evidence, both written and oral, to the commissioner. A supplementary memorandum of evidence was submitted by the BMA in London.

A good illustration of the activities of the overseas branches at this period was provided by the fifth annual meeting of the Middle East Branch, held at Damascus from 14 to 16 March 1955. Doctors from Syria, the Lebanon, Jordan, Iraq, and the Gulf States attended the meeting. Dr W M Ford Robertson of Beirut was elected President, and Dr E H R Altounyan of Aleppo was elected Honorary Secretary. The opening address of the scientific programme was given by the Minister of Health for Syria, and 22 papers were read and discussed, including three by distinguished visitors from London and Paris. The British Ambassador held a reception for all the doctors and their wives attending the meeting, and the annual dinner of the branch was held at the Orient Club. A special air excursion to Palmyra was organised on the day after the meeting.

In 1956 a serious dispute arose between the medical profession in Malta and the government of Mr Dom Mintoff. The principal issue was the Maltese Government's apparent intention to convert the Government medical service into a whole-time salaried service without private practice. The secretary of the Overseas Committee was sent out to Malta, and collective resignation of the Government medical staff was organised. Feeling ran high on both sides, and the situation became tense.

On 16 April 1956 the resignations of almost all Government medical officers came into effect, and an emergency medical service was set up by the doctors to provide essential medical attention by day or night. After some days a delegation from Malta came to London, and talks were held at BMA House to try to find a solution acceptable to both sides. A settlement of the dispute was finally reached late on 24 April 1956, when the Government of Malta agreed to an independent commission of inquiry and to the immediate reinstatement of all the Government doctors on the conditions obtaining at the time of resignation, including continuity of service and pension entitlements. The next day the Chairman of the Overseas Committee (Mr J L Gilks CMG, FRCSEd) flew to Malta to help the doctors during the phase immediately after the end of the dispute.

In due course the commission of inquiry entirely vindicated the stand taken by the medical profession. But animosities smouldered on and came to a head 21 years later, by which time Malta was an independent republic and the Malta Medical Association was fully independent of the BMA, although it worked closely with the BMA's Malta Branch which was still in existence. When Mr Mintoff was again in power in 1977 his Government interfered with the independence of the registration authority and the University Medical School, and imposed a measure of conscription on the medical profession — to such an extent that nearly all the professors and specialists resigned their appointments or were dismissed. The Malta Government proceeded to import doctors from the Communist world to staff its medical service. The BMA placed the Government of Malta in the "Important Notice" in the *BMJ*, and raised the plight of the medical profession of Malta twice in the General Assembly of the World Medical Association, which attempted to mediate.

But Mr Mintoff was undeterred. Many Maltese doctors and medical students came to Britain, and the BMA did its utmost to help these refugees from oppression. The BMA raised a fund of £27 000 to relieve distress, particularly among the displaced Maltese medical students. This is a tragic chapter in the long and distinguished medical history of Malta.

As more and more British colonies attained self-government, the careers of many expatriate medical officers were cut short, and in general these doctors experienced considerable difficulty in finding new medical employment on returning to the United Kingdom. This growing problem caused much concern to the BMA, which called a conference of distinguished people in November 1958 to debate a whole range of possible solutions. The President of the Association (Professor, later Sir, Arthur Thomson) took the chair, and the opening speakers included Sir Charles Jeffries (formerly of the Colonial Office), Mr (later Sir) Bernard Braine MP, Professor (later Sir) Alan Moncrieff, and Professor Charles Wells. Many interesting suggestions were discussed, such as the creation of a Commonwealth Medical Service, the linkage of the Colonial Medical Service with the Medical Branch of the Home Civil Service, and the establishment of some supernumerary appointments in UK universities and hospitals, to be held overseas; but no easy solution presented itself.

The BMA was also active in trying to solve the problem of recruitment to the Colonial Medical Service, later entitled the medical branch of HM Overseas Civil Service. The Association submitted proposals to the Platt Working Party on the Medical Staffing Structure of the Hospital Service, including exchanges, secondment, and the proleptic appointment of consultants in the NHS so that they could serve overseas for a period before taking up their consultant appointments. The BMA also established an overseas appointments fund, from which grants were made to help young doctors with those incidental expenses which might deter a young doctor from taking up a short-term post in one of the colonies or newly independent territories of the British Commonwealth.

But the BMA's efforts to safeguard the careers of doctors electing to work overseas encountered many difficulties. On 23 April 1960 the Chairman of the Overseas Committee (then Professor D E C Mekie) published a letter in the *BMJ* advising doctors not to apply for a permanent appointment advertised in British Honduras, because of the uncertain prospects there. He wrote: "... It is unfair to ask any individual doctor to accept the hazards and uncertainties of career appointments in the overseas services unless, and until, he can be assured that in the event of premature termination of his overseas post he can be guaranteed satisfactory reinstatement in this country." And in the *BMJ* of 16 May 1964 the chairman of the Overseas Committee published another strong letter, this time defending the BMA from an accusation that the Association had not done enough to safeguard the position of Government medical officers in the short-lived Federation of Rhodesia and Nyasaland. Professor Mekie gave chapter and verse of all the actions that the BMA had taken on their behalf.

In the late 1960s, the BMA started to hold annual clinical meetings outside the United Kingdom. These were outstandingly successful, attracting large contingents of members from the British Isles and other countries, and giving great enouragement to the local doctors hosting the meeting. Such meetings were held in Malta (1969), Cyprus (1972), Jamaica (1974), Denmark (1975), Holland (1977), Gibraltar (1978), Hong Kong (1979) and San Diego, USA (1981). Perhaps the most noteworthy of all these was Hong Kong. There was an enormous attendance from the British Isles, from Hong Kong itself (now the BMA's biggest overseas branch), and from other countries, and there was a high-ranking official delegation from the People's Republic of China. Never was there a better example of the important professional and diplomatic role which the BMA plays in the world of medicine.

FOREIGN AFFAIRS

Up to now this chapter has been almost entirely concerned with the BMA and the British Commonwealth. The BMA also has many dealings with foreign countries and foreign doctors. Even today, three of the BMA's overseas branches are in foreign countries: Lesotho, the Middle East, and the Sudan. Many international conferences have been held or entertained at BMA House, and innumerable foreign visitors (some very distinguished) have been received there.

As one of the celebrations of the centenary of the BMA in 1932, the Council created a new class of honorary membership — "foreign corresponding members." This was intended to be the highest compliment that the BMA could pay to a distinguished foreign doctor, and the first list included Calmette, Cushing, Flexner, and Pavlov. Later additions have included Ramon y Cajal, Bordet, Domagk, Houssay, Minot, Peyton Rous, and Olivecrona. The names of all the foreign corresponding members are inscribed in letters of gold outside the Great Hall at BMA House.

In 1967 a category of "Commonwealth corresponding membership" was created to enable the BMA to honour outstanding medical men and women in the Commonwealth. Only one Commonwealth corresponding member has so far been elected: Sir John Eccles of Australia.

In 1947 the BMA Council presented to the American Medical Association, on the occasion of its centenary, a gavel and block bearing the following inscription:

> To the American Medical Association on the occasion of its centenary, as a token of goodwill from the British Medical

Association, this gavel and block made from the mulberry tree which grew in the garden of Charles Dickens's home in London where the British Medical Association House now stands, June 1947.

There have been many other occasions in the past 50 years when the BMA has made presentations to other medical associations and to its own overseas branches to commemorate anniversaries or successful joint meetings, and the BMA in its turn has received many handsome gifts.

During the early postwar years a scheme was operated by the BMA (with the approval of the Bank of England) to enable British doctors to visit Canada or the USA or both for professional purposes, in exchange for Canadian and American doctors visiting Britain. The scheme was of real value in promoting contact between medicine in Britain and in North America at a time when the restrictions of exchange control made it almost impossible for British doctors to obtain any allowance of dollars.

In 1952 the BMA sent an invitation to the President of the Academy of Medical Sciences of the USSR for six Soviet doctors to pay a goodwill visit to Great Britain. The invitation had been sent with a little prompting from the Foreign Office, but it was declined. The next year, however, Stalin died and the BMA's invitation was renewed. This time it was accepted, and in October 1955 six distinguished representatives of the medical profession of the Soviet Union spent three weeks in Britain as guests of the BMA. In addition to many institutions visited in London, the tour included Edinburgh, Glasgow, Birmingham, Oxford, and Cambridge. The visit ended with a farewell dinner in the Great Hall of BMA House, at which compliments and gifts were exchanged. In due course, the Academy of Medical Sciences of the USSR invited six representatives of the BMA to pay a return visit to Russia, and this took place in August 1956. The BMA representatives were Dr Mary Esslemont, Mr Ian Fraser, Dr J G M Hamilton, Sir Geoffrey Jefferson, Dr Ralston Paterson, and Professor (later Sir) George Pickering, with Dr Alexander Duddington as interpreter.

These two visitations between the BMA and the Academy of Medical Sciences of the USSR were a manifestation of the "thaw" which took place in the Soviet Union's relations with the West after the death of Stalin. But the thaw was short-lived. In October 1956 Soviet troops moved into Hungary to crush a popular uprising against the communist regime. Some Hungarian doctors escaped to the West, and about 50 arrived in Britain. They were welcomed at BMA House and given financial and other help. The Chairman of Council launched an appeal fund, and some of the proceeds were sent to the Austrian Medical Association which was striving to relieve distress among the large number of Hungarian medical refugees in that country. The BMA has never been backward in helping colleagues in distress, whether British or foreign, such as the Czechoslovak refugees in 1968, the Ugandan Asians in 1972, the Maltese in 1977, and the Vietnamese in 1979. In addition, the BMA has frequently protested to the appropriate national or international authorities in proved cases of political oppression of individual doctors. The 1979 annual report of the International Medical Advisory Bureau included this passage: "From national publicity members will know of one happy event during 1979 which caused a great deal of delight to everyone, not least the staff of the bureau. This was the release from Russia of Misha Voikhansky to join his mother, Dr Marina Voikhanskaya, who has been in touch with the bureau for the past three years. . . . She is now working as a houseman in psychiatry and has proudly applied for membership of the British Medical Association."

THE BMA AND THE COMMONWEALTH MEDICAL ASSOCIATION

Alongside the steady march of the BMA's overseas branches towards self-government and then independence, the parent body turned its attention to a new kind of linkage.

In 1947 the BMA Council invited the affiliated associations or branches in the self-governing Dominions to co-operate in the establishment of a special council to be called the British Commonwealth Medical Council. The first meeting was held in September 1948 at BMA House, and was attended by delegates from Australia, Canada, Ceylon, Great Britain, India, Ireland, New Zealand, Pakistan, South Africa, and Southern Rhodesia. The chair was taken by the BMA President, Sir Lionel Whitby. It was evident that there was a general desire and need for some permanent liaison between the national medical associations in the countries of what was then called the British Commonwealth of Nations.

In 1959 the BMA hosted the fifth meeting of the British Commonwealth Medical Council. Delegates from ten countries (including the Republic of Ireland) attended. The subjects discussed included the relationship between the medical profession and the public, the filling of medical vacancies in the Commonwealth, and the health services in the countries represented. The meeting also considered the establishment of a Commonwealth medical association, with a permanent secretariat.

The Commonwealth Medical Association was duly founded in November 1962 in Colombo, and Professor D E C Mekie of the BMA was appointed Honorary Secretary-Treasurer. In 1964 the BMA hosted the second meeting of the council of the Commonwealth Medical Association at BMA House in London. Ten member associations were represented and the Canadian Medical Association sent observers. Sir Arthur (later Lord) Porritt presided. Apart from the business sessions, dinners were given in honour of the council by HM Government, the Royal College of Obstetricians and Gynaecologists, and the British Medical Association.

In recent years the BMA's commitment to the Commonwealth Medical Association has weakened. There is a feeling that in the 1980s the Commonwealth link is more sentimental than practical. It is also appreciated that if the BMA is to devote more of its energies and resources to the medical institutions of the European Community, the scale of the BMA's commitment to the Commonwealth Medical Association will have to be reduced. The BMA remains a founder member of the CMA, however, and the executive of the CMA met in London in 1981.

THE BMA AND THE WORLD MEDICAL ASSOCIATION

Besides fathering the Commonwealth Medical Association, the BMA also played a big part in creating the World Medical Association. Before the second world war the BMA was a member of the Association Professionnelle Internationale des Médecins (APIM), which had been founded in 1926 by Dr Alfred Cox (Secretary of the BMA) and Dr

Decourt. A report of its activities invariably appeared in the annual report of Council. By 1939, however, the Council had come to the conclusion that the BMA's membership of APIM should be discontinued on the grounds of cost and the amount of work needed: but the question was shelved because the outbreak of war put a stop to the activities of APIM.

In 1945 the BMA decided to arrange a conference with medical representatives of the Allied countries to explore ways and means of promoting closer relations between the BMA and the organised medical profession in other countries. This conference was held at BMA House on 6 June 1945, when doctors from Belgium, France, the Netherlands, Poland, Yugoslavia, the USA, and, of course, the UK were present, together with the Secretary of the APIM. The meeting decided that a second and larger conference should be held at BMA House in September 1946 to consider the formation of an international medical organisation with the following objects: (*1*) to undertake an exchange of information on medical affairs; (*2*) to promote closer ties among different national medical organisations; (*3*) to encourage better international relations generally by personal contact and otherwise; and (*4*) to embody, continue, and extend the work formerly undertaken by the APIM.

So the BMA's disillusionment with the APIM, evident in 1939, had evaporated in the fires of war, and here was the BMA taking the lead in forming what was soon to be launched as the World Medical Association.

The second conference was held at BMA House, London, on 25-27 September 1946, under the chairmanship of the BMA President, Sir Hugh Lett. There were 32 countries represented. A World Medical Association was formed with the following provisional objects: (*1*) to promote closer ties among the national medical organisations and among the doctors of the world by personal contact and all other means available in order to assist all peoples of the world to attain the highest possible level of health; (*2*) to study the professional problems which confront the medical profession in their different countries; (*3*) to organise an exchange of information on matters of interest to the medical profession; and (*4*) to establish relations with and to present the views of the medical profession to the World Health Organisation, UNESCO, and other appropriate bodies.

The BMA Secretary, Dr Charles Hill, was appointed provisional joint secretary with Dr Paul Cibrie of Paris.

At the conference in September 1946 delegates from the Continent spoke with great feeling of the crimes committed by medical practitioners in their countries during the war. Action was called for to prevent any repetition of such conduct, and the BMA drew up a statement on *War Crimes and Medicine*, which was adopted and published by the General Assembly of the World Medical Association in September 1947.

In October 1949 the 3rd General Assembly of the World Medical Association was held at BMA House in London. The President was Dr Charles Hill, who remarked beforehand to the organising secretary: "Let us show them how to run a meeting of this sort." The meeting was considered to be an outstanding success. The WMA returned to London in 1965 for its 19th General Assembly, and this was generally adjudged an even greater success.

In 1951 the BMA Council decided to raise no objection to the admission to the WMA of the medical associations of West Germany and Japan. The enmities of the war years had finally subsided.

The BMA hosted the First World Conference on Medical Education, held in London in August 1953 under the joint auspices of the World Medical Association and the World Health Organisation. The president of the conference was Sir Lionel Whitby, past President of the BMA and Regius Professor of Physic at Cambridge. Over 600 men and women from 62 countries attended the conference, and there was a list of brilliant speakers. The four vice-presidents, each responsible for a section of the agenda, were Professor A Hurtado (Peru), Dr Victor Johnson (USA), Sir A L Mudaliar (India), and Professor A Stampar (Yugoslavia). The Secretary of the Programme Committee was Dr Hugh Clegg (Editor of the *British Medical Journal*).

In 1957 the BMA Council received with dismay a report that the French Medical Confederation had decided to withdraw from the World Medical Association owing to an increase in its subscription. The French Medical Confederation, however, ultimately decided to remain a member. Also in 1957, the British Supporting Group for the WMA was inaugurated on the initiative of the BMA Council, and in it a small band of internationally minded people have continued to have faith in the World Medical Association in good times and in bad.

In 1968 the BMA Council itself became concerned at the rising cost of the BMA's membership of the World Medical Association, but accepted the advice of its Overseas Affairs Committee that the objectives of the WMA continued to be as desirable as before, and that it was very desirable that the BMA continue to give full support to the WMA. A feeling was beginning to arise that the World Medical Association had not yet emerged from the stage, common to all international organisations, of creating cordial personal relations, and was not moving on to the stage of effective action which would be of tangible benefit to the member associations, including the BMA.

From 1961 to 1966 a BMA member, Dr H S Gear, was Secretary-General of the World Medical Association. In June 1969 Dr Derek Stevenson, Secretary of the BMA, was elected Chairman of the council of the World Medical Association. The WMA began to include in its annual assemblies whole-day symposia on sociomedical topics.

The headquarters of the World Medical Association was moved in 1973 from New York to near Geneva, mainly for reasons of economy. Not long afterwards the USA withdrew from the WMA for some years.

At the 28th World Medical Assembly in 1974 the BMA undertook to prepare a report on the medical aspects of the interrogation and artificial feeding of prisoners. The BMA convened a special working party to undertake this delicate task, and the BMA's report was used by the World Medical Association as the basis of its Declaration of Tokyo (1975).

By 1977 serious doubts had arisen in the BMA Council as to whether continued membership of the World Medical Association was justified or worthwhile in view of the substantial cost and in view of the BMA's increasing responsibilities to the European medical institutions. A forceful speaker in the Council, Dr Brian Lewis, stated that "a World Medical Association which did not include the Soviet Union, China, and the United States was merely a grandiose title. . . ."; and the President (Mr Barry O'Donnell of Dublin) pointed out that out of 126 countries in the United Nations only 52 were members of the WMA. But other members of Council recalled that the BMA had played an important part in founding the WMA, and that the WMA had a vital role as the mouthpiece of the medical profession to Governmental bodies, such as the World Health Organisation, especially in matters traditionally assumed to be in the hands of the profession — such as medical ethics, medical education and standards. In the end the Council decided, with much heartburning, to recommend to the Representative Body that the BMA should withdraw from the WMA at the end of 1977: but the annual representative meeting declined to support the recommendation with the necessary majority. In fact, the BMA delegation played a prominent part in the 31st World Medical Assembly in Dublin in 1977 and Mr Walpole Lewin, immediate past-Chairman of the BMA Council, was elected Chairman of the WMA Council.

In 1979 the BMA Council, even more concerned at the rising cost of membership of the World Medical Association, again decided to recommend that the BMA should withdraw from the World Medical Association (and also from the Commonwealth Medical Association), but the representative meeting again rejected the recommendation. And so, despite recurrent doubts about its cost-effectiveness (which were first expressed in 1939, in relation to APIM), the BMA continues in membership of this international association of national medical associations, and has in fact made great contributions to its activities and to its personnel.

THE BMA AND THE EUROPEAN ECONOMIC COMMUNITY

In recent years a third important international linkage has claimed the attention of the BMA — the European Economic Community. In 1957 the Treaty of Rome was signed, and in July 1961 the Prime Minister (Mr Harold Macmillan) announced that his Government had decided to apply for accession to the treaty. The next day the Overseas Secretary of the BMA telephoned the Foreign Office to inquire what implications this might have for British medicine, and in February 1962 the BMA began discussions with the Ministry of Health about these implications. In that same year the BMA sought and obtained observer status on the recently created Standing Committee of Doctors of the EEC.

Britain's first application to join the EEC was vetoed by General de Gaulle, but the BMA prudently continued its observer membership of the European medical institutions. On 13 May 1967 the *BMJ* published an authoritative article by Mr N G C Hendry FRCSEd (one of the BMA's European observers) entitled "Medicine and the Treaty of Rome." And on the 23 July 1970 the other BMA European observer (Dr E Grey-Turner) published an article in the *BMJ* entitled "European Common Market and British Medicine." These two articles spelled out the medical implications of the Treaty of Rome for the information of the British medical profession: mutual recognition of European medical qualifications, free movement of doctors throughout the Community, and the accreditation and identification of specialists. The BMA Council also set up a special Committee on the European Economic Community, which contained not only representatives of all the main branches of the medical profession, but also (by invitation) representatives of the dental and nursing professions, of the General Medical Council, of the Health Departments, and of some other bodies.

In 1971 this committee drew the attention of the Department of Health and Social Security to several matters including "the desirability (if Britain joins the EEC) of the principle of free movement of doctors within the EEC applying to all doctors who are registered on the *Medical Register* of the United Kingdom, including those who are registered with Commonwealth, Irish, and foreign qualifications."

In February 1972 the BMA organised an informal conference of representatives of the health professions to discuss the implications for all those professions of the impending entry by Great Britain into the EEC. The views of the conference were conveyed to the Secretary of State for Social Services, Sir Keith Joseph. A month later the BMA formally submitted to the Government its comments on the draft medical directives of the EEC, and these comments were published in the *BMJ* of 13 May 1972. The United Kingdom entered the European Economic Community on 1 January 1973. The medical directives were still in draft form: the BMA continued to ponder them and focused attention on the criterion which they used to establish the mutual recognition of qualifications (both basic and postgraduate). Briefly, this criterion was the length of training, on an arithmetical basis, specified in years and even hours. The BMA Council commented: "The Council is of opinion (as are both the Department and the General Medical Council) that the line taken in the directives is too mechanistic. The quality of the instruction given to students is at least as important as the number of hours worked. The Council therefore supports the view that, in addition to harmonisation on a quantitative basis, there should be some form of quality control of basic medical training . . . by the creation of a supranational body charged with the maintenance of standards. . . ."

This BMA view gathered support in the Standing Committee of Doctors of the EEC. The European Commissioner for Research, Science, and Education, Professor Ralf Dahrendorf, took the bold and original initiative of convening a conference or "hearing" in Brussels in October 1973, to which he invited representatives of the medical profession, of the universities, of governments, of medical students, and of consumer interests. The BMA sent a full delegation. The outcome was that the draft directives were amended to provide for the establishment of an European Advisory Committee on Medical Training. In effect, this is an embryo General Medical Council for Europe.

The BMA accepted an invitation from the other eight countries to provide the presidency and secretariat for the Standing Committee of Doctors of the EEC for the years 1974, 1975, and 1976. Mr Walpole Lewin assumed the presidency, Dr Derek Stevenson became Secretary-General, and a special section of the BMA secretariat was formed to undertake the heavy and important new international commitment of running the Standing Committee of Doctors. The task of administering a large international body, whose members were spread over nine European countries and spoke six different languages, and whose many subcommittees met frequently between the twice-yearly meetings of the full committee, was not an easy one.

In the meantime the BMA's own Committee on the EEC (of which Dr Alan Rowe had become Chairman) continued to act as the main channel of communication between all branches of the medical profession in the UK and the

British Government on Common Market medical matters.

In 1975 the BMA Council stated: "Thus we are now (after a long preparatory period of 15 years) about to see the establishment of medical reciprocity and the free movement of doctors throughout the nine countries of the EEC. This is a dramatic development which ... will widen the horizens of British doctors and will confer upon them the opportunity to migrate freely throughout Europe and to practise their skills in other countries." Six years later, the word "dramatic" seems too strong: but the BMA's initial enthusiasm may yet prove to have been justified.

EPILOGUE

We must now attempt to sum up this chapter of the BMA's history. Until the second world war the BMA had active branches throughout the British Commonwealth (except Canada, but including the Irish Free State), and even in some foreign countries. The parent body kept closely in touch with its overseas branches and did much for them and for its overseas members. In the years after the war most of these branches evolved into independent medical associations, almost all of which entered into affiliation agreements with the BMA. The BMA is affiliated with 23 overseas medical associations, and relations with all of them are extremely cordial.

Running parallel with this process of "decolonisation," the BMA has played an important part in establishing new linkages of medical associations: the Commonwealth Medical Association, the World Medical Association, the Standing Committee of Doctors of the EEC, and the other medical institutions of the European Community. In recent years the BMA has tended to direct its overseas resources (which are by no means unlimited) towards the new Europe.

Although the BMA still has 15 overseas branches, it no longer undertakes regular and active negotiations with what used to be called the "Imperial Government" about its members overseas. The UK Government now has no control over the terms and conditions of service of doctors either in the Commonwealth or in foreign countries. Nevertheless, the BMA still keeps a watchful eye on the terms offered to British doctors by any employing authorities abroad — for example, multinational firms and foreign governments. Any grievance of a BMA member overseas is investigated and, if found to be justified, redress is sought by the BMA through whatever channel is judged to be the most suitable — for example, the Foreign and Commonwealth Office, an affiliated medical association, or an international organisation such as the World Medical Association or the World Health Organisation. The BMA's standing abroad is high. Relations with our remaining overseas branches, with the affiliated medical associations, and with foreign medical associations, are smooth and cordial, and at every annual general meeting a large contingent of Representatives and delegates from overseas branches and "kindred medical associations" is ceremonially received by the new President of the BMA. Like Great Britain itself, the British Medical Association has decolonised, but "hands across the sea" remain warmly outstretched and clasped.

An independent assessment of the BMA's achievements overseas was published in 1973 in the *Journal of Imperial and Commonwealth History*. Terence J Johnson and Marjorie Caygill wrote: "The Empire and Commonwealth role of the BMA has, then, been pervasive. Its overseas activities not only helped to shape professional organisation and politics throughout the world, but there has also been a feedback from these concerns affecting its prestige, organisation, and policies at home. The extent to which the BMA's early involvement with colonial governments influenced its developing medicopolitical role in Britain is still to be measured in detail, but that this influence existed, is clear."

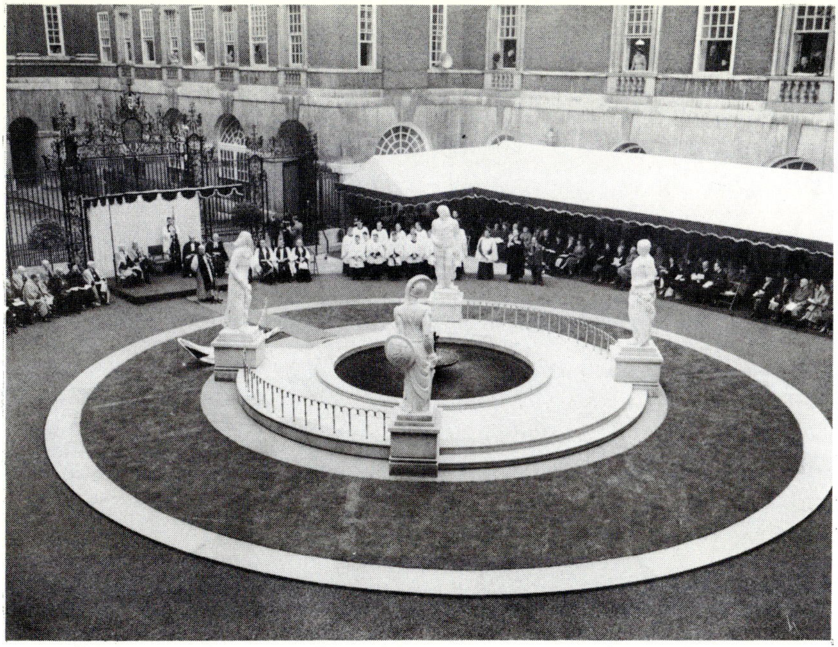

Dedication of the War Memorial by the Archbishop of Canterbury, Dr Fisher (2 November 1954).

(*Central Press Photos Ltd*)

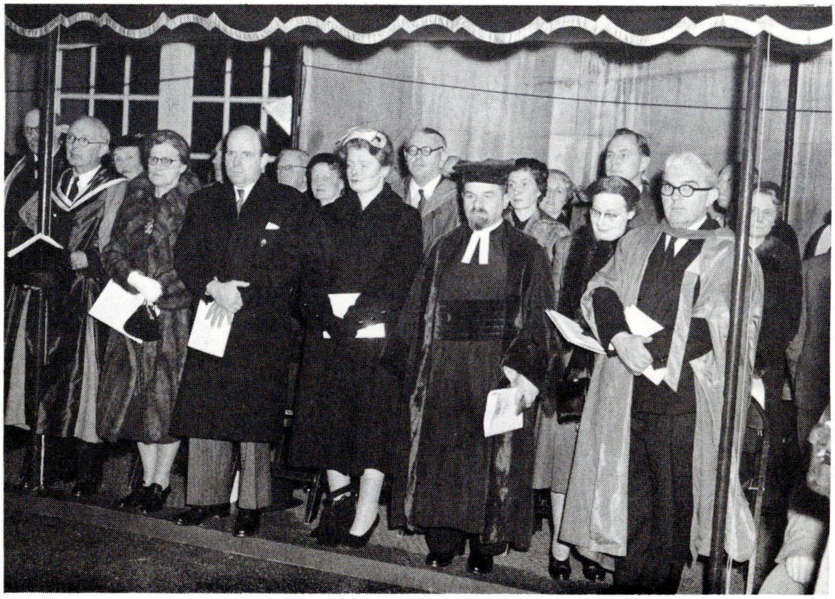

Some of the distinguished guests at the ceremony.
L to R: The Minister of Health (Mr Iain Macleod), the Chairman of the Labour Party (Dr Edith Summerskill), the Chief Rabbi (Dr Israel Brodie).

(*Fox Photos Ltd*)

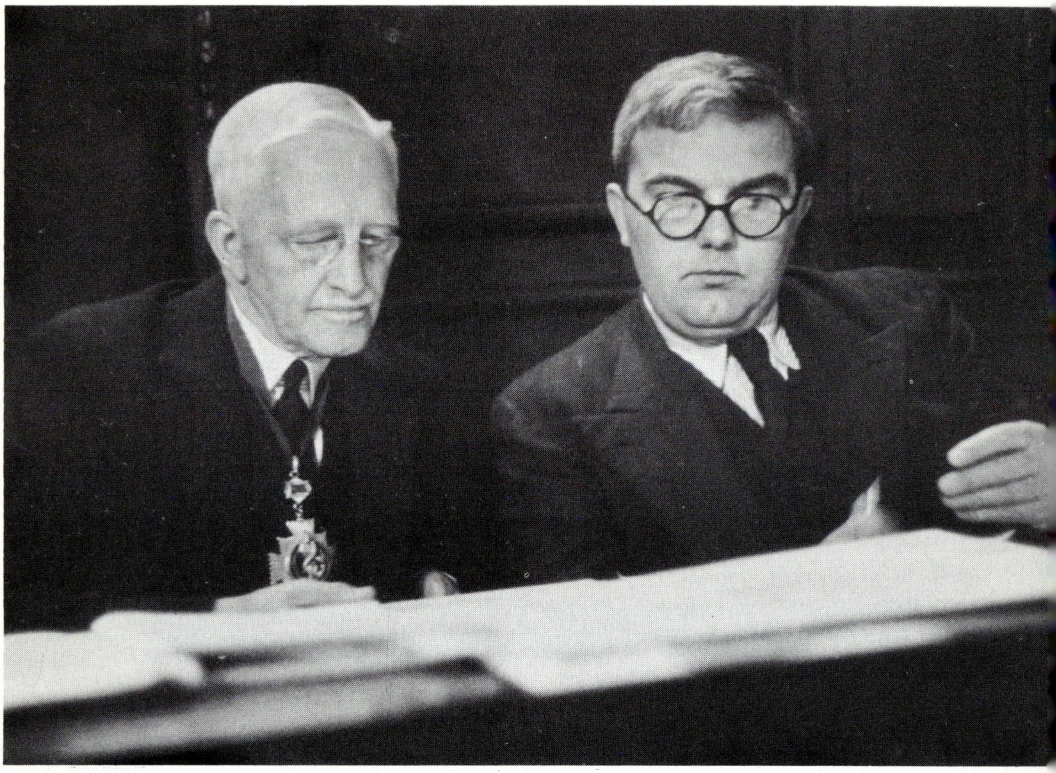

"The thin end of the wedge of a State-salaried service under local authorities."
The Chairman of Council (Dr Guy Dain) and the Secretary (Dr Charles Hill) study t
Coalition White Paper (1944).
(*BBC Hulton Picture Library*)

Chapter 5

Living with socialised medicine

> In politics, problems are rarely solved, they are only replaced by other, more pressing ones. — Lacey Baldwin Smith.

REMUNERATION: THE SPENS ERA

Those who remember the birth of the National Health Service will recall that the Service was just three months old when the first great dispute with the BMA erupted — on a subject which was destined to be a cause of almost continuous unrest: remuneration. The reason why this genteel 12-letter word was always used instead of the short and sharp word, pay, was that the first Spens Committee, appointed by the Coalition Government in February 1945, was officially entitled "The Inter-Departmental Committee on Remuneration of General Practitioners"; and the second Spens Committee, on the Remuneration of Consultants and Specialists, also had the word in its terms of reference.

The general practitioners received their first quarterly cheques from the National Health Service in October 1948, and at once there was an outburst of rage because the amounts were far less than they had been expecting. True, the Spens Report had been accepted by the BMA, but the Spens recommendations had been made in 1939 values and the committee had said: "We leave to others the problem of the necessary adjustment to present conditions, but we would observe in this connection that such adjustment should have direct regard not only to estimates of the change in the value of money but to the increases which have in fact taken place since 1939 in incomes in other professions." To make the adjustment, the Government had decided to add a "betterment factor" of 20% to the net remuneration recommended by Spens, and it soon became clear that this was grossly inadequate. A report by the General Medical Services Committee, published in the *British Medical Journal* on 19 February 1949, stated: "Many practitioners, notably those with lists of average and less than average size, are experiencing loss of income on such a scale as to spell hardship for themselves and their dependants." A leader in the *BMJ* said: "In the result, doctors generally have been grossly overworked and some of them have been on the brink of financial disaster."

It was scarcely surprising that the second immediate cause of dissatisfaction with the NHS was overwork. If the Government were to pass legislation by which on a certain date all public transport was provided "free," it would be no wonder if the public started to make many more journeys by bus and train, and if the transport staffs became overworked and dissatisfied with their pay and conditions. This is exactly what happened when the "free" health service was introduced.

The Annual Report of Council in 1949 used measured terms to describe events: "During the first six months of the Service evidence soon began to accumulate that the burden of work for the profession, particularly paper work, had greatly increased; that in many cases income had gone down; that private practice had diminished much more than was anticipated and in many cases had virtually disappeared; and that there were doubts whether the Spens recommendations were being fully applied. In general practice the ratio of visits to consultations tended to rise, and multiple consultations became more frequent. While it is possible that some of this increase is of a temporary nature, arising out of a desire to use the Service merely because it is free, there is good reason to believe that much of it has come to stay."

Meetings of indignant BMA members were held all over the country, and the Conference of Representatives of Local Medical Committees resolved unanimously: "That this Conference considers the present capitation fee to be grossly inadequate and calls upon the General Medical Services Committee, as a matter of the utmost urgency, to take immediate action to secure an adequate overall increase in order to relieve the serious hardship resulting from the new service." The GMS Committee produced a special report, in which it was contended (with expert advice) that the betterment factor in 1948, at the inception of the NHS, should have been 85%, not 20%. A special representative meeting was held on 29 March 1949 and voted overwhelmingly to support the general practitioners' case The meeting did not, however, support a motion calling for mass resignation of general practitioners from the Service if an adequate capitation fee was not quickly obtained.

The BMA and the Ministry of Health met to discuss the general practitioners' case on 14 April 1949. The BMA raised the possibility of arbitration, and received the following dusty answer: "It must not be assumed without further discussion that participation in the Whitley machinery necessarily involves, in the event of disagreement, the right to resort compulsorily to arbitration on all subjects." This was disturbing, because when the Government had persuaded the medical profession to take part in Whitley machinery for the new National Health Service (copied from the 30-year-old negotiating machinery for the Civil Service which was named after the Rt Hon J H Whitley*), the plan had provided for an arbitration agreement at the apex of the negotiating machinery.

To cope with the problems thrown up by the National Health Service, the BMA made certain constitutional adjustments. The old Insurance Acts Committee was replaced by a new General Medical Services Committee. Besides the new Central Consultants and Specialists Committee, a joint committee of the Royal Colleges, the Royal Scottish Corporations, and the British Medical Association was formed to speak with one voice for consultants and specialists "in the impending negotiations with the Government on matters arising out of the National Health Service Acts and the report of the Spens Committee on the Remuneration of Consultants and Specialists." The first Chairman of the new Joint Consultants Committee was the BMA President, Sir Lionel Whitby, and its members included the Presidents of the six Royal Colleges and Corporations.

At this time hospital doctors were on interim salaries and terms of service and provisional contracts, and the consul-

*Chairman of the Committee on the Relations of Employers and Employed, 1917-18, and afterwards Speaker of the House of Commons.

tants were by no means so dissatisfied with their pay as the general practitioners. But the BMA made representations to the Government about the financial position of hospital junior staff. Significantly, the registrars of the hospitals in the Bristol area announced in a letter to the *BMJ* that they had formed a registrars group. In 1950 the BMA itself set up a registrars group, under the machinery for the establishment of special groups of members. The Registrars Group Council became the recognised mouthpiece of hospital junior staff, and was the forerunner of the Hospital Junior Staffs Committee. The first concern of the registrars (senior, middle, and junior — there were three grades of them at that time) was not in fact their pay so much as their prospects of promotion to consultant, because of a growing imbalance between the numbers of registrars and consultant posts. This was the start of a long road, the search for a satisfactory staffing structure in the hospital service, about which much more will be said later in this chapter.

In July 1949 the Joint Consultants Committee advised consultants and specialists to enter into permanent contracts under the National Health Service, having obtained certain safeguards from the Ministry of Health, notably including an assurance that remuneration was a subject suitable for arbitration. This was qualified, however, by a statement that the conciliation machinery of Whitley must first be exhausted, and that any issues of remuneration remaining in dispute would go *either* to arbitration or for inquiry and report by a committee.

One thing that was already the cause of controversy and criticism among consultants was the system of distinction awards, which had been recommended by the Spens Committee on the Remuneration of Consultants and Specialists. They had made the fundamental recommendation that all specialties should be remunerated equally, saying that "in view of the standards of qualification and the length of training now proposed for the various special branches it would be unfair to recommend that any specialty should be relegated to a subordinate place in medicine. . . ." They had, however, balanced this important recommendation with another, that "any satisfactory system of remuneration must involve differentiation dependent on professional distinction." They had recommended that a hand-picked committee "should be empowered to recognise special contributions to medicine in the field of research or otherwise, exceptional ability, or any outstanding professional work (other than administrative) by the conferment on selected individuals of distinction awards in three grades." The President of the Royal College of Physicians, Lord Moran, was appointed the first chairman of the Advisory Committee on Distinction Awards, and this caused some comment. In a pungent letter to the *BMJ* (28 May 1949) Mr Reginald T Payne FRCS wrote: "Supposing the College had been asked to work out a design for patronage under the Health Act, how better could it have achieved this than by making the President the chairman of a Distinction Awards Committee?" By 1956, however, the Central Consultants and Specialists Committee was declaring its confidence in Lord Moran and his advisory committee, after he had appeared before them to explain his methods. Even so, the merit award system caused controversy for decades. As early as 1950 the BMA had suggested that regional awards committees should be set up to make recommendations to the Advisory Committee on Distinction Awards, and that the secrecy of the system should not be absolute. The BMA continued to press these and other suggestions for many years, and little by little they were adopted. In due course Lord Moran was succeeded as chairman by Lord Brain, who introduced some welcome changes, such as small regional committees to advise on potential candidates for C awards.

Jumping ahead in this particular story, in 1966 the ARM asked for a ballot to be conducted among the higher grades in the hospital service, in order to determine their attitude towards the distinction awards scheme. The ballot (in 1967) showed a 3 to 1 majority in favour of the principle of distinction awards. There was also a large majority who considered that some change was required in the existing system, but there was no unanimity about the kind of change desired. In 1972 another referendum on the distinction awards scheme produced much the same result.

Another thing that concerned the BMA at the very beginning of the NHS was the insistence of the Health Departments on creating a grade of specialists below the consultant grade — the senior hospital medical officers. This grade had not been envisaged by the Spens Committee, and the profession saw it as a device for getting the services of fully trained specialists on the cheap. The Central Consultants and Specialists Committee commented: "The creation of this grade, necessary as it may be for the appropriate classification of certain transferred officers, is fraught with danger in that it might lead to the establishment of two grades of specialist, involving a process of dilution which would be most undesirable." These measured words marked the start of a controversy which was to be a running sore in the profession for decades. Those specialists who were placed in the SHMO grade naturally felt hurt and aggrieved, and the BMA negotiated (not without difficulty) a series of appeal procedures which dragged on for many years. With the wisdom of hindsight, it may seem that the decision by the Government in 1948 to create the SHMO grade was a costly error: it would have saved endless appeals and ill feeling if all fully trained specialists — whether on the staff of teaching hospitals, non-teaching voluntary hospitals, local authority hospitals, or mental hospitals — had been transferred en bloc to the consultant grade.

Meanwhile, the case for an increase in pay for general practitioners was running into all the obstacles that were to become monotonously familiar in future years. The Minister of Health rejected the figures in the claim, and went on: "Moreover, quite apart from this clear conclusion, to which the analysis of the facts must lead him, the Minister would point out that the Association's proposals have to be seen also against the background of the general economic situation and the vital national need to avoid any unjustified raising of remuneration in any field." This was a refrain which was to be heard over and over again in the years to come, from governments of both political complexions.

January 1950 saw the first meeting of the Medical Whitley Council. The Council at once appointed three committees: Committee A to deal with general practitioners; Committee B for hospital medical and dental staff; and Committee C for public health medical officers. At this time considerable hopes were entertained about the future usefulness of the Whitley system of negotiation, but time was to show that it was too cumbersome, too slow, and too much inhibited by Government policy to give satisfaction to the doctors as a mechanism for negotiation of their pay and problems.

On 17 June 1950 the *BMJ* carried a detailed report from the General Medical Services Committee on all the steps which it had taken since the autumn of 1948 to secure an improvement in the pay of general practitioners. The Ministry had instituted a comprehensive inquiry into the amount each doctor was receiving from the NHS. The GMS Committee's report ended with six recommendations to a special conference to be held on 29 June 1950, including the following: "(C) That participation in the investigation into general practitioner income from NHS sources and practice expenses be made conditional upon a satisfactory assurance that remuneration will always be a matter for negotiation through Whitley machinery. (D) That the Conference instructs the General Medical Services Committee to make preparations for the withdrawal of general medical practitioners from the National Health Service in the event of the Minister failing to give the necessary assurance, sought in the previous resolution, or in the event of the investigations now under consideration not leading to a satisfactory settlement of general practitioner remuneration. (E) That, in the opinion of the Conference, one of the greatest dangers confronting general practitioners, and so the community, is the lowering of the status of the general practitioner." The special conference adopted the recommendations (with some slight amendments of wording), including the call for preparations to be made for general practitioners to withdraw from the National Health Service.

The start of 1951 was marked by an important political event. The Minister of Health, Mr Aneurin Bevan — the old antagonist of the medical profession — was transferred to the Ministry of Labour. (Three months later he resigned office, in protest at the imposition of new charges in the NHS.) He was succeeded by Mr Hilary Marquand, and representatives of the GMS Committee hastened to meet him on 28 February 1951. After that meeting a letter arrived saying: "The Minister himself is already convinced, as a result of his first discussion with the representatives — and the Secretary of State for Scotland agrees — that there is a good prima facie case for their reviewing, as a matter of urgency, both the adequacy of the total remuneration of general practitioners and its distribution. They will look without delay at the best way of speeding up that review."

Here indeed was a changed Government tune.

Meanwhile, the BMA was preparing its machinery for all eventualities. The Council had already created the British Medical Guild (see Chapter 9). Now two representatives of the Medical Practitioners Union were added to the General Medical Services Committee in order to ensure that no separate approach would be made to the Minister of Health by the union on general practitioner matters.

Negotiations with Mr Marquand continued, but without agreement. In July 1951 a special conference of Representatives of Local Medical Committees called on the Minister of Health to refer the general practitioners' claim to arbitration, and sharpened the request by deciding that the resignations of general practitioners should be collected unless a suitable form of arbitration was agreed by 25 September 1951. Shortly afterwards the Minister decided to refer the question to arbitration by an "independent adjudicator," and Mr Justice Danckwerts was appointed.

The hearing began on 18 March 1952, and lasted more than three days. Both sides were represented by eminent Counsel, the Attorney-General leading for the Government. The principal witness for the BMA was Professor R G D (later Sir Roy) Allen, Professor of Statistics in the University of London, who was to remain in the BMA's team of top-ranking advisers for the next 30 years. In a written memorandum Professor Allen said that a massive redistribution of purchasing power had taken place in the nation. The middle classes might have been impoverished to such an extent that they could no longer serve effectively in providing public service and cultural need. The Attorney-General probed this matter in oral evidence:

> Q: It is quite clear that general practitioners among other professional men have unfortunately suffered a loss of relative status since the war?
> PROFESSOR ALLEN: Yes.
> Q: You point out that the redistribution of the national income has favoured what you describe as the working class substantially at the expense of the professional classes?
> PROFESSOR ALLEN: Yes, including in "professional classes" salaried earners and particularly higher salary earners.

The Government called evidence from a senior official of the Inland Revenue, which was taken in camera.

Mr Justice Danckwerts made his award on 24 March

1952, and it amounted to an astounding vindication of the BMA's case for the general practitioners. Danckwerts applied a betterment factor of 85% for 1948 (the BMA's original claim) to the (1939) Spens recommendations, in place of the 20% that had been allowed by the Government; and 100% for the year 1950-1. The Danckwerts award amounted to an extra £10 million a year in remuneration (compared with the £2 million which had been offered by Mr Marquand) and cost the Government £40 million in increased pay and back pay. The BMA Council recorded its warm appreciation of the "stupendous exertions" of the Chairman of the GMS Committee, Dr S Wand, and the Secretary of the Committee, Dr D P Stevenson.

The Danckwerts award had a momentous consequence: never again would the Government agree to submit a claim from the doctors to arbitration by a High Court judge.

Not surprisingly, a claim was immediately prepared by the Joint Consultants Committee for the same betterment to be applied to hospital doctors as Danckwerts had awarded to general practitioners. The claim was lodged in June 1952, but on 2 July the new Chancellor of the Exchequer (the Conservative Party was now in power) stated in Parliament: "In accepting the results of the [Danckwerts] adjudication, which was of an exceptional nature, the Government have by no means adopted the view that similar adjustments in other fields should follow. In their view, there is no justification for any assumption that the appropriate standard of remuneration for the professional classes is a rate of 100% above that in force in 1939."

Lengthy negotiations followed, and eventually (with effect from 1 April 1954) improved rates of remuneration for hospital medical and dental staff were agreed in Committee B of the Medical Whitley Council. The minimum of the consultant scale was raised to £2100, which was 40% above the figure recommended (in 1939 values) by Spens. Other percentage rises were smaller; but it has already been remarked that in the early years of the National Health Service dissatisfaction with pay was less prominent in the hospital service than in general practice, probably because one-third of consultants were in receipt of distinction awards, and also because many consultants were part-timers with a continuing income from private practice. Accepting the settlement as a "payment on account," the BMA Council commented on it in these terms: "It appears to the Council that the result of the negotiations conducted so far in Committee B goes a long way to narrow the disparity between the remuneration of general practitioners and of hospital medical staff which was caused by the Danckwerts award." There was, however, a good deal of grumbling among consultants that their betterment had been pitched at a level so much lower than that achieved by the general practitioners, and the Chairman of the Joint Consultants Committee, Sir Russell (later Lord) Brain felt it necessary to write a strong letter to the *BMJ* calling for unity and declaring: "The settlement in no way ties our hands, and our claim to cost of living betterment is as valid as it was before — and as unenforceable."

Let us turn now to the third branch of doctors in the National Health Service, the public health medical officers. They were employed by the local health authorities (in England, county councils and county borough councils). The Askwith scales (originally negotiated by the BMA in 1929) were revised in 1946 and 1947. When the National Health Service was introduced the BMA set about trying to secure improved remuneration for public health medical officers, and in 1949 refused to accept advertisements for publication in the *BMJ* of vacancies with local authorities which did not comply with the Association's proposals. As soon as Committee C of the Medical Whitley Council was appointed in January 1950 negotiations began on the remuneration of public health medical officers, in order to apply the "Spens standards" to PHMOs. The negotiations reached a deadlock. Both sides agreed to arbitration by the Industrial Court, and the award of the court was accepted.

Some time after the Danckwerts award a further claim was lodged on behalf of all public health medical officers, but negotiations failed to produce a settlement and the claim was again referred to arbitration. The Industrial Court made an award in April 1955 which, although all scales were increased, fell well short of the claim. There was much dissatisfaction among public health medical officers, not only with the actual award but also with the Industrial Court itself, which insisted on comparing them with local government officers rather than with other doctors. On 7

April 1956 the BMA Council published a detailed and comprehensive report on remuneration policy, in which one of the recommendations was: "That the Government be urged to set up an independent committee of inquiry to consider what should be the range of remuneration of medical officers in the public health service, having regard to the remuneration of other sections of the profession and the desirability of the public health service maintaining its power to attract a suitable type of recruit."

Meanwhile, in February 1956 the Health Ministers had been informed that it was intended to submit a joint remuneration claim to them on behalf of consultants and general practitioners, and a joint negotiating committee had been set up with Sir Russell Brain (Chairman of the Joint Consultants Committee) and Dr A Talbot Rogers (Chairman of the General Medical Services Committee) as joint chairmen. The claim was submitted to Ministers on 14 June 1956. It was for an upward revision of the betterment factor (which was intended to take account of the rise in the cost of living, and changes in the remuneration of other professions) and was once more largely based on the expert advice of Professor R G D Allen. The claim was for an increase in net remuneration of not less than 24%.

Ministers replied that in present circumstances they would not feel justified in considering any claim for a general increase in medical remuneration. Meetings were held with Ministers, and a legal memorandum was submitted by the BMA arguing that the Government was under a contractual obligation to continue implementing the Spens Reports by making periodic adjustments of remuneration. The Government refused to accept this contention, and the BMA Council prepared for battle by overhauling the British Medical Guild machinery.

On 13 January 1957 Sir Anthony Eden resigned the Premiership and was succeeded by Mr Harold Macmillan. Mr Dennis Vosper (later Lord Runcorn) became Minister of Health. On 20 February 1957 representatives of the negotiating committee met Mr Vosper, who announced — out of the blue — that a royal commission was to be set up to conduct a full review of medical and dental remuneration. There had been no prior consultation about this with the medical profession, and the BMA regarded it as "a transparent device for shelving the Government's responsibility." These were the words used in a memorandum entitled "A Crisis of Confidence" which was sent by the BMA's public relations officer to Members of both Houses of Parliament. In the eyes of the BMA Council, the Government had refused to examine the profession's claim, refused to negotiate, and refused to go to arbitration. Instead, the Government had unilaterally decided to use the traditional stalling device of a royal commission.

The announcement of the royal commission had come as a complete bombshell. The GMS Committee decided to recommend the resignation of general practitioners from the National Health Service if the Government did not agree to an immediate and satisfactory settlement of the claim or, alternatively, to arbitration. The joint chairmen of the negotiating committee met the Minister of Health, and then met the Prime Minister. The Government offered some interim adjustment of remuneration, but the BMA was unimpressed. On 23 March 1957 the GMS Committee stated publicly: "Indeed, all the disastrous events of the past few months lead the Committee to the inevitable conclusion that the Government is determined by the device of a Royal Commission to rid itself of the embarrassment of the Spens Reports and the Danckwerts award and to replace them by a new basis of remuneration less favourable to the profession." On 27 March 1957 the BMA Council resolved that: "It is undesirable in present circumstances that the Association should co-operate in any way with the Royal Commission on the Remuneration of Doctors and Dentists," explaining that no disrespect to the chairman and members of the commission was intended, and still less any disrespect to the Crown. A special representative meeting was convened for 1 May 1957. A detailed plan for the progressive or phased withdrawal of general practitioners (area by area) from the NHS was published. There was a debate in the House of Lords (initiated by Lord Moran) on 5 April 1957, and a letter from the Chairman of Council (Dr S Wand) was published in *The Times* of 8 April 1957.

Now came a curious development. On 11 April 1957 the Royal College of Physicians issued the following statement: "The Royal College of Physicians at a special comitia today, after hearing the letters exchanged between Sir Russell Brain, their President, and the Prime Minister; and the President's account of his meetings with the Royal Commission and its Chairman, Sir Harry Pilkington, decided that they wished to co-operate with the Royal Commission on the remuneration of doctors and dentists." Thus it became apparent that the President of the Royal College of Physicians, who was also (as Chairman of the Joint Consultants Committee) joint chairman of the negotiating committee, had been in correspondence with the Prime Minister and the chairman of the royal commission. A critical letter from Dr John H Hunt (later Lord Hunt of Fawley) appeared in the *BMJ* of 27 April 1957: "Surely this reflects unfavourably on the capacity of the Royal College of Physicians to represent them [the Members and Licentiates of the College engaged in general practice] in medico-political matters, or to help in the future development of the general practice side of the National Health Service." Just at this moment Sir Russell Brain gave up the presidency of the college, and his successor, Sir Robert Platt (later Lord Platt), answered testily (*BMJ*, 4 May 1957): "The machinery of the British Medical Association has all the advantages and disadvantages of democracy. Surely there are times when one or the other will achieve the better result, and we should respect each other's opinions instead of descending to bickering and contumely."

There was bickering too in the other half of the profession's army, the General Medical Services Committee. At a special meeting on 17 April 1957 the GMS Committee asked Dr Talbot Rogers to relinquish the chairmanship of the committee, and Dr A B Davies was elected to succeed him. It was felt that Dr Rogers was not as hostile as they wanted to the idea of co-operation with the royal commission.

The same division of opinion was apparent at a meeting of the Council held on the morning of the special representative meeting on 1 May 1957, and at the SRM itself. The royal commission had issued a reassuring statement explaining that they intended to interpret their terms of reference as widely as possible, and the Minister of Health had also given assurances on certain points to the Chairman of Council. The plan for the phased withdrawal of general practitioners from the NHS was not universally popular. A leading article in the *BMJ* on 11 May 1957 said: "There can be little doubt that many general practitioners dislike the idea of withdrawal from the NHS to enforce a claim for more pay. Withdrawal has not been presented as a method of enforcing a claim for 24% increase in pay, but of securing the elementary rights of negotiation or arbitration. . . . It has been plainly stated to the profession's representatives that the Royal Commission is not an arbitrating or adjudicating body."

In all this confusion the Council and the Representative Body found it difficult to determine what attitude to adopt to the royal commission, and after a long and perplexed debate the SRM accepted a Council recommendation to defer decisions on the question of giving evidence to the royal commission, and withdrawal of service "until the next meeting of the Representative Body." Doctors were divided, furious with the Royal College of Physicians for intervening in the dispute, and critical of the indecision shown at the special representative meeting.

A further special meeting of the Representative Body was convened for 12 June 1957. This time the Council submitted a report on the position, but refrained from making any recommendation. The Council passed the buck to the Representative Body, inviting it "to take decisions in accordance with the prevailing views of the Association's members as ascertained in the Divisions and Branches."

The Representative Body decided: to submit evidence to the royal commission; to reiterate its strong disapproval of the exclusion of public health medical officers from the remit of the commission (they had been arbitrarily excluded by the Government, on the grounds that they were employed by the local authorities and not paid by the central government); and to defer any decision on withdrawal from the National Health Service. The first leading article in the *BMJ* of 22 June 1957 said: "It would be wrong to disguise the fact that the present controversy has revealed a profession divided in itself as it has never been before."

So ended the pre-Pilkington era of the National Health Service. Why was the profession so hesitant to accept the Royal Commission on Doctors' and Dentists' Remuneration? Before the war, doctors largely determined their own incomes by settling the level of the fees which they charged. They did not take kindly or comfortably to arguing publicly about their pay. The delicate question of what was a fair reward for medical skill and devotion, once the free market in medical services no longer operated, was settled by the Spens Reports. But the Spens recommendations were made in 1939 values of money, and the bitter argument about converting these to postwar values was not settled until the Danckwerts adjudication of 1952. Governments appeared to be more interested in making economies than in offering just rewards. When the profession applied for the Spens-Danckwerts values to be updated the Government suddenly (without any negotiation) appointed a royal commission. Small wonder that the BMA regarded this as at best a stalling device, and at worst a manoeuvre to get rid of the Spens-Danckwerts standards. It took 12 months of feverish discussion, commotion and reflection for the profession to come round to the view that the royal commission might turn out to be a blessing in disguise.

FINANCING THE NATIONAL HEALTH SERVICE

We shall continue the remuneration story later, but we must now turn to an even bigger subject which very soon caused concern in the NHS: how to find the money to pay for it. As early as February 1949 Dr Ffrangcon Roberts of Cambridge published a powerful article in the *British Medical Journal* on the cost of the National Health Service. He pointed out that the the Beveridge Report of 1942 had estimated the cost of a comprehensive health service for Great Britain at £170 million a year. The National Health Service Bill 1946 had estimated the cost for England and Wales at £152 million. In 1948 the Minister of Health gave an estimate of £230 million. Dr Roberts pungently criticised the premises of the Beveridge Report, notably its postulation of "a health service which will diminish disease by prevention and cure" and its forecast that "there will actually be some development of the service and as a consequence of this development a reduction in the number of cases requiring it." With remarkable foresight, he went on to say: "I believe that through ignorance and miscalculation in its preparation the cost of the Health Service has been grossly underestimated, that when in full operation it will be not less than £500 million, and that in future years it will rise to an even higher figure. ... In the twentieth century, civilisation is faced with a threat unique in its history, the existence of more ill-health than it can afford, due not to any temporary calamity but paradoxically to the advance of civilisation itself. Society has opened a new Pandora's box, releasing new diseases of its own creation and with them innumerable new methods of treating all the diseases which it cannot cure."

The actual cost of the Health Service in England and Wales in the first full financial year of the service (1949-50) was £385 million, that is 153% more than had been estimated in the Bill. Professor Harry Eckstein considered that the supplementary estimates which Mr Aneurin Bevan had to introduce lost him considerable face among his colleagues, and Eckstein wrote*: "There is no doubt that the supplementary estimates had first surprised, then shocked public opinion, the first reaction being, as it always is, that the request for additional funds must be due to mismanagement and waste."

In 1953 the Government appointed a small independent committee "to review the present and prospective cost of the National Health Service; to suggest means, whether by modifications in organisation or otherwise, of ensuring the most effective control and efficient use of such Exchequer funds as may be available; to advise how, in view of the burdens on the Exchequer, a rising charge upon it can be avoided, while providing for the maintenance of an adequate Service; and to make recommendations." The five members of the committee were non-medical. The chairman was a distinguished Cambridge economist, Mr C W Guillebaud.

The BMA gave written and oral evidence to the Guillebaud Committee, whose report appeared in January 1956. On the main issue, the committee reported that: "Expressed as a proportion of total national resources (the 'gross national product') the current net cost of the Service fell from 3¾% in 1949-50 to 3¼% in 1953-4." So the alarm about escalating cost was a chimera! "Any charge that there has been widespread extravagance in the National Health Service, whether in respect of the spending of money or the use of manpower, is not borne out by our evidence."

In addition to this conclusion, which astonished many, Mr Guillebaud and his colleagues made several other telling observations, among them the following.

* *The English Health Service* by Harry Eckstein (Harvard University Press, 1964).

> The rate of fixed capital expenditure on hospitals has averaged about one-third of the pre-war rate in real terms. Approximately 45% of all hospitals were originally erected before 1891; and many are regarded by expert opinion as seriously in need of replacement or radical reconstruction.
>
> We do not favour the suggestion that statutory ad hoc health authorities should be appointed to administer the hospital, family practitioner and local health authority services.
>
> We do not feel that a convincing case has been made out for transferring the hospital service to the local health authorities. Some form of regional authority will always be required for the efficient planning of a national hospital service. . . .
>
> We do not agree with the suggestion that a National Board or Corporation should be appointed to administer the National Health Service.
>
> It is still sometimes assumed that the Health Service can and should be self-limiting, in the sense that its own contribution to national health will limit the demands upon it to a volume which can be fully met. This, at least for the present, is an illusion.

The Guillebaud Report also urged that, whenever practicable, patients should be treated in their own homes by the general practitioner and the local health services, instead of being admitted to hospital; and that provision should be made for a new specialist grade, below the grade of consultant, in the career structure of the hospital service.

The report concluded that no convincing case had been made out for the imposition of new charges.

The Guillebaud Report's comments about the lack of new hospital building were strongly echoed by others, especially as conditions continued to deteriorate. In 1958 the Central Consultants and Specialists Committee invited two of its members, Mr A Lawrence Abel and Mr Walpole Lewin, to investigate the problem of the increasing inadequacy of hospital buildings. Their masterly report was published in the *BMJ* of 4 April 1959. They proposed a 10-year plan of greatly increased capital expenditure on hospital building. And in 1962 the Minister of Health (Mr Enoch Powell) published a Hospital Plan for England and Wales, which supported the concept of large district hospitals. Three years on, however, the BMA Council complained: "The profession is deeply concerned that the implementation of the Hospital Plan presented in 1962 is being seriously delayed. . . . It is urgently necessary that hospital building and modernisation should receive higher priority in the nation's construction programme." In May 1966 the Central Consultants and Specialists Committee continued the theme, with a special memorandum entitled "The Realities of Hospital Finance Today." This ended with some home truths: "If the public wishes to have an unrestricted Health Service, it must be prepared to pay for it, not only with money but with resources of manpower and equipment diverted from other activities. The alternative is to cut back, or contain, the Service and to *curtail demand.* If rationing by price is unacceptable, the alternative is rationing by allocation — in the crudest form, through "queueing" — which means longer waiting for hospital treatment." In the same month the Ministry of Health published "The Hospital Building Programme," which was a revision of the 1962 Hospital Plan for England and Wales. But hospital replacement has continued to the present day to be one of the most glaring failures of the National Health Service. Parliament itself looks out on St Thomas's Hospital, whose modernisation and reconstruction were stopped half-way through. It must be added that views on the effectiveness of very big hospitals are now more sceptical than when Mr Enoch Powell's 1962 plan was announced.

In 1967 the BMA submitted to the Health Ministers a Memorandum on the Current Problems of Hospital Medical Staff (nicknamed the "hospital doctors' charter"). On finance it said: "The nation has not provided the necessary funds to realise the concept on which the National Health Service was founded ... vast new sums of money are urgently needed; and if the Exchequer is unable to provide them it is the duty of the Government to order an independent inquiry into alternative sources and to publish its findings." Ten years were to elapse before the Government adopted something resembling this proposal, in a royal commission (see below).

In the same year (1967) the ARM called for the preparation of an alternative health service in which financial provision would be less dependent on taxation. The task was entrusted to a special committee (or Advisory Panel) chaired by Dr Ivor M Jones. Their report, which was entitled *Health Services Financing,* was published in 1970 in a volume of 600 pages and was seen on the desks of many top civil servants soon after publication. The report concluded that there was insufficient finance for the health services and that this was likely to continue and even deteriorate in the future. The proposal in the report was a scheme, spelled out in detail, by which health services in the future would be financed partly out of taxation, and partly by a separate insurance system, paid for direct by consumers. The act of insurance would be compulsory, but each person would have the opportunity to contract out of the "compulsory" insurance and into a "voluntary" insurance with additional premiums and higher benefits (roughly speaking, the higher benefits associated with the private sector of medical care — a greater choice of the time of treatment, a personal choice of the doctor who was to attend the patient, and some additional privacy and other physical amenities. There would be no question of two standards of clinical care). Despite the work which had gone into its preparation, the Ivor Jones report did not make the impact which it deserved: partly perhaps because it aroused controversy within the BMA itself, but mainly because the public were broadly satisfied with the care provided by a tax-based National Health Service.

The ARM 1974 deplored "the current limitation of NHS expenditure, the lower standard of care which will be an inevitable consequence, and the lack of public awareness about this danger facing the NHS." On 31 July 1974 the Chairman of Council (Mr Walpole Lewin) led a deputation, representing the medical, dental, nursing, and midwifery professions, to express grave concern to the Prime Minister (Mr Harold Wilson) about the chronic underfinancing of the NHS and to ask that the Government should institute a top-level inquiry into methods of providing the necessary finance for the Service. The Prime Minister declined to set up an inquiry, but gave an assurance that the Service would be buffered against inflation, and, in fact, £480 million of new money was injected into the Health Service. The BMA continued its campaign, however, and submitted a memorandum to the Prime Minister, in which it was shown that an injection of £900 million was required in the next five years to save the NHS from collapse; and the memorandum again proposed that the time had come for a high-level independent inquiry into the financing of the NHS.

At last, in May 1976, the Government relented, partly no doubt because of other problems, such as the acrimonious negotiations between Mrs Barbara Castle and the hospital doctors about contracts and pay-beds. A royal commission was appointed under the chairmanship of Sir Alec Merrison FRS, Vice-Chancellor of the University of Bristol, who had successfully chaired the Committee of Inquiry into the Regulation of the Medical Profession (see Chapter 6). Even so, the terms of reference given to the royal commission were to consider "the best use and management of the financial and manpower resources of the National Health Service," phraseology which did not cover the *provision* of the necessary financial resources. Nevertheless, the royal commission indicated that it would range widely over its remit.

The BMA went to enormous trouble to compile comprehensive evidence to the royal commission. The BMA's main memorandum of evidence was 52 pages long and, of course, included a chapter on finance. This described eloquently the chronic underfinancing of the Health Service, but was less convincing in its proposals for remedying matters. These were (*a*) a separate fund to be earmarked for the National Health Service (*b*) payments into the fund to be made by the Government, and also by the public ("a basic compulsory payment to be paid regularly by or on behalf of every member of the population"); and (c) payments to be made by patients for use of the Service ("hotel" charges in hospital and prescription charges). Perhaps the most important suggestion was contained in the words: "We do, however, urge the Royal Commission to consider the whole question of the provision of medical services on a fee-paying basis with subsequent reimbursement by the National Health Service to the patient, as in other EEC countries."

If the BMA's evidence on an alternative way of financing the NHS was unimpressive, the royal commission's answer (1979) was even more so: "We do not think that the NHS should be funded by health insurance . . . it will be apparent that we are not enthusiastic about charges . . . there is a good case for their gradual but complete extinction. ... The external issues of how tax or charges affect the public and public policy are certainly not our concern and must lie in the hands of the government." So the top-level inquiry into methods of providing the necessary finance for the Service, for which the BMA had been pressing since 1974 and earlier, came up with nothing. When chided about this, the royal commission pointed out (quite correctly) that their terms of reference did not include the *provision* of funds for the Service. Nevertheless, their report was received with widespread disappointment inside and outside the profession.

Since then the BMA has brooded over the question how the National Health Service can cut its coat according to its cloth. There has been agonised cogitation about priorities in health care, redistribution of resources, and living within Government-imposed "cash limits." These are thorny topics. Dr Ffrangcon Roberts was right. No solution is in sight to the problem of how the nation can provide the vast sums which are necessary, on a steeply rising scale, to enable the National Health Service to supply the quantity and quality of medical care which modern medical science makes possible.

ORGANISATION OF THE NATIONAL HEALTH SERVICE

In the early days of the National Health Service, the criticisms of the medical profession were not often directed at its structure, and eight years after the Service was launched the Guillebaud Committee said that it would be "altogether premature" to propose any fundamental change in structure.

There was, however, plenty of general discontent with the NHS, which found expression within the BMA in the Amending Acts Committee. The Committee prepared a First Interim Report on the Reform of the National Health Service, which was debated by a special representative meeting on 13 December 1951. The committee, and the Representative Body, showed themselves to be chiefly concerned about (*a*) the absence of legally binding arbitration machinery in the NHS; (*b*) the extent of the Minister's powers (for example, to make changes by regulation in the pay and conditions of service of any section of the profession); and (*c*) the contention that a patient who elected to receive treatment privately should be entitled to drugs and appliances at public expense. This last issue became known as "drugs for private patients," and remained in the forefront of the BMA's mind for many years. Significantly, in 1949 the name of the General Practice Committee was changed to Private Practice Committee, partly because the affairs of general practitioners within the NHS were now taken care of by the General Medical Services Committee, but also because it was appreciated that under socialised medicine private practice would need a strong representative committee of its own. In the event, the Private Practice Committee soon ranged widely over all kinds of affairs outside the ambit of the National Health Service.

The campaign to secure the unilateral right to arbitration in disputes was strongly fought for several years, but in 1955 and 1956 the Council gradually came to the conclusion that it would be a mixed blessing, because the employing authorities would also have the right to take the BMA to arbitration, and there might be some issues — for example, the question of a permanent sub-consultant grade in the hospital service — in which this could be highly inconvenient. So the campaign was quietly dropped.

In 1957, during the furore created by the appointment of the Pilkington Royal Commission, the BMA Council instituted an inquiry by a special committee into "the whole field of publicly administered medical services in the light of the experience gained of the National Health Service since 1948." The *BMJ* commented: "It will in effect complete the investigation begun in 1941-2 of the BMA Planning Commission. This commission, it may be recalled, produced a draft interim report, but at the time allowed itself to be diverted from this by the publication in 1942 of the Beveridge Report which inaugurated the Welfare State in this country."

The special committee was eventually composed of members nominated by the BMA, the Royal Colleges, the College of General Practitioners, and the Society of Medical Officers of Health. Sir Arthur Porritt, President-Elect of the BMA, future President of the Royal College of Surgeons, and Sergeant-Surgeon to the Queen, accepted an invitation to be Chairman of the committee, which was entitled the Medical Services Review Committee.

The Porritt Committee took evidence from many sources, and fulfilled its task thoroughly and conscientiously. Its report (of 266 pages) was published in 1962.

There were 223 recommendations, the most important being: "(*13*) We recommend that the responsibility for the administration and co-ordination of all the medical and ancillary services in any area should be in the hands of one authority only — the Area Health Board." The main body of the report stated in heavy type: "We have concluded that in future one administrative unit should become the focal point for all the medical services of an appropriate area, and that doctors and other personnel in all branches of the Service should be under contract with this one authority."

This important recommendation was received with mixed feelings by the BMA Council, briefed as always by its Standing Committees. In a guarded comment, the Council indicated that it had considerable reservations about the suggestion that family doctoring should be placed under the same administration as hospital interests, but felt that teaching hospitals should not be excluded from administration by area health boards. This was a characteristic BMA view: pro-family doctoring, and anti-teaching hospital! The Porritt Report was fully debated at the ARM in Oxford in July 1963, and, by chance, Sir Arthur Porritt entered the hall at the psychological moment and was invited to speak by the Chairman, Dr R G Gibson. Sir Arthur's eloquent and firm lead carried all before him, and the meeting resolved: "That this Representative Body instructs Council to support the setting up of area health boards as this would increase co-ordination and co-operation between the three parts of the Service."

The Porritt Report stimulated a good deal of discussion within the standing committees of the BMA, and with the Government, about the structure and efficiency of the NHS. Yet in 1966 the BMA Council decided that the Amending Acts Committee, which one might have expected to be principally concerned, had exhausted its usefulness and should be wound up. This decision showed how far the profession's attitude had moved since the emotional ARM of 1950. By now the BMA (like Professor Higgins) had grown accustomed to the face of socialised medicine, and enthusiasm for major reform had waned. Moreover, within the BMA the so-called "craft committees," which represented the different branches or "crafts" of the profession working in the National Health Service, had become so well-established that they resented the interference of the Amending Acts Committee. The power of the craft committees was destined to go on growing.

In 1968 the Ministries of Health and of Social Security were merged under a new overlord entitled the Secretary of State for Social Services. The first was Mr Richard Crossman. Just before the merger, the Minister of Health (Mr Kenneth Robinson, the best Minister of Health in the 50 years covered by this book) had announced his intention of issuing a Green Paper (a pre-White Paper) on the administrative structure of the medical and related services. This Green Paper followed the recommendation of the Porritt Report and proposed that area health authorities should replace the existing regional hospital boards, boards of governors, executive councils, and local health authorities (in so far as their health functions were concerned). To promote integration, the Government advocated a clean break from the existing divisions between the three branches of the NHS, and there would be no committees to deal with particular services.

This was not to the taste of the BMA's powerful craft committees, which had not much liked the Porritt Report, and the BMA Council put its finger on the tender spot: "The Green Paper is in direct conflict with the Porritt Report, which recommended that each of its proposed area health boards should have a number of subsidiary councils responsible for the administration of individual services. . . . The Green Paper on the other hand proposes an area board with an internal organisation consisting of four or five major departments, each of which would deal with different aspects of the medical services *as a whole.* There would be no committees of the board representing any particular sectional interest."

With more emotion than logic, the BMA Council declared that "the main proposals enunciated in the Green Paper are unacceptable to the profession as a means of achieving unification of the National Health Service." The Council paid lip service to the principle of unification of the administration of the Health Services, but stated "that there should be adequate financing of the Health Service, and that separate provision for each branch of the Service should be a prerequisite to any change in the administrative structure." The Council also affirmed that the independent contractor status of the family doctor must be maintained, that there must be medical supervision of all social work services with a predominantly health content, and that occupational health services should be included in any new administrative pattern for the NHS.

The Council's views were backed by a special representative meeting on 30 January 1969. Shortly after the Council had forwarded the views of the Representative Body to the Department, the Secretary of State (Mr Richard Crossman) announced that he had noted the criticisms he had received and proposed to issue another Green Paper.

In due course this document appeared, and was examined line by line by the committees and Council of the BMA. Divergences of view became apparent between the main branches of the profession. The *BMJ* reported that "the differences between the opinions of hospital doctors and those of general practitioners and public health doctors on quite fundamental matters are, if not extreme, certainly wide." Dissatisfaction was greatest in the Central Committee for Hospital Medical Services. The Council described it thus: "For 22 years the hospitals have been organised in large regions, of a kind appropriate for the administration of the most sophisticated and expensive branch of medical care, and each (except Wessex) having at least one 'centre of excellence' in the form of a medical school with associated hospitals. The Green Paper threatens the destruction of this concept altogether, and the fragmentation of the hospital service into much smaller, utilitarian units, most of which will be deprived of the beneficial influence of a medical school. The Central Committee for Hospital Medical Services would regard such a reorganisation as disastrous for the hospital service. . . ."

A special representative meeting was held in May 1970 to consider the second Green Paper. It voted for "enlarged executive powers for the regional health councils or authorities, especially in relation to regional planning, to the hospital service and to medical teaching and research." A consultant from Cornwall said that it was not sensible to try to run the hospital services without some form of regional planning. To run the hospital service properly there must be a device on a regional basis which could co-ordinate, advise, and plan the various schemes of the area health boards. This regional "device" must be able to take executive action and to budget. The GMS Committee opposed this view, but the SRM approved it.

The general election of 1970 brought a change of government, and the new (Conservative) Secretary of State for Social Services (Sir Keith Joseph) announced that the Government intended to proceed with the unification of the administration of the NHS in England, on the same date as the projected changes in the structure of local government — that is, April 1974. Meanwhile, the Hunter Working Party, which had been set up by the previous Government to consider the functions and training of medical administrators in a reorganised Health Service, continued its inquiry. The BMA gave evidence, but this was an occasion when the Council found itself unable to present a single, co-ordinated Association viewpoint, contenting itself with forwarding to the Hunter Working Party the memoranda prepared by the craft committees. Nevertheless, the Council distilled three fundamental points from the separate craft comments.

> (*1*) There is a need for medically qualified administrators in the health services at national, regional and area levels, and with functions that are more than advisory.
>
> (*2*) At regional and area levels there should be a designated chief executive of each authority who must be medically qualified. . . .
>
> (*3*) For the training of medical administrators, there should be a career training programme, comparable with the programme for training in a clinical specialty. . . .

When the report of the Hunter Working Party appeared, the BMA's Public Health Committee considered that the specialist training required in community medicine merited a career grade of consultant, equivalent in status and pay to the grade of clinical consultant, and with an allocation of distinction awards. These views encountered opposition from the Central Committee for Hospital Medical Services, but after an uncomfortable debate the BMA Council came down on the Public Health Committee's side.

Sir Keith Joseph's consultative document on NHS reorganisation in England was published in May 1971. The BMA welcomed the proposal to restore the regional tier, but commented: "The profession is faced not with integration of the three branches of the National Health Service, but with complete reorganisation, involving a concept of management taken from industry. . . ." It must be said, however, that the BMA Council's comments as a whole were indecisive, again reflecting divisions between the crafts. In 1972 the National Health Service Reorganisation Bill was introduced in Parliament, and the *BMJ* commented, perhaps more in hope than in expectation: "The important thing now for the profession, which started the march to integration over ten years ago, is to ensure that the detailed management arrangements, still open to discussion, can be so moulded as to help doctors give the best possible care to their patients."

In due course the BMA welcomed the decision to create district management teams, half of whose members would be medical. This was probably one of the most successful of the 1974 innovations, bringing clinicians (consultants and general practitioners) into the day-to-day management of the Service. The Association also laboured hard to devise model constitutions for medical advisory committees at district, area, and regional levels, to ensure that the profession had a strong voice in the reorganised NHS. But time was to show that the complexity of these constitutions (with their punctilious determination to give appropriate representation to all the crafts) was self-defeating, and, in its evidence in 1977 to the Royal Commission on the National Health Service, the BMA said that the medical advisory machinery should be streamlined and made less time-consuming and more effective. The royal commission heartily agreed, and recommended that "the Health Departments should urgently consider with the professions concerned the best way of simplifying the present structure." In due course the Chief Medical Officer (Sir Henry Yellowlees) convened a joint working party to do just that.

The BMA had been worried that the royal commission might recommend a salaried service for general practitioners, and a chapter was included in the BMA's evidence putting the case for the independent contractor status of the general practitioners. The royal commission said that "it would be pointless to depart from existing arrangements to which many GPs are plainly much attached," but they recommended the abolition of the family practitioner committees which administer the independent contractors in England and Wales. This recommendation was not adopted by the Government, which presumably decided that a head-on clash with the general practitioners would be to nobody's benefit.

One major reform proposed by the BMA (and others) was to remove one tier of the four tiers of management created by the 1974 reorganisation, for there was a universal feeling that the administration was top-heavy. This submission was accepted by the royal commission, and by the Government and was implemented in the Health Services Act 1980.

THE RESCUE OF GENERAL PRACTICE

Other things besides cost and remuneration troubled the National Health Service in its early days. The status and the future well-being of general practice caused concern. In March 1950 *The Lancet* published a report entitled "General Practice in England Today: A Reconnaissance" by an Australian research fellow from Harvard, Dr J S Collings, who described it as a "grim analysis of the present position and future prospects." In the same year (1950) the BMA published a report on "General Practice and the Training of the General Practitioner," written by a special committee under the chairmanship of Sir Henry Cohen (later Lord Cohen of Birkenhead).

Soon afterwards, the BMA Council appointed a committee under Dr C W Walker of Cambridge, "To review the present position in general practice, its difficulties and its trends, both generally and with reference to the two years' experience of the National Health Service Acts, and to the BMA Report on 'General Practice and the Training of the General Practitioner' and to make recommendations." The Council decided that the secretary of Dr Walker's special committee, who was Dr S J Hadfield (an assistant secretary of the Association), should personally visit about 200 practices, selected at random. And in 1951, the Central Health Services Council also set up a special committee to study general practice, a move which provoked suspicion at BMA House (even though the chairman of the special committee was Sir Henry Cohen, who was now President of the BMA), because the first row about general practitioner remuneration was by then at its climax.

The fact that all these investigations were set in train shows that there was a widespread feeling that the continuance of general practice was in the melting pot. The report of Dr Hadfield's "Field Survey of General Practice 1951-52" was published in September 1953 and covered 24 pages of the *BMJ.* It was a thorough and conscientious report, and some of Dr Hadfield's conclusions offset to some extent the strictures of the Collings Report and placed it in a wider perspective:

> Ninety-two per cent of practitioners seen at work were adequate or something better. Some were harassed by a considerable amount of overwork and sometimes by financial anxieties. . . . The general practitioner, the consultant, and the public health medical officer need to get to know each other and then to learn to work in concert. There is growing up a new generation of consultants, and a still newer one of those who will become consultants. These know little of the general practitioner and are unaware of his difficulties. . . . The NHS is crying out for a unified administration. . . . There seem to be two courses for general practice to take. The first is to make such adjustments to meet the new situation as will stimulate clinical interest anew and give scope for its exercise. The other course is towards the impersonal health service. . . . A number of practitioners expressed their sensation of being dragged down to a lower level, a feeling of being disregarded and in bondage.

In 1954 the Nuffield Provincial Hospitals Trust published a report by Dr Stephen Taylor (later Lord Taylor) entitled *Good General Practice.* It was a survey of 30 selected general practices in England and Wales. The *BMJ* commented: "Taken in conjunction with Dr Hadfield's survey, to which in many important respects it is complementary and in broad agreement, this latest Nuffield Report will do much to restore confidence in the future of general practice. . . ."

Also in 1954, the BMA Council published a detailed and well thought out scheme for the restoration of the right to buy and sell goodwill. Many general practitioners still felt that the loss of this right in 1948 had dealt a severe blow to the independence of the general practitioner. The scheme came to nothing, however, and goodwill is no longer a medicopolitical issue.

A development which was to have far-reaching effects on general practice occurred in 1956. With society moving towards the five-day week and more leisure, the first emergency call service, organised on commercial lines, began offering general practitioners a relief from their 24 hours a day, seven days a week NHS commitment. Initially some doubts were felt about the legality of such a service, and the GMS Committee set up a special subcommittee to examine the problems of deputising arrangements. There was general understanding that the interests of general practice and the public are best served by providing general practitioners with reasonable off-duty periods and leisure time. Group partnerships and rota schemes could provide these, but in some circumstances an emergency call service might constitute a suitable supplementary method. Guidelines were suggested for the organisation of such a service, and in 1966 the BMA itself, in conjunction with a commercial firm, organised a deputising service in Sheffield. By 1967 the BMA Emergency Treatment Service (as it was at first entitled) was operating successfully, guided by national and local medical advisory committees, in seven centres, and by 1981 in 19 centres. Indeed, the success of deputising services has prompted the Review Body to examine their implications for general practitioner remuneration.

In 1961 the Standing Medical Advisory Committee of the Central Health Services Council set up a special subcommittee to advise on the future field of work of the family doctor. The chairman was Dr (later Dame) Annis Gillie. The subcommittee included some BMA nominees, and the BMA gave evidence. The Gillie Report appeared in 1963 and drew attention to "the scarcity of objective studies of what the general practitioner does today or of alternative methods of organisation for doing it." The report also said: "The economic difficulties of the family doctor in carrying out his work are fundamental and have recurred at every stage of our investigation. . . . The present method of remuneration offers scant encouragement to good doctoring. . . ." But the main conclusion of the Gillie Report was that the function of the family doctor in co-ordinating the resources of hospital and community care on behalf of his patient was potentially greater than ever before.

In 1964, at the time when the general practice section of the BMA was in turmoil over the "pool method" of remuneration (as will be described later in this chapter), the Minister of Health set up a joint working party under the chairmanship of Sir Bruce Fraser, his very able Permanent Secretary, with the following terms of reference: "Having regard to the importance of securing the best possible standards of general medical practice, to consider the report and recommendations of the Annis Gillie Committee and any other methods relevant to the work of the general practitioner in the National Health Service, apart from the quantum of remuneration." The *BMJ* commented: "There are two problems rather than one. The first is general practice in the National Health Service. The second is general practice in the context of modern medical science and its application." The Chairman of the GMS Committee, Dr J C (later Sir James) Cameron, considered that the setting up of the Fraser Working Party had come as a great opportunity. It got down to its task with a will, and was making great progress, when it was engulfed in the volcanic eruption which followed the Review Body's special award of February 1965. This is described later in this chapter.

This same eruption of discontent prompted the production (at a hectic week-end working party in Hove) of one of the most important memoranda ever produced by the BMA, "A Charter for the Family Doctor Service." Though written under intense medicopolitical pressure, the charter was soundly based on the work done in the profession for the Gillie inquiry and for the Fraser working party. Some of its ideas came from the Medical Practitioners Union. On 17 February 1965 the BMA Council resolved that immediate negotiations should be opened with the Minister of Health "with a view to devising an entirely new contract for general practitioners involving a fundamental change in the method of remuneration and terms and conditions of service."

The BMA's proposals for a new contract were set out in the 41 paragraphs of the Charter, some of which are quoted here:

> All medical schools should include departments of general practice which should also organise vocational postgraduate training.
>
> An independent corporation should be set up with adequate public funds to finance the purchase and modernisation of premises and equipment.
>
> We therefore recommend that the family doctor's contractual obligation should be limited to: (*1*) a reasonable working day (we see no reason to perpetuate the anachronism of late evening surgeries); (*2*) a $5\frac{1}{2}$-day working week; (*3*) 46 weeks

in the year. This would give every family doctor sufficient time for postgraduate education and leisure.

The whole range of medical certification requires urgent reform. But the first immediate step must be to reduce to a minimum the burden of certification for National Insurance purposes.

It is essential that the Government should provide greater inducements in under-doctored and special areas. The evidence gathered by the Association for the Fraser Working Party suggests that the majority of family doctors wish to keep the capitation fee method of payment. But this evidence also suggests that a by no means inconsiderable number of doctors favour payment by item-of-service. Others, a smaller number, favour payment by some form of salary. We see no reason why any one system should be imposed to the exclusion of others. Since the National Health Service began there has been too little flexibility in the method of paying family doctors.

[There were a number of other proposals about remuneration, which were submitted to the Review Body.]

We believe that these proposed arrangements would provide a great stimulus to better general medical practice. . . . they lay down a firm basis on which we can confidently build the general practice of the future.

Propelled by the discontent seething among general practitioners, negotiations on the charter proceeded swiftly with the Minister of Health and his officials, and at a special representative meeting on 23 June 1965 progress was approved and it was decided that negotiations, ably led by Dr James Cameron, should continue "on the basis of the Charter."

In due course the proposals about pay were put to the Review Body, and on 4 May 1966 it published its momentous Seventh Report. This did much to restore the status and the morale of general practice, and the Council recommended: "That the Seventh Report of the Review Body, taken in conjunction with the three reports of the joint discussions on the Charter for the Family Doctor Service, represents a substantial advance, and be accepted as the basis of a new contract."

The effects of the "charter revolution" were epitomised by Dr Andrew Smith of Newcastle upon Tyne who wrote (in the *BMJ* of 11 April 1970): "A new situation has arisen in the National Health Service. The revised pay structure, the burgeoning of group practice and health centres, the Royal Commission's recognition that special training is as necessary for family doctors as for skin specialists or surgeons, have changed the image of general practice, and many broadly educated young doctors see in it an attractive career."

The BMA was not concerned just with the remuneration and terms of service of general practitioners: in concert with the Royal College of General Practitioners it took a lively interest in their education. By 1972 there was general agreement with the Health Departments on a broad outline for vocational training of three years for general practice. In 1975 a Joint Committee on Postgraduate Training in General Practice was set up with the college to advise on the standards required for vocational training programmes and to recognise those programmes which were of the required standard. The final stage of the vocational training reforms is due to come into force in the BMA's 150th anniversary year.

TRIBULATIONS OF HOSPITAL MEDICINE

The early days of the National Health Service saw far less discontent and turbulence in the hospital service than in general practice. But hospital doctors had their problems: the first to arise was the "registrar bulge" — an excess of registrars and senior registrars in relation to the prospects of promotion to consultant. This "career structure" distortion has bedevilled the Health Service since the start. Everyone knows that the most junior appointments in the hospital hierarchy must be filled by newly or recently qualified doctors, who receive essential early experience under close supervision in resident posts; and it is generally agreed that the top of the hospital hierarchy must be the consultant grade, filled by fully trained and widely experienced specialists who carry ultimate responsibility for all the patients in hospital. The controversy, which has so far defied solution, surrounds the intermediate work: who should do it, and on what terms?

At the end of the war, as part of the arrangements for the reabsorption into civil practice of the large numbers of young doctors who had been conscripted into the Forces, "demobilisation registrarships" were created. In 1952 the Registrars Group Council addressed the Minister of Health in these words: "It can be seen that there is need for a revised senior registrar establishment, and also that there are some senior registrars who are unlikely to achieve their ambitions because they do not come up to the required standards. It is not felt, however, that any plan is fair if it fails to recognise the special position of the post-war generation of senior registrars and proposes a precipitate reduction of posts ... such an immediate reaction ... would certainly release on to the medical 'labour market' a flood of doctors whose chances of immediate re-employment would be small."

The BMA (through the Joint Consultants Committee) urged upon the Ministry of Health that the ultimate solution to the surplus of senior registrars lay in an expansion of the consultant establishment, particularly in medicine and surgery. In order to meet the immediate difficulties of the existing senior registrars the BMA argued that they should be allowed, on completion of their appointments (the Spens Committee had recommended that a senior registrar appointment should be for three years) to be reappointed for a further period of two years, and the Ministry agreed to this. Such reappointed senior registrars were known as "time-expired."

By 1954 the BMA was worried that a surplus of doctors might be developing in the profession as a whole. Back in 1943 the BMA had given evidence to the Inter-departmental Committee on Medical Schools (the Goodenough Committee) suggesting that a substantially increased number of general practitioners would be required after the war. But that was over ten years ago, and times had changed. In an important démarche, which was to have far-reaching effects, the BMA asked the Minister of Health to set up a working party to review the whole problem. The BMA suggested that the working party should include representatives not only of the Association and the Health Departments, but also of the Colonial Office and the Ministry of Defence.

Paradoxically, there was simultaneous concern about the shortage of hospital junior staff, especially in the non-teaching hospitals. The BMA Council commented: "Another aspect of this problem is the breakdown of the old custom whereby a practitioner combined an appointment on the staff of the local hospital with a general practice. This has led young practitioners to doubt whether anything is to be gained by remaining in the hospital service longer than absolutely necessary if they intend ultimately to enter general practice." The influx of hospital junior staff from overseas had not yet begun.

The Central Consultants and Specialists Committee set up a special subcommittee, under Professor G I Strachan FRCP, FRCS, FRCOG of Cardiff, to examine the problem of shortage of junior staff, and they came to a conclusion which was to be repeated by several subsequent inquiries: that there was a need for a permanent career grade in the hospital service below the consultant grade. This proposal touched a sensitive nerve in the profession, and whenever put forward it provoked a howl of opposition. The reasons for this were twofold: firstly, the suspicion that such a grade would be exploited by the Government as a form of "cheap consultant labour"; and, secondly, the fear among hospital junior staff that many of them might find themselves shunted into this grade as "failed consultants." The Strachan Report had to be redrafted because of these objections; even so, the revised report (published in the *BMJ* of 23 April 1955) declared: "The subcommittee therefore suggests that there is still a need for an intermediate grade of hospital officer who shall bear responsibilities consistent with the performance of much of the regular medical, surgical, and other treatment which makes up the work of the hospital, while he is preparing for a consultant post." The report proposed the name of medical (or surgical) assistant for this grade.

Meanwhile, the Health Departments had accepted the advice of the BMA and had appointed a committee, under the chairmanship of the Rt Hon Henry Willink KC, Master of Magdalene College, Cambridge, who had been Minister of Health from 1943 to 1945, to estimate the future requirement of medical practitioners and the appropriate intake of medical students. The BMA gave evidence, and the Willink Committee reported in 1957. Their general conclusion was that after the year 1961 "a reduced output will suffice. Our estimates suggest that the reduction of the student intake by about a tenth from as early a date as is practicable would meet the case." Subsequent events were to show that the Willink Committee had misjudged the trend in the birth rate, and their proposal to reduce the intake of medical students (which was implemented) came in for much criticism in later years.

If career structure and medical manpower caused concern, so too did hospital administration. In the pre-NHS negotiations the medical leaders had, wisely or unwisely, thrown their influence against the system of medical superintendents — which had obtained in the local authority hospitals — in favour of a lay administration, which was the pattern in the voluntary hospitals. But soon after the nationalisation of the hospitals in 1948, doctors began to have second thoughts and suspicion of the lay administration took root. It was destined to last a long time. In 1950 the Central Health Services Council appointed a committee, under the chairmanship of Alderman A F Bradbeer, to consider the internal administration of hospitals. Its report appeared in 1954 and suggested an administrative troika: medical, nursing, and lay administrators acting in partnership. But the ARM 1955 considered that "equal tripartite administration . . . is not in the interest of the patient" and expressed the opinion that the "lay and ancillary services" should be subordinated to the medical. Indeed, the ARM went much further, affirming "that under no circumstances shall the medical and nursing personnel of hospitals be under the control of lay administrators."

In 1958 the continuing controversy about hospital staffing structure was referred to a special working party chaired by the President of the Royal College of Physicians, Sir Robert Platt. Their report appeared in March 1961. They were the third committee of inquiry to advocate a permanent sub-consultant grade, which they entitled the medical assistant grade. The proposed medical assistant grade was not accepted by the profession until 1964, and then only with stringent safeguards about the control of the growth of the grade in consultation with the profession.

The Platt Report also recommended increases in consultant establishments. Because the requests from the regions for additional consultant posts had far exceeded the available number of "appropriately qualified candidates" (these were the words used in the Annual Report of the BMA Council), it was agreed with the profession that the increases in consultant establishments should be held down to "the median" — that is, the middle figure of the proposals received from all hospital boards. Later attempts over the years, both by the profession and the Government, to expand the consultant grade were frustrated by two other obstacles: the cost of providing the necessary supporting facilities (such as theatre time, and laboratory back-up) for each new consultant post; and a second (unspoken) consideration — the reluctance of some existing consultants to see the limited sector of private practice invaded by an influx of new consultants.

All the many problems of the hospital service were reviewed, and remedies suggested, in an important memorandum published by the BMA in June 1965. This was entitled "An Appraisal of the Hospital Service," nicknamed the Richmond Document because it had been drafted by a small handpicked working party in an intensive weekend at Richmond, Surrey. The decision by the Central Consultants and Specialists Committee to produce the document had been prompted by the publication of the GMS Committee's "Charter for the Family Doctor Service." Imitation is the sincerest form of flattery!

The Richmond Document contained 74 paragraphs and was comprehensive in its scope. It opened with the words: "The demands which the nation is making upon its hospital service are greater than the present resources of the service can meet. . . . For at least 17 years, the hospitals have been starved of money, buildings, equipment and staff: at the same time the population has grown, the standard of living has risen, and the public has demanded ever more plentiful and sophisticated hospital medicine. For 17 years the gap between dwindling resources and increasing demands has been bridged, more or less successfully, by goodwill — the willingness of hospital staffs to tolerate unsatisfactory conditions and to overcome shortages by exertion beyond the call of duty. This fund of goodwill is being steadily depleted."

There was a large section about the pay and conditions of hospital junior staff: "The tradition whereby service in the house officer grade is regarded as an apprenticeship for which only a nominal salary is paid is outdated. . . . Where a hospital authority decides that it is essential, for the needs of the Service, that a doctor be compulsorily resident, he should be charged nothing for his accommodation. . . . In the case of compulsory residence the hospital is the doctor's home for the duration of his appointment: his accommodation should therefore be as comfortable and as private as the home of any other young professional man. . . . It is not only quite unreasonable, but against the best interests of the patients, that a young doctor should ever be on call for 168 hours in a week, and on active duty for 80 hours or more."

There was also an important section about consultants, in which the first hint was dropped about a new contract, based on a 10-session (or five-day) week. Other matters dealt with were private practice ("There are sound social and economic reasons for allowing the continuance of private practice in hospitals and, indeed, for extending the meagre facilities at present available"), and study leave ("Regular study leave is essential to hospital doctors if the hospital service is to maintain the highest standards, and this must be recognised by hospital authorities").

On 3 September 1966 an important development occurred. The Central Consultants and Specialists Committee held a special meeting and announced its readiness and its desire to assume responsibility for all negotiations on remuneration and terms of service for hospital doctors, in place of the Joint Consultants Committee. This was the culmination of years of suspicion, particularly among junior staff and non-teaching hospital consultants, of the influence of the Royal Colleges in such matters, but it came at a time when the colleges were ready to agree to the change, because the Royal College of Surgeons of England had raised legal doubts as to whether it was consistent with the charters and charitable status of the colleges to play any part, directly or even indirectly, in negotiations on pay and terms of service. So the change was made. A new negotiating subcommittee of the Central Consultants and Specialists Committee was set up and the BMA changed the name of the parent committee to the Central Committee for Hospital Medical Services.

On the same day (3 September 1966) the committee announced its intention to prepare a "charter" for hospital doctors. Another working party met at Richmond and drafted a "Memorandum on the Current Problems of Hospital Medical Staff." This was an even more detailed and comprehensive review of the problems and grievances of hospital doctors than the first Richmond Document. It opened with the words: "Never before have hospital doctors been so disenchanted with the conditions under which they are called upon to practise." Other pungent sentiments were: "The nation has not provided the necessary funds to realise the concept on which the National Health Service was founded. . . . The recent statement by the Ministry of Health on hospital building shows how slow and inadequate is the current rate of progress. . . . The chief financial attraction of a career in hospital medicine is the scale of consultant remuneration. If this is unattractive to doctors of the highest quality the whole of hospital medicine will suffer. . . . At a time when it is vitally necessary to expand the output from the medical schools, it is folly to allow the attractions of a career in medical teaching to fall behind those of a career in the hospital service."

The memorandum included a section on work load. In view of the subsequent negotiation of a work-sensitive contract for junior staff, and of the later unsuccessful attempt to negotiate a similar new contract for consultants, it is worth quoting the following passage: "Nearly all of the junior hospital staff and a large proportion of the senior staff are on 'whole-time' contracts. 'Whole-time' service means continuous availability, with unlimited hours of work, upon a fixed salary. When the level of staffing is adequate, this is acceptable: but when the staff are seriously short and 'whole-time' begins to mean being on duty the *whole of the time*, the situation becomes intolerable. If the disparity between medical manpower and the medical needs of the population continues to widen, the time will come when the concept of 'whole-time' service has to be abandoned. The maximum contractual week might then be defined as one of ten notional half-days, and any service provided over and above this would require a separate (additional) contract."

When subsequently the BMA began to negotiate "closed-ended" contracts, with a defined working week and special payments for overtime or "supertime," the Association came in for a great deal of criticism from many different quarters. It is therefore important to record the origin of this development, in the words quoted above.

The BMA's Memorandum on the Current Problems of Hospital Medical Staff was submitted to the Minister of Health (then Mr Kenneth Robinson) in January 1967 and was used by a team of negotiators as the basis for an intensive round of negotiations with the Health Ministers which led to many improvements, but also much controversy. The outcome of the negotiations was reported by the BMA Council in 1968, as follows: "Intensive negotiations, based upon the 'charter' memorandum, have continued throughout the year with the Health Departments. Eleven plenary sessions were held, with the Minister of Health in the chair. . . . Three joint reports have been issued. . . ." There followed a list of 16 hospital memoranda in which the new agreements had been promulgated, on topics that included minimum time off duty, professional and study leave, postgraduate medical education, and residential accommodation for hospital junior staff. But the most important product of these intensive and high-level negotiations was a report on career structure and career planning (called the Panel 1 Report). This made a large number of cogent and valuable observations, but its principal solution to the problem of career structure was to make much wider use of an enhanced medical assistant grade. The profession's instinctive emotional objection to a sub-consultant grade erupted once again at the subsequent ARM at Eastbourne. The meeting could not stomach "the idea that the medical assistant grade should form any part of a progressive consultant career structure," and the Panel 1 Report was to all intents and purposes summarily rejected.

The same year (1968) saw the publication of the two "Cogwheel" reports by joint working parties on the organisation of medical work in hospitals in England and Wales, and in Scotland. Their nicknames derived from the jacket of the English report, which showed a series of interlocking cogwheels. The chairmen of the joint working parties were the two distinguished chief medical officers, Sir George Godber and Dr (later Sir) John Brotherston. The reports advocated the divisional system of medical administration.

In 1969 yet another report, on the responsibilities of the consultant grade, came from a special working party chaired by Sir George Godber, which he had convened after the summary rejection of the Panel 1 Report in 1968. This latest report (colloquially known as the "tomato sauce" report from its jacket colour) suffered the same fate, because it was thought by many regional consultants to devalue the quality and the status of the consultant grade. The report had suggested that not all consultants were necessarily equal and that there could be junior consultants and senior consultants, as had existed in every "firm" in the teaching hospitals before the NHS. But it made a proposal which bore fruit: the creation of a part-time sub-consultant grade, the hospital practitioner grade. This was to be filled exclusively by general practitioners. The hospital committees took exception to this restriction, however, and thus exposed their tacit recognition of the need for a sub-consultant grade in the hospital hierarchy, even if only part time.

In 1971-2 a new Central Manpower Committee was established, to advise the Health Departments on planning targets for staffing in the different grades and specialties in the hospital service. Ten of its 17 members were BMA nominees. In addition, regional manpower committees were set up in each region.

The BMA Council reported in 1972 that the Central Committee for Hospital Medical Services had set up a special working party to devise a new consultant contract, based on a 10-session week, with a specified content, and extra remuneration for work over and above this basic commitment. The National Conference of Hospital Medical Staffs — hospital doctors had emulated the general practitioners' annual conference of local medical committees — approved proposals made by the working party, but Mr D E Bolt, who was later to labour like Hercules in trying to negotiate the new contract, remarked with foresight that "several doctors had expressed doubts about it. They did not think it right to negotiate a contract which might produce gains in pay but losses in professional freedom. Furthermore, they had grave doubts about the air of optimism on the financial consequences of the proposed changes." Prophetic words! A new model contract for consultants was published in the *BMJ* on 15 July 1972, and negotiations were opened with the Health Departments. At a later date the BMA Council explained: "The existing form of consultants' contracts has been basically unchanged since the National Health Service began. There are three main objections to it. (*a*) It is based upon a five and a half day week which is out of tune with accepted conditions today. (*b*) It involves a burden of work which is undefined and unlimited. (*c*) In recent years, the Government has shown itself progressively more determined to exploit the undefined nature of the contract to its own advantage and it has become clear that, without a definition of what work is covered by their salaries, consultants have little hope of securing rewards commensurate with their work load." Briefly, the aim was to replace the existing full-time contract of 11 half-days a week by a contract covering 10 half-days — that is, a five-day week — all consultants having the right to engage additionally in non-contractual work (such as extra NHS sessions, or private practice) for additional reward.

Negotiations made little progress until the change of Government in February 1974, when the new Secretary of State for Social Services (Mrs Barbara Castle) set up a special joint working party under the chairmanship of her Minister of State, Dr David Owen. But willingness to discuss the contract was part of a less congenial Government strategy. In 1965-8 the Minister of Health (Mr Kenneth Robinson) had reviewed the distribution of pay-beds and reduced their total by a quarter, in return for which he abolished the control over the level of professional fees which had been in force since 1948. Matters now went much further. It was part of Labour Party policy that pay-beds should be "phased out" (this was the expression used) from NHS hospitals, and the terms of reference of the Owen Working Party included consideration of arrangements for doing this.

If pay-beds and private work were to be phased out of NHS hospitals, the part-time consultants would suffer a unilateral alteration of their terms of service and would also face a substantial loss of income. The wholly natural concern of the consultant body at this prospect was greatly aggravated by the action of certain Health Service trade unions which decided to withdraw the labour of their members from private patients in certain hospitals. The BMA Council commented: "This was an unwholesome development. If trade unions can withdraw labour from a certain category of patients (for example, paying patients) they can equally well decide to withdraw labour from other categories on political or racial grounds. Interference of this sort with the care of particular categories of patients should not be tolerated in a National Health Service and the

Council was shocked and dismayed that the Secretary of State reacted so ineffectually . . ."

In fact, the BMA suspected that the Health Service unions' strikes against pay-beds were not unwelcome to Mrs Castle. It is significant that she wrote in her diary* (on 5 February 1975): "A delegation from the TUC about pay beds. Their representations were very low key. . . . I suspect they were not more ferocious because we are busy fixing up a secret dinner with them to discuss how we can best implement our policy."

Despite all these snags, discussions on a new consultant contract made considerable progress in the Owen Working Party until 20 December 1974, when Mrs Barbara Castle suddenly intervened and presented the profession with a memorandum of Government proposals, on a "take it or leave it" basis. The proposals amounted to a thinly disguised attempt to induce all NHS consultants to become whole time and to abandon private practice. They were rejected by the hospital doctors' negotiators, who decided to embark on a programme of sanctions. Consultants were recommended to withdraw from the administration of the NHS and to "work to rule" — in other words, to suspend all those services and facilities which consultants normally provide by goodwill beyond the extent of their NHS contracts.

This state of cold war dragged on until April 1975, when the profession was on tenterhooks awaiting a Review Body report. In an all-night negotiating session Mrs Castle "clarified misunderstandings" and the consultants called off their sanctions. Negotiations on the new contract were then resumed. But in August 1975 the Government published a consultative document on the separation of private practice from the NHS, which the BMA described as "perhaps the greatest threat to the independence of the medical profession since the controversy associated with the introduction of the NHS 30 years ago." The profession reacted promptly: in September 1975 the BMA and 15 other medical and dental organisations (including the Royal Colleges and the Hospital Consultants and Specialists Association) sent to Mrs Castle a detailed critical commentary on the Government's policy of complete separation

---

* *The Castle Diaries, 1974-76* (Weidenfeld and Nicolson, 1980).

("apartheid") of public and private medicine. In October the Prime Minister announced the appointment of the Royal Commission on the National Health Service, and the profession represented to Mr Wilson that the whole question of the private sector in the NHS should be referred to the royal commission and that in the meantime legislation for "separation" should be withheld. This request was flatly refused, so the BMA decided that consultants should again apply sanctions.

This time consultants were recommended to limit their work to the treatment of emergencies and other urgent cases and to the continuing care of patients already in their wards. Mrs Castle wrote in her diary: "The BMA's response was to call on all senior hospital doctors, from consultants downwards, to ban all NHS work except emergencies. Similar action by the juniors was made official at the same time.* Some people in the Cabinet began to get cold feet. Harold Wilson schemed with his old friend, Arnold Goodman, to force a compromise."

Lord Goodman exercised his famous skills as a mediator and produced what became known as "the Goodman proposals." In effect, these consisted of acceptance of the ultimate separation of private practice from NHS hospitals, with the transfer of the control of the process (after the initial phasing-out of 1000 pay-beds) from the Secretary of State to an independent board. The BMA balloted the consultants, who voted (in a regrettably low poll) overwhelmingly for rejection of Mrs Castle's consultative document, and by two to one in favour of the Goodman proposals. So sanctions were suspended and discussions continued with the Government on the Goodman proposals, which were eventually enacted in the Health Services Act 1976.

The negotiations at this period between Government and the profession were among the toughest and most tense that had ever taken place in the National Health Service. In her diary for 5 December 1975, Mrs Barbara Castle paid an unsolicited compliment to a BMA leader who was destined to become Chairman of Council: "In the discussion which followed Grabham made all the running: he is by far the ablest (and toughest) negotiator they have got."

*The hospital junior staff were concurrently in dispute with Mrs Castle about the implementation of their new contract.

With the pay-bed problem temporarily out of the way (it was solved in 1980, when the Conservative Government reversed the previous Government's policy), negotiations were resumed on a new consultant contract. Detailed proposals were published in the *BMJ* on 11 September 1976, and attracted support and also much criticism, particularly from whole-time consultants who considered that the proposals were biased in favour of part-timers. But a ballot of consultants and senior registrars in May 1978 produced a vote of 70% in support of the new contract, and so the proposals were submitted to the Review Body for "pricing." Everything was made ready for the introduction of the new contract: a job description under the new contract was agreed with the Health Departments, and a draft implementation circular was sent to the health authorities. But the Review Body's award of 1979 produced a débacle: the pricing of the new proposals was such that the new contract would attract no more remuneration than the old. The Review Body had carried out a redistribution exercise: 11 half-days under the old contract were equated with 13 half-days under the new. The consultant leaders were enraged, and the pricing of the new consultant contract was unanimously rejected.

This was a bitter pill for the BMA to swallow, given the great effort which had been put into negotiating a new consultant contract over a period of seven years. But no time was spent crying over spilt milk. The consultant leaders, notably the tireless Mr David Bolt, at once approached the new Secretary of State — Mr Patrick Jenkin had succeeded Mr David Ennals when the Conservatives came to power — to secure improvements to the existing contract. Modifications were quickly agreed, including a limited right to private practice for whole-time consultants, the payment of 10/11ths of the whole-time salary to maximum part-timers, instead of 9/11ths, and an additional paid session for whole-timers and maximum part-timers where the needs of the Service required this extra work. With these improvements, much was saved from the wreckage.

Another subject which caused gradually increasing concern to the BMA was the mounting demand in Parliament and among the public for the introduction of wider powers to investigate complaints in the hospital service. Despite pre-1948 misgivings, clinical freedom had survived astonishingly well, but the growing consumerism and pressure groups of the 'sixties turned their eyes on the National Health Service. A special committee of inquiry under Mr Michael Davies QC had sat for two years; the 1974 NHS reorganisation had included the creation of a Health Service Commissioner (or "Ombudsman"); and a Parliamentary Select Committee recommended in December 1977 that the remit of the Health Service Commissioner should be widened to include complaints concerning clinical judgment. The BMA consistently and doggedly argued that undue emphasis on complaints procedures would inevitably compel doctors to practise defensive medicine. This would unbalance clinical judgment and impair the doctor's initiative, and would be against the patient's best interests.

The late 1970s brought a recrudescence of the BMA's concern about medical manpower. There was a strong body of opinion (not unanimous, however) that too many doctors were being trained and that medical unemployment would follow. The BMA's evidence to the Royal Commission on the NHS said (in 1977): "A major review of the medical manpower situation should be instituted forthwith, and an impartial body, upon which the BMA would be represented, should be set up to monitor the situation annually." The next year the Hospital Junior Staff Committee again expressed alarm at the prospect of widespread medical unemployment, and recommended an immediate reduction in medical school intake and an annual review of medical manpower. But the royal commission were unimpressed. They reviewed the available information about numbers, and quoted the evidence of the Royal College of Surgeons of England which had written (very truly) that "Previous attempts to forecast the staffing needs of the NHS have not met with conspicuous success and the most important lesson to be learnt from the past is that the future is unpredictable." The royal commission then reported rather lamely: "Nonetheless we chance our arm here. We think that the planned output of medical graduates is about right at present, and that there is unlikely to be medical unemployment this century."

It must be conceded that there are many imponderables in forecasting medical manpower. One need only mention financial constraints, the proportion of women practising medicine, and future trends in medical emigration and immigration. In 1980 the BMA set up a permanent Manpower Committee to grapple with this subject.

REMUNERATION: THE PILKINGTON ERA

We must now return to the chequered story of doctors' pay. The Royal Commission on Doctors' and Dentists' Remuneration was appointed on 27 March 1957. The chairman was Sir Harry Pilkington, a top-level industrialist, and there were eight other members, including one woman, none of them medically or dentally qualified. Two were lawyers, one (Professor John Jewkes) was an economist, one (Mr J H Gunlake) was an actuary, and one was a nominee of the TUC. Their terms of reference were "to consider: (*a*) How the levels of professional remuneration from all sources now received by doctors and dentists taking any part in the National Health Service compare with the remuneration received by members of other professions, by other members of the medical and dental professions, and by people engaged in connected occupations; (*b*) What, in the light of the foregoing, should be the proper current levels of remuneration of such doctors and dentists by the National Health Service; (*c*) Whether, and if so what, arrangements should be made to keep that remuneration under review; and to make recommendations."

The Commission sat for three years, belying the Prime Minister's optimistic assurance at the outset that they would complete their task within a year. During that time the Government made three interim increases in the pay of the medical and dental professions. After overcoming its initial hesitation about co-operating with the royal commission — a special representative meeting having finally decided on 12 June 1957 that the Association should give evidence — the BMA entered with great energy and thoroughness into the daunting task of preparing and presenting comprehensive evidence on behalf of the medical profession. A special evidence committee was appointed, great pains were taken to correlate the views of all the different sections of the profession, and close liaison was maintained with the other professional bodies which were known to be giving evidence to the commission. Five memoranda of evidence were submitted by the BMA, and oral evidence was given on several occasions, at which the BMA witnesses were accompanied by Professor R G D Allen, Mr S B R Cooke (of Counsel), and Mr N Leigh Taylor (solicitor to the Association).

In its second memorandum of evidence the BMA proposed a new procedure for reviewing medical remuneration in the future. The BMA recommended "that medical remuneration should be the subject of an annual review and report by a standing committee appointed by the Prime Minister whose terms of reference and composition should be agreed with the profession. Both the Government and the profession would have the right to make representations to the standing committee. . . . It would be agreed that the findings of the standing committee would be accepted by both sides. A procedure of this kind would eliminate the protracted disputes which have been so unfortunate a feature of the past."

In another of its memoranda of evidence the BMA dealt with the position of the public health doctors and proposed radically revised salary scales for them. One of the reasons why the BMA had been so hesitant at the outset about co-operating with the royal commission was that, although its terms of reference covered "doctors and dentists taking any part in the National Health Service," the public health medical officers had been excluded by the Government. The BMA protested vehemently against this arbitrary exclusion, but the Minister of Health explained that if PHMOs were included the royal commission would inescapably find itself conducting an investigation into the pay of the whole of the higher staff of local government, and this would enormously prolong its task. Nevertheless, the royal commission itself said: "The Commission are not asked to recommend remuneration for doctors and dentists employed by local authorities; but these doctors and dentists are among the 'other members of the medical and dental professions' on whose remuneration evidence will be received for purposes of comparison." So the BMA gave evidence about this important branch of the profession. There remained, however, a great deal of bitterness among public health medical officers at the acquiescence by the BMA in their arbitrary exclusion from the full scope of the royal commission's inquiry.

The Pilkington Report was published on 10 February 1960. Briefly, the report recommended an average increase of 23% in remuneration (compared with the BMA's original claim of 24%, which had subsequently been increased to 29%). And the royal commission recommended the establishment of a Review Body system for the future. The full report (of 346 pages, including a 26-page Memorandum of Dissent by Professor John Jewkes) is an important document in the history of the National Health Service, and indeed of the development of pay negotiations in the UK. Here are a few, a very few, of its salient passages:

> We were appointed nearly three years ago to carry out a task that was then expected to be simple, and short. It has turned out to be neither.
>
> We recommend the setting up of a Review Body . . . to watch the levels and spread of medical and dental remuneration, and to make recommendations to the Prime Minister. The main task of this Body will be the exercise of the faculty of good judgment, and it must be composed of individuals whose standing and reputation will command the confidence of the professions, the Government, and the public. . . . While the Government cannot abrogate its functions and responsibility for ultimate decisions, we are insistent that the recommendations of the Review Body must only very rarely and for most obviously compelling reasons be rejected.
>
> Doctors and dentists in the public service should not be used as a regulator of the national economy. Their earnings should not be prevented from rising because of a fear that others might follow.
>
> We recommend that the terms of reference should be: To advise the Prime Minister on the remuneration of doctors and dentists taking any part in the National Health Service.

By far the most important recommendation of the Pilkington Royal Commission was this creation of the Review Body system, which had been suggested by the BMA in its evidence. Another especially important paragraph (number 166) of the Pilkington Report threw Spens out of the window: "The professions, in giving evidence to us, laid great emphasis on what was sometimes called 'proper implementation of the Spens Reports.' We have studied all three reports with great care, but . . . we state emphatically that the remuneration of two great professions in the National Health Service can no longer be governed by their recommendations."

The royal commission made one recommendation (in

paragraph 348) which was to be an apple of discord: "We accordingly recommend that, over and above the finance needed to meet our other recommendations, a special fund of £500 000 per annum be provided expressly to recognise distinguished general practice by additional remuneration. We recommend that this sum be applied in accordance with a scheme to be agreed between the profession and the Government, and that until a scheme is agreed, the money should revert permanently to the Exchequer."

Apart from this suggestion of merit awards in general practice, the Pilkington Report was well received. The Council decided to recommend to the Representative Body that the commission's recommendations should be accepted "as a whole as they stand." These were the words which had already been used by the Government in announcing its readiness to accept the report. A special representative meeting on 19 May 1960 resolved to accept the report, and to enter at once into detailed discussion on its implementation with the Health Departments. The *BMJ* first leading article said: "All those who gave evidence for the profession to the commission deserve the congratulations of their colleagues in the NHS." And the SRM passed a euphoric resolution expressing gratification at the way the Government had readily accepted the report of the royal commission, and expressing hopes of a similar happy relationship in the future with any Government in office.

In September 1960 another SRM was held to consider the results of the detailed negotiations on the implementation of the royal commission's report. After a good deal of debate the Representative Body agreed to accept the Government's "package deal" — that is, the royal commission's recommendations "as a whole as they stand." All was not sweetness and light, however. Dr P S Byrne, of Westmorland (later to become President of the Royal College of General Practitioners) said that the package deal should be labelled "fragile, not to be handled by the SRM," and was in many ways an unlucky dip. As the wrapping was removed there emerged not an odour of sanctity and honour, but the sour scent of rosin from a Government fiddle — and not a first or second. Dr C M Scott, of Barnet, led a strong attack on one of the decisions made by the general practitioner joint working party, to hold back temporarily £1 million of the award to general practitioners in order to continue the difficult negotiations on some new proposals from the Ministry of Health for distributing remuneration in order to provide incentives to good practice. And there was anxiety and disappointment that the Government had not so far agreed that public health medical officers should be covered by the new Review Body. In the end, however, the "package deal" as implemented by the reports of joint working parties was accepted.

So ended the Spens/Danckwerts era of NHS remuneration, and the Pilkington era began. Early in 1962 the BMA Council and the Joint Consultants Committee decided to set up a small joint committee to act for the profession in all matters relating to the new review machinery. This soon became known as the Joint Evidence Committee, and continued to be so called even after the Joint Consultants Committee had withdrawn from all matters concerning pay. (Thereafter the correct title of the committee, which was then purely a BMA committee, was the Review Body Evidence Committee.)

In 1962 the first Review Body was appointed by the Prime Minister. The chairman was Lord Kindersley, a patrician and captain of industry, who had won a Military Cross in the first world war and commanded a Guards brigade in the second. The profession soon developed the fullest confidence in Lord Kindersley, and respect tinged with affection. The other members were a lawyer, an economist, an actuary (Mr J H Gunlake, who had also served on the royal commission), an academic, an industrialist, and a banker. The Joint Evidence Committee soon began what was to become a regular and onerous task: the careful preparation, with much expert economic, statistical, and legal advice, of written evidence to the Review Body.

In April 1962 the report was published of a joint working party that had dealt with the suggestion by the royal commission that £500 000 might be provided annually to recognise distinguished general practice. The joint working party produced a scheme for selecting certain general practitioners for differential payments. But the ARM 1962 rejected "the principle of differential payments for general practitioners based on merit awards," and that was that.

On the issue of the reserved £1 million, a second joint working party recommended the creation of a postgraduate education fund and increased loading on the capitation fee for the patients between 1000 and 1500 on a doctor's list, with the object of encouraging lists of moderate size. These proposals were approved by the ARM 1962.

The BMA had continued to press that public health medical officers should be covered by the Review Body, but in September 1962 the Review Body informed the Association that they did not regard as within their remit doctors in the employment of local health authorities, or of nationalised industries, or of universities. The BMA Council was deeply disappointed with this decision and took legal advice on whether the decision could be challenged at law. Opinion of two eminent Counsel stated that: "We have no doubt whatever that public health medical officers are excluded from the terms of reference of the Review Body as recommended by the Royal Commission." In the light of this legal advice (subsequently confirmed by eminent Counsel in Scotland), the Council reluctantly decided to abandon its campaign, but this caused much bitterness among public health medical officers.

The general practitioners were now showing signs of dissatisfaction with the "pool" method of settling their remuneration, which had been accepted since the Danckwerts award of 1952 and had been endorsed by the royal commission. Briefly, an average individual income settled by negotiation or by arbitration — for example, Danckwerts — was multiplied by the number of principals in general practice, and this calculation yielded a "pool" of money, which was then distributed in capitation fees and other payments to the general practitioners. But payments to general practitioners for any work performed in hospitals, or for services to local authorities, were a first charge on the pool and reduced the amount that was left for the remuneration of family practice itself.

The First Report of the Review Body was published in February 1963. It awarded a straight increase of 14%. This was a simple matter in the case of hospital doctors. In the case of general practitioners, the global pool was increased by 14% and a joint working party decided how the increase should be distributed. The proposed distribution was approved by the Representative Body at Oxford, but owing to the pool system many individual general practitioners received less than the 14% increase in their net remuneration and were correspondingly disappointed and angry. Dissatisfaction with the pool method of remuneration grew apace. On 25 January 1964 the first leader in the *BMJ* stated: "The pool method of paying general practitioners has got to be radically altered. At long last the mounting criticism of this has come to a head. General practitioners will no longer tolerate a system which means that those who are paid for their work for government and local authorities, for maternity services, and, for example, for smallpox vaccination should receive these payments at the expense of their fellow practitioners. . . . It seems, indeed, that at long last a system of paying general practitioners which has with modification been in force since 1911 is being sharply and openly challenged by a body — the BMA — which by and large has supported it through the years of the NHI and the NHS up to date."

Another criticism of the pool system was that practice expenses were distributed on an averaged basis that generally benefited practitioners who provided substandard accommodation and staff for their patients, at the expense of those who provided the best.

There was a second main grievance among general practitioners, and that was "the differential." This dissatisfaction had been expressed in a resolution by the ARM 1963 which drew attention to the disparity between the career earnings of general medical practitioners and consultants, quoting the figures of £79 000 and £117 000 respectively, culled from the royal commission report, Table 9.

Alarmed by the anger expressed by general practitioners at the ARM 1963, the Council decided to submit a case to the Review Body for a substantial improvement both in the remuneration and in the terms of service of general practice. The hospital branch of the profession might well have resented a special case being presented on behalf of general practitioners, and the Council took great pains to keep the Central Consultants and Specialists Committee and the Joint Consultants Committee fully informed at all stages of the preparation of the case.

The Council's Memorandum of Evidence was published in the *BMJ* of 25 January 1964. Some of its salient passages are worth quoting: "The case is supported by the whole profession. . . . Those who have had long experience of representing the interests of general practitioners cannot remember a time when dissatisfaction was so widespread, vehement, or vociferous. . . . The principal object of this memorandum of evidence is to secure the correction of what are now seen to be inherent defects in the pool system. . . . The distribution of that award [the first award of the Review Body] has caused bitter disillusionment to general practitioners. . . . The proposed increase in the remuneration of general practitioners is intended to secure . . . that general practice shall receive its fair share of the limited recruitment to the profession, and that the standard of service is as high as can be obtained."

There had been some hard-hitting debate in Council before the memorandum was approved, and there was even more controversy and acrimony when it came before a special representative meeting held at Church House, Westminster (the Great Hall at BMA House was being redecorated) on 25 March 1964. The BMA leaders were desperately anxious to maintain a united front within the profession, because Lord Kindersley had intimated that the Review Body would not be willing to adjudicate any dispute between one branch of the profession and another. But some prominent general practitioners, such as Dr Ivor Jones of Sunderland, were determined to pull no punches in criticising "the differential," and argued their point of view with great force and eloquence. This clash of tactics came to a head between the meeting of Council and the special representative meeting, when a special Conference of Representatives of Local Medical Committees recommended that Dr Ivor Jones should be added to the Joint Evidence Committee. The Chairman of the General Medical Services Committee, Dr A B Davies, who was of course the chief representative of general practice on the Joint Evidence Committee, took this as a personal affront and resigned. He was succeeded by Dr James Cameron.

The special representative meeting at Church House was bad-tempered and unhappy. Great heat was engendered about "the differential" and Mr Robin Blackburne, speaking for the consultants, was almost shouted down. A motion of no confidence in the GMS Committee was defeated. East Yorkshire had submitted a rival (euphemistically called "additional") memorandum of evidence. At the end of the day, the Council's memorandum was approved, but with some amendments and additions. The Chairman of Council (Mr J R Nicholson-Lailey) paid a warm and well-deserved tribute to Dr A B Davies, and the meeting unanimously agreed to send him a telegram of deepest regret at his resignation and sincere thanks for all his work in the past. The revised memorandum of evidence was supported by the Joint Consultants Committee, and submitted to the Review Body.

The award of the Review Body on this special case for general practitioners sparked off a volcanic eruption. Briefly, the Review Body agreed that payments to general practitioners by hospital authorities, local authorities, and Government departments should be excluded from the pool. So far so good. But in response to the profession's claim for an increase of £18 million, the Review Body awarded £5½ million with a recommendation that the bulk of this money should be used for new schemes for the partial reimbursement of the cost of ancillary help and of maintaining practice premises. Further, the Review Body rejected a claim for seniority payments and recommended instead that the profession and the Ministry should try to devise an acceptable scheme of merit payments for general practitioners.

All this was more than general practitioners could stomach. As the *BMJ* stated: "This action to the most unbiased observer seemed to go beyond the terms of reference of the Review Body. It was not only making an award but was deciding how the money should be distributed." The BMA Council, in its other guise as the British Medical Guild Trustees, collected undated resignations of general practitioners from the National Health Service. Urgent discussions took place with the Minister of Health, and the Review Body was induced to "clarify" its award by saying that the £5½ million could be added unconditionally to the pool.

This additional sum was distributed in the form of increased capitation fees from 1 April 1965. In the meantime, as has already been related, a charter for general practice was drawn up during a weekend at Hove by six negotiators for general practitioners. On 24 March 1965 a special combined meeting of the Representative Body and of the Conference of Representatives of Local Medical Committees decided that the British Medical Guild should be advised to hold the resignations in its hands until 30 June while intensive negotiations on the charter proceeded with the Minister of Health, Mr Kenneth Robinson.

On 23 June another SRM was held. By then, 18 000 general practitioners had sent in their undated resignations. The main debate of the day was on an amendment by Croydon to the effect that, as progress in the negotiations on the charter had not proceeded fast enough, the resignations should be submitted on 1 July. After a long and acrimonious debate this was defeated by 281 votes to 143. The meeting then resolved that the undated resignations should continue to be held by the British Medical Guild and that the negotiations on the charter should continue.

The negotiations with Mr Kenneth Robinson reached a successful conclusion, and one of the tasks of the Review Body in its second major review (in 1966) was to price the agreed general practitioners' charter. Hence this report of the Review Body (the seventh — there had been intervening reports on dental pay, the pay of senior hospital medical officers, and the numbers of distinction awards for consultants) was of particular importance.

The award was a differential one. For hospital doctors, the average increase recommended was 13·4%, ranging from 43% for a first house officer to 10% for a basic consultant — that is, a consultant without a distinction award. For general practitioners, whose case had been brilliantly put by Mr Desmond Ackner QC (now Lord Justice Ackner), the average increase recommended was 33·3%, a figure which accrued from the pricing of the new charter. But there was a fly in the ointment. Because of the size of the award to general practitioners — at the time of another national economic crisis — the Government announced that payment of the increase would be "phased": half would be paid on 1 April 1966, and the balance on 1 April 1967.

Despite this, the General Medical Services Committee recommended that the award and the phasing be accepted (though the latter was "deplored"), and that the guild should "withdraw the undated resignations of general practitioners which it holds." The Council reported: "The advances offered in the terms and conditions of service, and financially, could lead to a renaissance of general practice"

— a forecast that proved to be true despite the traumatic events which were about to ensue.

Much more difficult was the situation facing the hospital leaders. The Chairman of the Joint Consultants Committee was Sir Thomas Holmes Sellors, a wise and experienced medical statesman, who at once advised his team to accept the award with a good grace. Not surprisingly, however, the junior staff representatives were irritated by an award of 11-16% for senior registrars and registrars, compared with $33\frac{1}{3}\%$ for general practitioners. They raised such strong objections that the Council felt itself inhibited from immediately accepting the award, and convened a special representative meeting for 21 June 1966, seven weeks after the publication of the Review Body's award.

At the SRM, great annoyance was expressed at the relatively small award to hospital doctors, and also at the "phasing" of the award to general practitioners, but in the end the Representative Body agreed to accept the Seventh Report of the Review Body and the "phasing," together with the reports of the negotiations on the charter for the family doctor service, and to advise the British Medical Guild to "withdraw" the undated resignations.

About a fortnight later ugly whispers began to circulate at BMA House that the country's financial position had deteriorated further and that the Government was preparing some form of drastic action. The rumours proved to be true. On 20 July 1966 the Government imposed a prices and incomes standstill, under which pay increases, even those already awarded or negotiated, were frozen for six months if they were not actually in payment. Thus the pay rises due to be received from the Seventh Report of the Review Body, both those for general practitioners and those for hospital doctors, were compulsorily deferred from 1 April to 1 October 1966, and six months' increases were lost by the profession forever. This was the dire consequence of the profession's delay in accepting the Review Body's report, a lesson the BMA did not forget.

The Seventh Report of the Review Body, followed closely by the Government's pay standstill, caused tremendous turmoil in the medical profession. But the worsening economic position and the application of the "freeze" to everyone, led the BMA to conclude that doctors, as responsible citizens, must accept the Government's decision. Indeed, there was no alternative: the Government held the purse-strings in the National Health Service, and total resignation from the Service and a return to private practice was scarcely a practical proposition in a time of economic crisis.

And how was the third branch of the National Health Service faring at this time? After the Seventh Report of the Review Body, a detailed and closely reasoned claim was lodged on behalf of public health medical officers. The management side of Whitley C refused to consider the claim until the increases due to other chief officers had been settled, so in 1967 the BMA imposed a ban on the advertisement of vacancies in the Public Health Service, and advised doctors not to apply for posts in it. The BMA published a detailed account of the background to the dispute in *The Medical Officer*, a journal with a big circulation in the Public Health Service, and sent a 23-point statement to local authorities explaining why it had been found necessary to impose sanctions.

The ban lasted seven months. During this period only two large authorities were able to fill posts of medical officer of health. In some cases loyalty to the policy of the BMA had serious consequences for the careers of public health medical officers, but a settlement was reached and new salary scales came into effect on 1 July 1967. Many public health medical officers expressed their appreciation of the BMA's efforts throughout a difficult year of negotiation.

In 1969 a new claim was lodged on behalf of public health medical officers. The employing authorities offered a much smaller increase and deadlock ensued, but this time both sides agreed to refer the dispute to a single arbitrator. Hitherto, such disputes had been referred to the Industrial Court, but the BMA had long felt that the Industrial Court was biased in favour of the local authorities' fundamental thesis that public health medical officers were first and foremost local government officers, and doctors only secondarily. In one of its awards (No 2692) the court had stated bluntly that "the claimants [ie, public health medical officers] must be considered as being members of the local authority hierarchy." As things turned out, however, arbitration did not prove to be necessary: the local authorities made an improved offer which was accepted. Another claim was submitted to take effect from 1 April

1970, and this also was settled without open warfare or recourse to arbitration.

The BMA was now seriously concerned at the relative decline in the remuneration of hospital doctors. The evidence to the Review Body on behalf of hospital doctors and dentists for the 1968 review covered 38 pages. Twenty-three supplementary memoranda were submitted, and the oral case was presented by eminent Counsel (the Rt Hon Quintin Hogg QC, MP, now Lord Chancellor). And in 1970 the BMA Council reported: "The basic consultant rate of remuneration is now standing at a totally unrealistic level. . . . In the event of a substantial improvement in remuneration not being forthcoming there could be only one course open, namely, to review the existing contractual obligations of hospital doctors and to renegotiate their contracts."

The Wilson Government delayed publication of the 1970 award (the Twelfth Report) of the Review Body, and this caused unease in the BMA, which sent a letter of inquiry to the Prime Minister. The BMA's unease was greatly magnified on 18 May, when the dissolution of Parliament was announced. A request for a meeting was addressed to the Prime Minister. On Friday 22 May 1970, the Chairman of Council (Dr Ronald Gibson) and other BMA leaders were at a meeting of the Brynmor Jones working party on the GMC (see Chapter 6) when a message came from BMA House that an envelope had arrived from 10 Downing Street. Although it was the start of a bank holiday weekend, the messenger was told that some of the staff were to be retained on duty at BMA House, in case of emergency.

When the Chairman of Council and his colleagues got back to BMA House, they read the letter from the Prime Minister, which stated: "The Government have concluded that it would not be right to continue with the consideration of the [Review Body's] Report during the election period.... In the light of the Government's decision, you may agree that there would be no advantage in a meeting with your representatives at this stage."

The Government had had the report of the Review Body in its possession for seven weeks before the dissolution was announced. The BMA immediately issued a press statement saying: "Doctors will have no doubt that they are once again to be made the victims of political expediency, the very thing which with the agreement of the Government the Review Body was set up to avoid." The Chairman of Council set up a small action committee to examine a list of possible "sanctions" which had already been drawn up, and a clarion call was issued to all BMA honorary secretaries immediately after the bank holiday.

On 28 May 1970 the leaders of the BMA and the British Dental Association met the Prime Minister and the Secretary of State for Social Services (Mr Richard Crossman) at 10 Downing Street. At this stage the professions were pressing for the immediate publication of the Review Body's report. A Downing Street statement said: "In view of the strength of the representations made by the professions, the Government had decided to bring forward the date of publication, with the announcement of its decisions, to Thursday June 4."

This was some advance, but the BMA had long suspected that the Government's reluctance to publish the report indicated an intention not to implement it. The Association therefore pressed ahead with emergency meetings of the Council and committees, and with a printed circular to the whole profession.

Early in the morning of 4 June 1970 the BMA leaders met Mr Crossman, and their worst suspicions were confirmed. The Review Body's award was extremely simple: an across-the-board increase of 30%. Thus all Mr Crossman's talk during the waiting period about an "extremely complicated and important report"* was seen to have been bluff. The Government's decision was to pay the 30% in full to the junior hospital doctors, but to pay only half to consultants and general practitioners and to ask the National Board for Prices and Incomes to advise how much of the balance of 30% awarded by the Review Body should be paid to those grades!

The BMA found this intolerable. Everyone knew that the Government had the right, under the terms of the Pilkington Royal Commission report, to reject the recommendations of the Review Body "for most obviously compelling reasons"; but to refer the report of the Review Body to another tribunal for emasculation made a mockery of the independence of the Review Body. Lord Kindersley

*See, for example, *Hansard* for 27 May 1970, column 1784.

and his colleagues of the Review Body promptly resigned en bloc, and the BMA declared war. The whole profession was warned to get ready to apply sanctions, and full statements of the BMA's view of the crisis were issued to the profession, to the press and broadcasting organisations, and to Parliamentary candidates — the election campaign was now in full swing. On the same day (4 June 1970) the Chairman of the Conservative Party (Mr Anthony (later Lord) Barber), said at Watford: "The Conservative Government set up the Review Body. . . . For the [Labour] Government now to refer the recommendations to the Prices and Incomes Board is to make a farce of the existing independent Review Body. The professions have every reason to be angry."

The BMA activated the British Medical Guild machinery and energetically organised a programme of collective protest actions (including the withholding of National Insurance Certificates) which is fully described in Chapter 9. On 9 June 1970 *The Times* carried a letter from the Chairman of Council, which ended: "I make this appeal to the Prime Minister: let him call us to the conference table before further damage is done to a vital public service which we doctors have loyally served for so many years." But Dr Gibson's letter was sandwiched between a letter from the Presidents of six of the Royal Colleges (but not including the Royal College of Surgeons of England) in which they wrote: "This is surely a time when the profession should remain calm and it is more likely to receive public support if it retains its dignity," and a letter from a former Labour MP, Dr David Kerr, in which he said: "The Government cannot escape severe censure for its handling not of the Kindersley Committee's award, but of the committee itself. We may now find ourselves back in the wretched days ... before Mr Macmillan set up the Royal Commission on Doctors' and Dentists' Pay."

On 13 June the *Economist* published a letter from Mr J H Gunlake strongly defending the Review Body's award and stating that, whether from ignorance or by design, the report of the Royal Commission was being brushed aside. On 16 June the first leading article in *World Medicine* was headed "Well done," and said: "Few doctors would regard this magazine as an uncritical admirer of the BMA. We are certain, however, that most of our readers will join us in congratulating the BMA on its action over the Review Body report."

On that same day Mr Crossman wrote in his diary: "Some 75% of the GPs are refusing to sign sickness certificates, far more than the Ministry expected, but far fewer than the doctors had hoped." But his Party's election campaign was not helped by the dispute with the doctors.

On 19 June 1970 there was a change of Government and the Conservatives came into power. On 23 June the new Cabinet held its first meeting. The new Secretary of State for Social Services (Sir Keith Joseph) invited the BMA leaders to meet him and the Prime Minister (Mr Edward Heath) on 26 June. After that meeting, Sir Keith Joseph wrote to Dr Gibson: "I told you that the Government was willing ... to withdraw the previous Government's reference to the National Board for Prices and Incomes ... and to arrange for the re-establishment of an independent review body to advise them on doctors' and dentists' pay. The recommendations of this body would not be referred to any other body."

The Representative Body, which was in session at Harrogate, welcomed the new Government's offer, which assured the continuance of an independent Review Body and withdrew the reference to the Prices and Incomes Board. These had been the objectives of the BMA's campaign of sanctions, and so the Representative Body requested the British Medical Guild to discontinue them.

On 29 June the BMA sent a "diary of the dispute" to the whole profession. In thanking the vast number of doctors who had loyally supported the stand taken by the BMA, the letter said that "the resolute stand taken by the BMA on behalf of the whole profession has saved the concept of an independent Review Body for the future: a body which will remain impartial and not be subordinated to any other body. Without this there could have been no future security for the profession."

The new Government did not in the end pay the whole of the balance of the twelfth award, but it carried out its promise to establish a new independent Review Body whose reports would not be referred to any other body for consideration. The first chairman was the Earl of Halsbury FRS. At the same time the Government established two other review bodies, one for the armed Forces in general, and the other for the highest ranks of the judiciary, the Civil Service, and the Forces, and for certain other earners of "top salaries." The secretariat of the Doctors' and Dentists' Review Body was transferred from the Cabinet office to a new Office of Manpower Economics, established to serve all three review bodies.

In November 1972 the Government imposed a total freeze on wages and salaries as the first part of a three-stage incomes policy. This was introduced by the Government after discussions with the Trades Union Congress, the Confederation of British Industry, and the Civil Service. The BMA protested to the Prime Minister about the lack of consultation with the medical profession, and a request was made that the BMA should be included in any future talks on the Government's economic programme. As a result, the Secretary of State for Social Services invited the BMA and the British Dental Association to meet him. The BMA's view was that the medical profession did not expect to receive special treatment at a time when the Government was enacting a statutory control of incomes; but the Association required to be satisfied that the policy was being applied fairly across the board. When, in February 1974, the Heath Government fell as a result of the miners' strike, the new Labour Government promoted a settlement with the miners without reference to the incomes policy established by the previous Government. The BMA immediately told the new Secretary of State for Social Services that the medical profession's willingness to comply with an incomes policy was dependent on it being applied equally and fairly to all sections of the community.

In 1973 the BMA, for the first time, gave evidence to the Review Body on behalf of community physicians, because the unified administration of the NHS was to come into operation in 1974 and it was necessary to settle the salaries of the new community medicine posts so that they could be advertised. Thus ended a long-standing grievance. The BMA had tried hard but unsuccessfully to get public health medical officers covered by the Pilkington Royal Commission and then by the Review Body — even to the extent of proposing that the terms of reference of the Review Body should be suitably amended. Now at last the problem was solved by NHS reorganisation.

A subject which grew more and more important as the

years went by, especially when inflation gathered momentum, was NHS superannuation. The BMA worked hard on this, often in conjunction with the other staff organisations, and achieved much. So much, in fact, that the Review Body said in its 1981 report that the value of the pension scheme for doctors and dentists was "noticeably greater than the value of schemes which apply at comparable levels" and compensated fully for the value of pensions and other benefits, taken together, at equivalent levels elsewhere.

The 1978 Review Body award was 30·4% but staged over three years in order to comply with Government pay policy. The Government accepted and implemented the award. But in 1981 the Government found "compelling reasons" for reducing that year's award from 9% to 6% — the third time since the inception of the Review Body system 20 years previously that a Government had exercised its right, conferred by the Pilkington Royal Commission, to reject an award. The two earlier occasions had been in 1966 (when the BMA acquiesced under protest) and in 1970 when the BMA went to war, not because of the reduction of the award but because of the Government's flagrant violation of the independence of the Review Body.

MEDICINE AND POLITICS

This is a long and eventful chapter of BMA history. The National Health Service is 33 years old. Very briefly and superficially, the NHS is popular with the public but not with the doctors. Medicine and politics do not mix well. In the first half of its existence, it was the general practitioners who found the most difficulty in living with socialised medicine, and, in the second half, the chief problems and discontents have arisen in the hospital service and among hospital doctors.

Aneurin Bevan said in 1948 that the National Health Service "is being watched by every country in the world. There will come over here a stream of visitors to find out how it works and how its difficulties are being resolved." Thirty-three years later, he would have to admit that some of its principal difficulties have not been resolved.

Chapter 6

Not everything was nationalised

The condition upon which God hath given liberty to man is eternal vigilance. — John Philpot Curran.

MEDICAL EDUCATION, AND RELATIONS WITH THE GENERAL MEDICAL COUNCIL

A common misconception among the general public is that the whole of medical practice was nationalised in 1948. One of the BMA's criticisms of the Government's proposals for a National Health Service was that the Service was not going to be sufficiently comprehensive, but we now deem it fortunate that a considerable proportion of medical work was left outside it.

The most important segments excluded were medical education and medical research. In these, the BMA has fulfilled its traditional dual function: it has endeavoured to promote medical education and research, and it has striven to maintain the honour and interests of medical teachers and research workers.

In 1934 the BMA published a report on undergraduate medical education, prepared by a special committee chaired by Sir Henry Brackenbury. The Association also had a special Postgraduate Subcommittee and was represented on the council charged with the organisation of the new postgraduate medical school established under the auspices of the University of London and the London County Council at Hammersmith. This was opened in 1935, and quickly became internationally famous as the British (now Royal) Postgraduate Medical School.

Soon afterwards the BMA founded the Board of Registration of Medical Auxiliaries to promote higher standards of training for the burgeoning professions supplementary to medicine, and to confer medical recognition upon properly trained auxiliaries.

The BMA gave evidence to the Interdepartmental Committee on Medical Schools (the Goodenough Committee), which reported in 1944. The next year, the BMA supported the Royal Colleges in representations to the Privy Council against a proposal by the GMC for the establishment of a statutory list of consultants and specialists.

Prompted by a resolution of the ARM, the Council also set up a special committee to review the working of the Medical Acts, with special reference to the composition, functions, and procedure of the General Medical Council. The BMA had been instrumental in persuading Parliament to create the GMC in 1858, and always kept a watchful eye on it.

Learning that the Government intended to bring in a Bill to give effect to the recommendation of the Goodenough Committee (previously suggested by the Medical Planning Commission) that a preregistration year should be introduced, the BMA, after conferring with the GMC itself and with the defence societies, put forward a list of 25 proposals for inclusion in the Bill, relating to the composition, functions, and procedure of the GMC. These included proposals that the GMC should be required to establish two distinct and separate committees, a Penal Cases Committee and a Disciplinary Committee; that the number of directly elected representatives of the profession on the GMC should be increased from seven to 12; and that visitors should be appointed by the GMC to visit medical schools. Most of these proposals were implemented in the Medical Act 1950.

In 1954 the GMC invited observations on its "Recommendations as to the Medical Curriculum," which had been published in 1947 and were under review. The BMA offered several comments — chiefly, that the recommendations were too rigid and too detailed, and therefore obstructed educational experiment. The special committee which drafted the BMA's comments also considered other matters, such as the Proceedings of the First World Conference on Medical Education (1953). It was a distinguished committee, chaired by Sir Lionel Whitby (Regius Professor of Physic at Cambridge), and including the

President of the GMC itself and the Presidents of three Royal Colleges.

In 1956-8 the BMA examined the working of the Medical Acts (consolidated in the Medical Act 1956) "with special reference to the difficulties attendant upon provisional registration, disciplinary procedure, and elective representation of the profession." The report was published in the *British Medical Journal* of 19 April 1958 and included the following passage: "There are 11 direct representatives of the profession on the General Medical Council. . . . After comparing the present ratio of elected members to the number entitled to vote with the ratio in some previous years, the [BMA] Council has come to the conclusion that there is insufficient evidence at present for an increase in the number of elected members. The Council is, however, of the opinion that this question should be kept under review. . . ." The BMA report went on to recommend improvements in the Association's procedure for proposing and supporting candidates for election to the GMC. The procedure existing at that time dated from 1935, and two unsuccessful candidates in the 1956 election had issued a memorandum criticising the part played by the BMA in supporting candidates.

We must now turn for a time to the BMA's second function, that of maintaining the material interests of the medical profession. In 1949 the Council appointed a special committee to consider the application of the "Spens standards" of remuneration to medical teachers, and other full-time salaried doctors not remunerated wholly through the NHS. Concurrently, the University Grants Committee recognised the implications of the Spens Report on consultants' pay and informed universities of new ranges of salaries for medical teachers. The BMA went further and recommended four grades, each with its own salary scale — higher for clinical than for non-clinical posts. A situation then arose which was to become familiar: the University Grants Committee pointed out that the actual salary scales implemented by each particular university were a matter in which the University Grants Committee could not intervene. The BMA then approached the Committee of Vice-Chancellors and Principals, and individual universities, and embarked on years of struggle to achieve satisfactory remuneration for full-time medical teachers.

The BMA was dissatisfied with the salary scales that were announced for university medical teachers after the report of the Pilkington Royal Commission, and in 1962 affirmed the Association's policy, which was that clinical teachers should have their remuneration equated with that of hospital medical staff of equivalent status, and that the remuneration of medically qualified preclinical teachers should be closely related. For years the BMA persisted in urging this policy on the relevant Government departments, the University Grants Committee, the Committee of Vice-Chancellors and Principals, the National Incomes Commission, the National Board for Prices and Incomes, and (not least) the Association of University Teachers. It was an uphill task, because of the doctrine of "equality of prime stipend" to which both the universities and the Association of University Teachers were deeply committed. This was the doctrine that remuneration in all university faculties should basically be the same.

In the early years of the Review Body system the BMA tried to get medical teachers included within its scope. These efforts were unsuccessful, but in 1967 the Government decided that the remuneration of all university teachers should be made a standing reference to the National Board for Prices and Incomes. Accordingly, the BMA (together with the British Dental Association) submitted a comprehensive memorandum to the board on behalf of medical and dental teachers. It covered eight pages, and included an appendix on medical emigration.*

The main case was simply that clinical professors, senior lecturers, and lecturers should receive salaries comparable with those of their consultant colleagues in the NHS; and that preclinical teachers should be placed on scales not more than 10% below the corresponding clinical scales. The memorandum stated: "This is the least that can be done effectively to stem the loss of staff from preclinical departments."

The Prices and Incomes Board reported in December 1968 recommending that clinical teachers with honorary consultant contracts should receive the same rates of pay as

*In 1962 Dr John Seale had startled the country — and angered the then Minister of Health, Mr Enoch Powell — by publishing an estimate that the equivalent of a quarter of the output of the medical schools was lost each year by emigration. This estimate was confirmed by studies in 1964 and 1966.

their NHS hospital colleagues. This was a major victory for the BMA. Unfortunately, however, the position of preclinical medical teachers remained unsatisfactory, being complicated by the fact that the Association of University Teachers was recognised by the universities and by the Medical Research Council* as the representative organ of non-clinical medical teachers and research workers, and the Association of University Teachers was firmly opposed to "subject differentials." In 1972, however, the BMA Council forthrightly stated: "The Council . . . is determined that the future of medical education in this country should no longer be endangered by the universities' doctrinaire policy of 'equality of prime stipend.'" Even the great University of Cambridge was blacklisted for some years by the BMA, because it refused to introduce the scales recommended by the University Grants Committee for clinical academic staff.

In 1977 the BMA reconstituted its Full-time Medical Teachers and Research Workers Committee as a new "craft committee" entitled the Medical Academic Staff Committee, the better to continue the fight for the interests of medical teachers and research workers, both clinical and non-clinical. The committee is backed by an annual craft conference, and has shown itself to be an energetic reinforcement of the BMA's armament.

Let us now return to the content of medical education. In 1966 the BMA submitted a memorandum of evidence to a subcommittee set up by the General Medical Council "to review medical education." The BMA said: "We would stress that the undergraduate course and immediate post-qualification time is only the initial period of instruction in a continuing education. It should be followed by planned vocational training for all branches of medicine, including general practice."

Shortly before this the GMC had made a fateful announcement: that the gap between its expenditure and the yield from initial registration fees was widening year by

* The Association of Scientific, Technical, and Managerial Staffs (ASTMS) had made an initially successful bid to be recognised as the sole bargaining agent for the non-clinical staff of the Medical Research Council. The BMA and the Association of University Teachers both opposed this, and in the end the Association of University Teachers was recognised on the understanding that the BMA would be consulted whenever medically qualified non-clinical staff were concerned. The BMA's right to represent clinical MRC staff was never questioned.

year, and that it proposed to seek statutory authority to impose an annual registration, or retention, fee. The BMA Council assumed that the Privy Council would need to be satisfied as to the necessity for the proposed changes. Subject to this assumption, however, the BMA Council expressed its agreement with the proposal that "the load should be spread throughout the whole profession." This decision by the BMA Council was destined to incur much criticism.

Another important event was the appointment by the BMA Council of a special committee under the chairmanship of Sir John Richardson (later Lord Richardson, President of the BMA and President of the GMC) to prepare the Association's evidence to the Royal Commission on Medical Education. The BMA's evidence, submitted in June 1966, was highly regarded by the royal commission. Among many other things, the BMA suggested that postgraduate centres should be established throughout the United Kingdom; that two central committees should be set up to oversee postgraduate training; and that married women doctors should, by various practical arrangements, be encouraged to continue practising medicine.

On 4 April 1968 the Report of the Royal Commission on Medical Education (the Todd Report) was published. The BMA was chiefly concerned with its views on postgraduate training. The report recommended that, after the intern year, there should be three years of general professional training, during which there would be progressive assessment culminating in the award of a certificate. The report recommended that possession of this certificate should make the holder eligible for membership of the appropriate Royal College (including the Royal College of General Practitioners), and, as a corollary, the royal commission recommended that the Royal Colleges of Surgeons should redefine their membership to match the completion of the three-year period of general professional training.

After general professional training, the Todd report recommended, there should be a further period of specialised training leading to vocational (or specialist) registration, and the GMC should maintain the register of vocationally trained doctors. The royal commission proposed that there should be a grade in the hospital service for registered specialists in which a doctor could remain for the rest of his career if he wished. The assessment of individuals or of programmes of training would not be the concern of the GMC but of a new Central Council for Postgraduate Medical Education and Training.

On medical manpower the royal commission forecast that there would be a shortfall of 10 000 doctors by 1976 and recommended the creation of three new undergraduate medical schools. But the report also suggested that the plethora of medical schools in London should be reduced to six, by combinations or amalgamations of existing schools.

The report gave a new name — "community medicine" — to the specialty practised by epidemiologists and medical administrators, and by the staffs of corresponding academic departments.

The Todd Report contained in its 400 pages far more than what is indicated here. The first leading article in the *BMJ* of 13 April 1968 commented: "A particularly commendable feature of this vision of the future is that the present barriers between the main branches of the profession would be cut down to size and at least be no more formidable than garden fences across which neighbours may chat and even occasionally leap." Some of the royal commission's recommendations, however, were bound to cause controversy. In August 1968 the BMA's Medical Education Committee wrote to the Ministry of Health: "In its evidence to the Royal Commission, the Association firmly opposed any idea of a two-tier medical profession. At first sight this danger appears to be inherent in the proposals for vocational registers."

The GMC then entered the fray. In January 1969 they issued a statement about the way in which vocational registration could be carried out, and in the following July the Government announced that it intended to introduce legislation as soon as possible to enable the GMC to undertake the registration of specialists. In September the Government informed the BMA that the GMC had proposed "that the opportunity should be taken to include in the legislation . . . certain other provisions." There were six additional proposals,* on which the BMA Council later

*Set out in the *BMJ*, 21 March 1970, Supplement p. 92.

commented: "It was at once apparent that these proposals went very much further than had been envisaged from a study of the Todd Report, and in some unforeseen directions." The BMA immediately protested to the Secretary of State for Social Services and to the President of the GMC — Lord Cohen of Birkenhead. At a meeting with Lord Cohen, the BMA expressed the opinion that "before anything else, the meeting should discuss the functions and structure of the GMC. It should be so constructed that a majority of its members would be elected by the profession and be responsible to the profession." As a result of the BMA's objections, the Government decided to postpone the introduction of the Bill on specialist registration. The postponement has continued until the present day.

The Todd Report was difficult to digest, and did not include a summary of recommendations. The BMA therefore prepared its own summary of the Todd recommendations — 130 of them — and this was published in the *BMJ* of 21 March 1970, together with a commentary by the BMA Council which evoked congratulations and thanks from a special representative meeting. The BMA's main conclusions on the Todd Report were: (*1*) that any concept of a rigid or compulsory programme of general professional training after full registration should be rejected; (*2*) that any legislation to introduce vocational or specialist registration would be premature; (*3*) that the proposal to create a council for postgraduate medical education and training should be supported; and (*4*) that the money necessary for the planning and implementation of proper postgraduate medical education and training must be provided by the Government over and above the moneys allocated to the National Health Service.

At this point we must return to the GMC's proposal, first made four years before, to introduce an annual retention fee. The BMA Council and Representative Body originally acquiesced in the proposal, but this decision came under fire in both of those bodies in 1967, and in March 1968 the President of the GMC (who was a past President of the BMA) appeared before the BMA Council to explain the urgency of the financial crisis facing the GMC. After debate, the BMA Council again acquiesced (albeit reluctantly) in the principle of an annual retention fee, but expressed the wish that the lowest possible fee should be negotiated.

Parliament then voted the necessary legislation (in the Medical Act 1969) to enable an annual retention fee to be introduced. Meanwhile, opposition in the profession was mounting. In July 1969 the Representative Body stated that it appreciated the necessity for instituting an annual retention fee by the GMC, but felt that it should be paid only by those who were admitted to the Medical Register after the legislation became effective. Fuel was poured on the smouldering fire by the GMC's proposal (of September 1969) that multiple fees should be payable by applicants for specialist registration, in order to meet the substantial administrative costs that would be involved.

The BMA staff worked out that if the retention fee were paid only by new registrants, they would have to pay about £50 initially and then £20 per annum, so the BMA Council agreed with the GMC that the fee should more appropriately be £2 spread across the board. This action by the BMA Council was subsequently challenged, but the Council refused to reconsider its decision. Tension was now so high, however, that the members of Council were summoned by telegram to an emergency meeting on 17 January 1970, when it was decided to convene a special representative meeting on 12 February. The signs pointed to a fight between the Council and the Representative Body, which would show up in stark relief the defect in the constitution of the BMA which vested power in two controlling bodies (see Chapter 9).

At the SRM on 12 February 1970 emotion boiled over and there was a great deal of criticism of both the GMC and the BMA Council. There were four causes for the Representatives' anger:

(*1*) the natural irritation of the profession at the prospect of being saddled with a new annual subscription, and a compulsory one at that;

(*2*) the feeling that the prospective imposition of this new subscription justified a demand for an elected majority in the GMC (Lord Camden said in 1765: "Taxation and representation are inseparably united");

(*3*) an uneasy suspicion that the GMC, under the cloak of the Todd Report, was seeking to increase its control over the profession, particularly in regard to postgraduate education and vocational training; and

(*4*) a feeling (not universal) that the GMC was too autocratic and too distant from the rank and file of the profession, and deserved to be humbled.

The BMA Council was accused of not standing up to the GMC. Both a motion of censure on, and a motion of no confidence in, the BMA Council were moved, but neither was carried. On the main issue, the SRM passed a long and much amended resolution, the gist of which was: "That the Representative Body is not opposed to the introduction of an annual retention fee of £2 . . . provided that . . . the GMC shall contain a majority of members who have been directly elected by the profession . . . [and] the Representative Body shall agree with the GMC and the Government on the functions and composition of the GMC following an immediate review thereof. . . ."

The meeting also passed another and more ominous resolution: "That in the event of an annual retention fee being imposed against the medical profession's wishes the BMA should advise members of the medical profession to withhold payment." In the meantime, the meeting decided that doctors should be advised to make a single contribution of £2 for 1970-1, without prejudice to the future.

The regulations instituting the retention fee were made by the Privy Council in March 1970, and in the same month it was agreed between the Government, the GMC, the BMA, the Royal Colleges, and the universities to set up a special working party to review the composition of the GMC. (The functions of the GMC would be tackled afterwards.) So a working party consisting of a non-medical chairman nominated by the GMC (Sir Brynmor Jones, Vice-Chancellor of the University of Hull), and three representatives each from the BMA, the Royal Colleges, and the universities was established, and published a unanimous report on 6 March 1971. The essence of the report was that there were three elements represented in the composition of the GMC: (*1*) the medical educational institutions; (*2*) the practising profession (represented by the directly elected members); and (*3*) the general public (represented by the Crown nominees); and that no one of these three elements should be put in a position to dominate the other two. Hence the Brynmor Jones Working Party did not accept the contention that there should be an absolute majority of directly elected members on the

GMC, but recommended that the number of directly elected members should be increased and maintained at a strength that would always exceed by one the number of representatives of the academic institutions. The *BMJ* commented: "The working party's conclusions are supported with detailed arguments which show that its members examined the problems thoroughly. Especially important was the attention paid to the public interest . . . should the reforms be rejected then a totally new situation would arise in which an independent public inquiry might be the only course; and the outcome of this could be very different from the present proposals."

The Brynmor Jones Report was accepted by the ARM 1971, and the BMA advised doctors to make a second contribution to the GMC (for 1971-2) while a review was conducted of the GMC's functions. The GMC's financial procedures were also to be examined by an independent firm of accountants, because the annual retention fee was already being raised substantially (to £5). The GMC agreed to all this, so anxious was it to secure the backing of the BMA for its annual retention fee. Meanwhile, the Government made known its intention to introduce a Bill to reconstitute the GMC along the lines recommended by the Brynmor Jones Report.

The review of the GMC's functions was carried out by a joint working party of the BMA and GMC, under the chairmanship of Professor Sir Ronald Tunbridge (President-Elect of the BMA). It published an interim report in November 1972, of which the main conclusions were: "(*a*) that there is a continuing need for a statutory body such as the GMC (reconstituted in accordance with the Brynmor Jones proposals) to control basic medical education, registration, and discipline, (*b*) that although in certain areas substantial differences of opinion have emerged from these joint discussions, they should be capable of resolution by further detailed discussions."

But all the while a time bomb was ticking away. Led by some militant objectors, about 5000 doctors had so far withheld payment of any annual fee to the GMC, and in mid-1972 the GMC announced its intention to erase these doctors from the Medical Register. This unpalatable announcement was badly received at the ARM 1972, and the BMA Council appealed to the GMC to stay its hand while the joint talks continued in the Tunbridge Working Party. On 9 November 1972, however, the GMC decided that those doctors who had received a final warning notice and had still refused to pay the fee should be erased from the register. The decision caused great resentment within the profession, and was widely criticised in the press, both medical and lay. *The Times* referred to "the [General Medical] Council's capacity for misjudgment." Pressure for a public inquiry was mounting, and the GMC was the subject of an adjournment debate in the House of Commons.

The BMA Council, however, was still trying desperately to solve the crisis within the profession and avoid a public inquiry, being fearful that such an inquiry might recommend revolutionary changes, such as a lay majority on the GMC and regular requalification for doctors. The BMA therefore appealed to the Secretary of State for Social Services to find a formula to defer the erasures. He replied that he had no power to intervene. The very next day he announced that he had decided to set up a committee of inquiry "to consider what changes need to be made in the existing provisions for the regulation of the medical profession," and to examine both the functions and the constitution of the GMC. The chairman of the inquiry was to be Dr A W (later Sir Alec) Merrison FRS.

We are now nearing the end of this tiresome episode. The "fee strike" petered out. The BMA swallowed its reservations about a public inquiry and agreed to co-operate fully. The Association went to its customary trouble to prepare detailed and well-reasoned evidence, approved by the ARM at Folkestone in June 1973. Briefly, the ARM voted for a large GMC with an absolute majority of directly elected members. Great reservations were still expressed about specialist registration, though it was recognised that future EEC agreements might make such registration necessary; and the opinion was expressed that the medical profession should set up its own inquiry into the maintenance of standards of competence to practise and of patient care.

The Merrison Committee reported in April 1975. Its chief conclusions were:

> The medical profession should be largely self-regulated and should be regulated by an independent body.

A specialist register should be instituted. The specialist register should be indicative in character.

The GMC should issue further guidance on the nature of professional misconduct.

The GMC should have the power to order the immediate suspension of a doctor's right to practise in certain circumstances.

There should be ten more elected members on the Council than all other members.

The medical profession's financial support of the GMC should be provided mainly by way of an annual fee for the retention of doctors' names on the medical Register.

Doctors' registration should continue to be withdrawn for failing to pay the annual retention fee.

The Merrison Report received a warm welcome in the profession. The *BMJ* called it "A Good Report." After some delay the Government (in November 1977) introduced a Bill to change the constitution and functions of the GMC along the lines recommended by Merrison (but *not* to introduce specialist registration) and the Bill was much strengthened and improved by the efforts of Lord Hunt of Fawley in the House of Lords.

Relations between the GMC and the BMA returned to the harmonious and mutually respectful level which had prevailed before 1966. Much of the credit for this should go to Lord Richardson, who had become President of the GMC in 1973. His distinguished predecessor (Lord Cohen) had been subjected to much unfair criticism in some quarters of the medical profession, and Lord Richardson (who was also a past President of the BMA) took on the presidency of the GMC in difficult circumstances. His great statesmanship, tact, and diplomacy made him entirely equal to the task.

This unhappy wrangle about the finances, composition, and functions of the General Medical Council had lasted a decade. Perhaps the best epitaph on it is to be found in the first leader in the *BMJ* of 13 March 1971: "One of the least satisfactory aspects of the GMC crisis has been the amount of emotional and often ill-informed comment which has accompanied it."

OCCUPATIONAL HEALTH

In several countries, notably those of the Communist world, medical care is based on place of work rather than place of residence. In Britain, the latter system is traditional but health at work has long been recognised as important. Much of the health legislation of the nineteenth century was concerned with health at work, starting with the Factory Act of 1833. In 1925 James Mackenzie (not to be confused with the famous physician of the same name) founded the Industrial Health Education Society in Edinburgh. Its office soon moved to London, where it was welcomed by the BMA and accommodated in BMA House. When Mackenzie died in 1944 the BMA instituted a James Mackenzie Lectureship on the relation of health to industry, but this was discontinued in 1981 on economy grounds.

In 1936 the General Practice Committee of the BMA appointed a subcommittee to deal with industrial medical matters. In 1941 the Council appointed a special committee in industrial health (later called occupational health), in view of the "increasing importance of medicine in the industrial field." The committee included members nominated by the Association of Certifying Factory Surgeons and the Association of Industrial Medical Officers. In all the years since then, the Occupational Health Committee has played an important, if sometimes underestimated, part in promoting occupational health, and improving the status and remuneration of those doctors engaged in occupational medicine.

The BMA published a report entitled *First Aid in Industry* in 1939 and two years later published a report on industrial health in factories, a topic of obvious importance in war-time. An appendix contained a statement (first promulgated by the BMA in 1937) of the duties of, and ethical rules for, industrial medical officers. This was published because the demarcation line between the spheres of the family doctor and of the "works doctor" was a sensitive one. Just after the war the BMA published a report on rehabilitation, emphasising the need for closer liaison between the general practitioner, the hospital medical staff, and the industrial medical officer.

In 1947 the BMA joined forces with the Society of Medical Officers of Health and the Association of Industrial Medical Officers to submit evidence to a Government committee on the health, welfare, and safety of persons in places of employment. At the 1948 annual meeting, Sir

George Schuster (a distinguished banker who was a member of a Government committee on industrial productivity, and chairman of its panel on human relations) opened a discussion on the contribution that the medical profession could make to industrial productivity through human relations — a subject that is still of the highest national importance.

As has already been related (in Chapter 3) one of the BMA's criticisms of the nascent National Health Service was that it did not include industrial medical services. In 1949 the ARM approved a report on "A Comprehensive Occupational Health Service" and the BMA gave evidence to the Dale Committee on Industrial Health Services. Briefly, the BMA expressed its conviction of the value of occupational health services; considered that full provision to meet the special health needs of occupational groups was not made under the existing National Health Service and that additional arrangements, closely integrated with the NHS, should be made; and expressed its belief that the State should assume responsibility for developing a national occupational health service and providing "at least in part" the necessary financial resources.

The *BMJ* of 27 March 1954 contained three memoranda by the BMA on occupational health topics: one which had been submitted to the Ministry of Labour and National Service on the future of occupational health services; another to the Ministry of Transport on medical standards for road, rail, and air transport; and a third to a Government committee on the National Insurance (Industrial Injuries) Act.

The BMA recommended rates of remuneration and terms of service for industrial medical officers in a statement published in 1958, which was later entitled *The Doctor in Industry*. This was revised after the publication of the Pilkington Royal Commission Report, and in the light of each Review Body report thereafter. In 1963 a section on training was added with this explanation: "The Council believes that employers and doctors would welcome guidance on this important aspect, as there is no clearly defined portal of entry to this field of medicine."

The BMA regularly negotiated with the boards of the nationalised industries (such as the National Coal Board, the British Railways Board, and the National Dock Labour

Board) about the salaries and conditions of service of their medical officers.

In 1969 the BMA pursued further its longstanding campaign to secure the creation of a comprehensive national occupational health service. Representatives of the Association and of the Society of Occupational Medicine argued the case with the Secretary of State for Employment (Mrs Barbara Castle), who countered by putting forward the concept of the Employment Medical Advisory Service to replace the existing Appointed Factory Doctor Scheme. The BMA was unenthusiastic, because it felt that this concept might reduce the likelihood of the Government introducing a fully comprehensive national occupational health service. The proposal was discussed, however, in the joint committee of the BMA and the TUC, and both bodies decided to go along with the Employment Medical Advisory Service, without prejudice to the long-term objective.

In its comments on the second Green Paper on National Health Service reorganisation in England, the BMA Council said on 1 April 1970: "The Council regrets that occupational health was not mentioned at all in the first Green Paper, and has been relegated to an appendix in the second. About 1000 doctors are engaged full time in occupational health. The population spend about a third of their working lives at their places of work, and no national health service can be regarded as comprehensive which fails to cover the provision of medical care at work."

The work of the BMA's Occupational Health Committee has always fallen under three main headings: questions relating to the organisation of occupational health services; negotiations on behalf of doctors engaged (whether in groups or singly) in occupational medicine; and consideration of official documents, a steady stream of which has reached the BMA over the years. In the session 1977-8, for example, the BMA commented on: a draft circular from the Department of Health and Social Security on an occupational health service for NHS staff; a paper on the training of sick-bay attendants on oil rigs (a subject of special interest to the Scottish Council); proposals for an industrial medical advisory service in Northern Ireland; a pamphlet by the Health and Safety Executive on "the way ahead" in occupational health services; and a government paper on the diagnosis of occupational diseases.

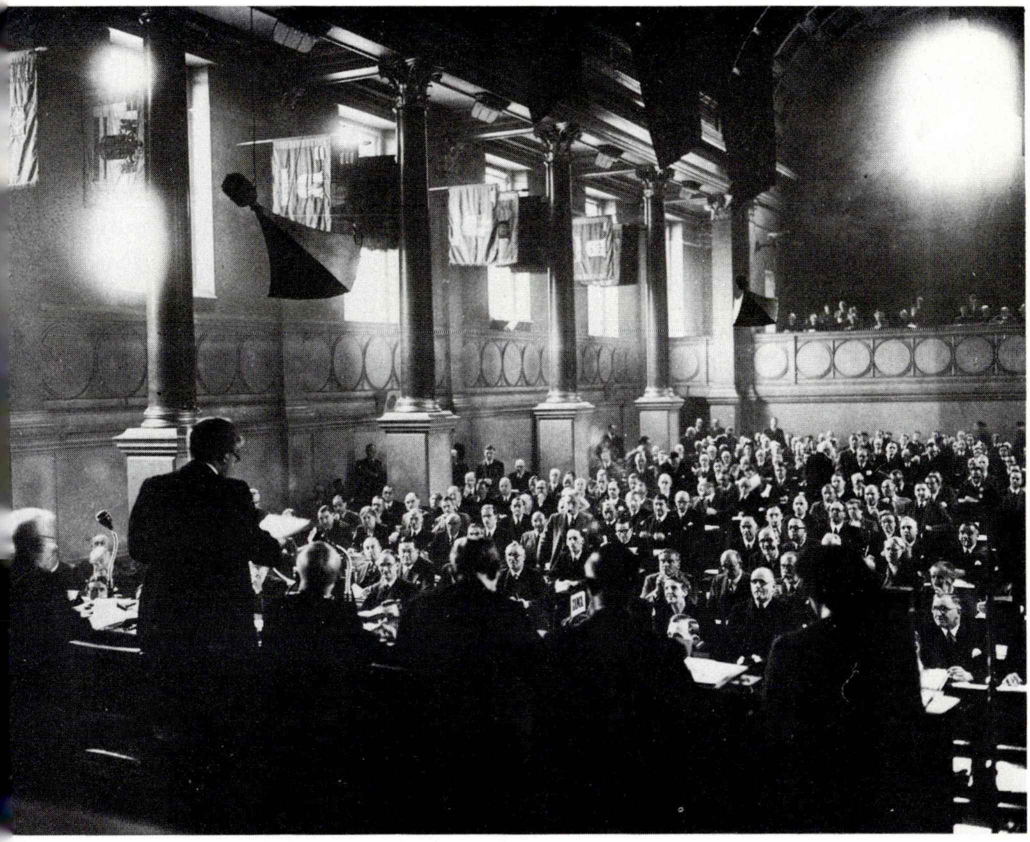

May 1948: The Representative Body decides to advise the medical profession to co-operate in the new National Health Service.

(*Topix*)

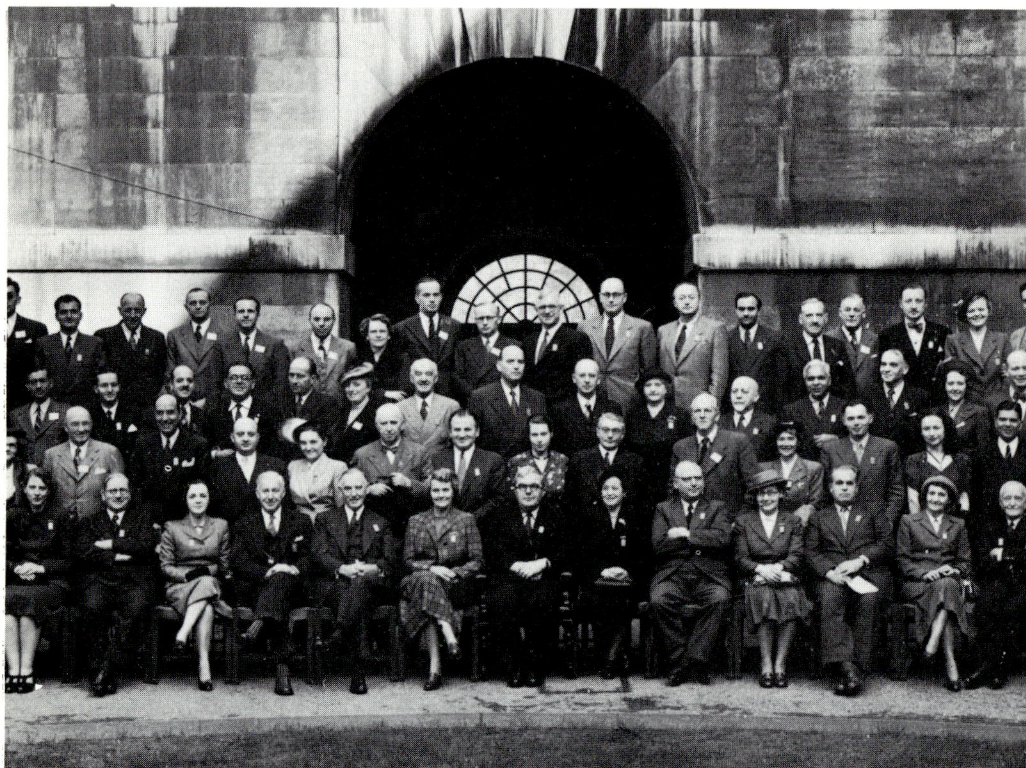

1949: Some of the delegates at the 3rd General Assembly of the World Medi
Association, at BMA House, London.

Front row, L to R: Miss M Natwick, Dr J A Pridham, Miss M Gregg, Dr Louis Bauer,
Clarence Routley, Mrs Knutson, Dr Charles Hill, Mrs Leuch, Dr Otto Leuch, M
Hill, Dr Dag Knutson, Mrs Pridham, Dr Guy Dain.

The BMA has always been firmly opposed to any threat of a State monopoly (or any other kind of monopoly) of medical care. The Association believes that a patient should be free to seek medical attention privately if he so desires and is willing to meet the cost, and that a doctor should be free to practise privately, for some or all of his time, if he so wishes.

The BMA's annual report in 1933 included the following paragraph: "The Council regards the provision, by insurance, for the medical and institutional needs of the middle-class patient as a problem of the highest importance. While contributory schemes have enabled the working classes to obtain adequate hospital provision, there is little provision of this kind for the middle classes. The Council has accordingly convened a conference of representatives of organisations interested in provident schemes in order to consider the lines upon which approval might be given to principles governing provident schemes to assist middle-class patients (that is, those above the usually recognised hospital income limits) in providing the cost of hospital and/or nursing home services and the associated necessary medical services."

In 1938 the King's Fund (King Edward's Hospital Fund for London) initiated the formation of a committee to devise a provident scheme for middle-income earners in the London area. The committee included the Secretary of the BMA (Dr G C Anderson). Two years later the BMA joined with the three Royal Colleges and the King's Fund to found the London Association for Hospital Services, which was incorporated as a non-profit-making company limited by guarantee, without share capital. The London Association launched the Hospital Service Plan on 1 January 1943. Twenty years later the name was changed to Private Patients Plan. In 1960 the BMA negotiated with the Hospital Service Plan a group scheme for BMA members on specially favourable terms, and 20 years afterwards the BMA did the same with the British United Provident Association, which had started in 1947.

In the 1960s the Private Practice Committee (which had been formed in 1949) was very active under the vigorous chairmanship of Dr Ivor M Jones, ably supported by Dr J D J Havard as committee secretary. In the session 1964-5, for example, the committee negotiated fees for a variety of services (such as attendance at law courts, medical reports for life assurance, lectures on advanced first-aid for civil defence authorities); pursued the BMA's campaign that drugs at public expense should be available to private patients; prepared an insurance scheme for patients to obtain family doctor care in the event of general practitioners withdrawing from the NHS; and carried out various tasks not exclusively concerned with private practice but entrusted for convenience to the Private Practice Committee. These included: giving evidence to a Departmental Committee on Death Certification and Coroners; making representations to the Home Office about revision of the cremation regulations; negotiating suitable remuneration for ships' surgeons; and holding discussions with the Ministry of Transport and local authorities about car parking concessions for doctors on professional duty. The problem of car parking had first reared its ugly head in 1947. It grew more acute as the years went by, and the BMA designed a special car-parking badge for doctors which was officially recognised in many places.

An important event took place in 1966. This was a time when collective resignation from the NHS was much talked about. The BMA Council promoted the establishment of a limited liability company, Independent Medical Services Ltd, to provide an alternative to the National Health Service for patients and to enable doctors to move into private practice. The chairman of the board of directors was Dr Ivor Jones, and the *BMJ* commented: "Dr Jones has worked hard and long to get IMS Ltd off the ground, and is to be congratulated on his pertinacity." But the response from the profession was half-hearted: far fewer doctors joined the scheme than had been hoped. In order to increase the attractions of the scheme, Independent Medical Services Ltd embarked on discount trading: the company made an arrangement with a discount trading organisation by which its members (who were also members of the BMA) might obtain a wide variety of branded goods at a substantial discount. This was a mistake: a scheme to provide an alternative to the National Health Service should not be linked with discount trading. But credit must be given to IMS Ltd for providing a scheme of private general practitioner cover, which the provident associations (PPP, BUPA, etc) found difficulty in doing. Even so after some years IMS Ltd stopped operating.

Private fees were caught up (like everything else) in Government pay policy. "Fees" were mostly classified as prices, not as pay. In 1977 the BMA negotiated with the Price Commission an increase of 32% in all medical fees except those paid from public sources, which were deemed by the Government to come within pay policy. The BMA regarded this distinction as illogical and worked towards parity between the public and private sector fees for part-time work. This was broadly achieved in 1979 and 1980.

The BMA regularly published a fees guide to help members with this very complicated subject, and in 1981 this was issued as a loose-leaf section for inclusion in the *Members Handbook.* Interestingly enough, the BMA Fees Guide was also much sought after by non-members.

ABORTION LAW REFORM

In 1934 the BMA Council published a report on the law relating to abortion, which concluded that although the Association would be willing to contribute evidence to any committee set up by the Government "to examine the various relations of the practice of abortion . . . the initiation of the proposed inquiry does not properly fall within the responsibilities of the medical profession." But this was to be the start of a long road. In 1936 the BMA published a report on the *Medical Aspects of Abortion,* which recommended "not only the clarification of the legal position, but also the institution of some system of authorisation of abortion in the individual case." In 1938 a distinguished obstetrician and gynaecologist, Mr Aleck Bourne, was acquitted of unlawful termination of pregnancy in a case which aroused much public interest, the judge saying: "If the doctor is of opinion . . . that the probable consequence of the continuance of the pregnancy will be to make the mother a physical or mental wreck, the jury are quite entitled to take the view that the doctor . . . is operating for the purpose of preserving the life of the mother." In 1939 an Interdepartmental Committee on Abortion issued a report (the Birkett Report) which recommended that the law should be amended "to make unmistakably clear that a medical practitioner is acting legally when in good faith he procures the abortion of a pregnant woman in circumstances which satisfy him that continuance of the pregnancy is likely to endanger her life or seriously impair her health." The war inhibited the Government from introducing any legislation to implement this recommendation.

The subject lay dormant until 1952, when Mr Joseph Reeves introduced the first of a long line of Private Members' Bills. In 1961 Mr Kenneth Robinson introduced a Private Member's Bill to bring statute law into line with case law, as enunciated in Rex versus Bourne 1938, but the Bill made no progress beyond a debate on Second Reading. In 1966 the BMA commented on Lord Silkin's Bill and also published the report of a BMA special committee, chaired by Dr E A Gerrard FRCOG (a past President of the Association) on therapeutic abortion. This called for some amendments to the law but also said: "Whether or not a pregnancy should be terminated is a question which can be decided only in the circumstances of each particular case. The ultimate decision to advise termination of pregnancy rests with the doctors in charge of the case and . . . the law should not seek to influence this decision. . . ."

At this precise time, however, Mr David Steel was sponsoring a fresh Private Member's Bill in the Commons, with support from all the political parties. In conjunction with the Royal College of Obstetricians and Gynaecologists, the BMA commented closely on Mr Steel's Bill at all its stages, both to Mr Steel himself and to Government Ministers. Mr Steel's Bill was passed by Parliament as the Abortion Act 1967. The BMA expressed two criticisms of it. Firstly, it permits termination in certain cases where there is neither risk to the health of the mother nor risk of serious abnormality of the fetus. Secondly, the Act does not require either of the two doctors concerned with the authorisation of an abortion to be of consultant status.

By 1971 public opinion was concerned about the huge increase in the number of terminations of pregnancy and at the number of foreign women coming to Britain for abortions, and the Government was considering setting up a review of the Abortion Act. The BMA published a memorandum on the working of the Act. One of the criticisms made by the BMA was of the "tremendous pressure on available resources (outpatient, theatre time, laboratories) affecting the waiting time of outpatients and putting strain on personnel even where services are reasonably adequate." This was not the first, or the last, time that Members of Parliament passed an Act to provide an extra service without a moment's thought about providing additional consultants, nurses, and operating theatres. The Government set up a committee to review the operation of the Abortion Act 1967, and the BMA gave evidence.

The chairman of the reviewing committee was the Hon Mrs Justice Lane (Dame Elizabeth Lane), and the members included Miss (later Dame) Josephine Barnes FRCP, FRCS, FRCOG, who was to be the first woman President of the BMA. The Lane Report appeared in April 1974 in three volumes. The essence of its conclusions was:

> The Act has relieved a vast amount of individual suffering. It has helped also to focus attention on the paramount need for preventive action. . . . It has served to stimulate research into all aspects of abortion and the development of safer operative techniques. These have been undeniably great benefits.
>
> On the other hand, the passing of the Act, resulting in a greatly increased number of those seeking legal abortions, has imposed considerable strain on the NHS.
>
> For the reasons we have outlined above, and which are much more fully dealt with in the body of the Report, we are unanimous in supporting the Act and its provisions. We have no doubt that the gains facilitated by the Act have much outweighed any disadvantages for which it has been criticised. The problems which we have identified in its working, and they are admittedly considerable, are problems for which solutions should be sought by administrative and professional action, and by better education of the public.

The Lane committee made some specific recommendations, including recommendations that doctors should continue to make the decisions as to abortion, that there should be an upper time-limit for abortion of 24 weeks' gestation, and that all medical referral agencies which charged fees should be licensed and controlled.

The BMA gave its support to the Lane Report, but in 1974 another private Member, Mr James White, introduced a bill to amend the Abortion Act 1967. It was referred to a select committee, to which the BMA gave evidence — opposing the legal changes proposed in the Bill and expressing the opinion that the current abuses arising out of the 1967 Act could be controlled by a simple change in the regulations. The Bill lapsed at the end of the session, but the select committee was reappointed and continued its investigation.

In 1977 another Private Member's Bill was introduced (by Mr William Benyon) seeking to amend the 1967 Act. The BMA again expressed the opinion that any further changes in the control of abortion "could best be effected by the more flexible system of administrative control, rather than by further legislation." Even so, in 1978 another private Member (Sir Bernard Braine) introduced a Bill, and in 1979 yet another private Member (Mr John Corrie) did likewise. Neither of these Bills succeeded. Meanwhile, the ARM 1978 deplored the persistent attacks on the Abortion Act 1967 and declared its belief that it was a "practical and humane piece of legislation."

THE MOUTHPIECE OF THE MEDICAL PROFESSION

One of the BMA's most onerous functions is to give evidence on behalf of the medical profession to Parliament and to every kind of commission of inquiry. The BMA's usual method has been to assemble a distinguished committee to prepare the evidence, consisting not only of experts in the subject concerned but also of representatives of the main branches of the practising profession. The evidence drafted by this committee has been submitted for approval to the Council of the Association, and sometimes also to the the Representative Body, although everyone recognises that a body of 500 Representatives is hardly suitable for settling a memorandum. The written evidence has usually been supported by oral evidence, given by a carefully chosen team of eminent witnesses. Several important occasions when this function has been discharged have been described elsewhere in this book. Some of the other occasions in the past 50 years are mentioned here.

In 1935 the BMA gave detailed evidence on the theory, technique, and practice of osteopathy to a select committee of the House of Lords, which was considering a Bill for the registration of osteopaths. The Select Committee recommended "that the Bill be not further proceeded with." Many years later, in 1964, the BMA gave a fair hearing at the Annual Representative Meeting to a petition for the formation of a special group of medical osteopaths, but rejected it.

In 1952 the BMA gave evidence to the Royal Commission on Marriage and Divorce. The evidence was published in the *BMJ* of 19 April 1952. Two of the proposals in the BMA's evidence were: "Separation by agreement, where there is no prospect of reconciliation, should be a ground of divorce, and it should be possible for the petition to be presented by either party, or, if they are agreed, by both partners jointly"; and "Where there are grounds for divorce but the offended party refuses to take action, the offending party should after a period be able to sue for divorce." Criticism began almost at once, alleging that the BMA was advocating easier divorce. It so happened that the annual meeting in 1952 was to be held in Dublin, the capital of a strongly Catholic country. It became apparent that the BMA's evidence was repugnant to many doctors in Ireland (and perhaps elsewhere). A special meeting of the Council was convened in Dublin on the eve of the annual meeting, and the Council decided to withdraw the BMA's evidence from the Royal Commission on Marriage and Divorce. This was a humiliating episode for the BMA.

In 1954 the BMA gave evidence to the Royal Commission on the Civil Service. At that time doctors in the Civil Service were represented by a joint committee of the Institution of Professional Civil Servants, the Ministry of Health Medical Staff Association, and the BMA. This arrangement did not give the BMA full scope to negotiate on behalf of Civil Service doctors, but the Institution of Professional Civil Servants expressed its cordial thanks for the "powerful assistance" of the Association. A joint committee with the Institution of Professional Civil Servants has continued over the years, but not very effectively. Relations between the BMA and the medical staff of the Civil Service have always been good. It is recognised that the doctors in the Civil Service are loyal servants of the Government, but they are also loyal members of the medical profession and are, indeed, the spokesmen of the profession within the Government machine.

In 1955 the BMA submitted evidence, including 70 recommendations, to the Royal Commission on the Law relating to Mental Illness and Mental Deficiency.

The Association commented to the Government on the Report of the Royal Commission on Local Government in Greater London in 1961, and, in due course, when extensive reorganisation of London local government took place, the BMA was active in safeguarding the interests of the medical staff and medical services concerned. On 8 May 1965 the *BMJ* published a leading article headed "End of an Epoch" which paid a warm tribute to the achievements of the medical departments of the London and Middlesex County Councils, which had been abolished in the reorganisation.

In 1965 the BMA gave evidence to the Royal Commission on the Penal System, and the next year to the Committee on the Age of Majority (the Latey Committee), and to the Committee of Enquiry into the Relationship of the Pharmaceutical Industry with the National Health Service (the Sainsbury Committee).

The BMA played an important part in drawing attention to the link between alcohol and road accidents, and the first "breathalyser" was demonstrated at a press conference at BMA House. In 1966 and 1967 the Association commented in detail on the Road Safety Bill as it made its way through Parliament, and in 1975 gave evidence to the Blennerhassett Committee, which was reviewing the law on drinking and driving.

In 1967 the BMA submitted a memorandum of evidence to the Royal Commission on Local Government in England, in which perhaps the most important sentence was: "It is recommended that the health and social welfare functions should be administered in one department, under the direction of the medical officer of health." The Association also gave evidence to the Committee on Local Authority and Allied Personal Social Services (the Seebohm Committee). The Seebohm Report was badly received by the BMA, which complained that it tended towards "an undesirable separation of social work from health services."

In 1968 the BMA gave evidence to the Monopolies Commission, which was investigating some of the practices of the professions. This was one of the few occasions when the organisations representing the leading professions got together to meet a common threat. (See Chapter 9.)

When the Welsh Council of the Association gave evidence to the Royal Commission on the Constitution in

1971, they called for the continuation of a single standard of medical registration throughout the United Kingdom, and a common standard of provision, or at least intended provision, of medical services. These same aims caused the BMA to object in 1977 to plans for devolution in Scotland and in Wales.

The Annual Report of Council in 1975 recorded that the BMA had given evidence to no fewer than three Royal Commissions — on the Press, on Civil Liability and Compensation for Personal Injury, and on the Distribution of Income and Wealth. A good example to end this section is the session 1976-7, when the BMA considered and commented on: the Court Report on child health services; a consultative document from the DHSS on priorities for health and personal social services; the McCarthy Report on the Whitley machinery of the NHS; the Bullock Report on industrial democracy; the report of a joint working party of the Royal Colleges and the BMA on the ethics of "industrial action" by doctors; and a report by the Standing Medical Advisory Committee of the Central Health Services Council on the standardisation of cancer records. Truly, the BMA's role as the principal spokesman of the medical profession is a lively one.

AND OTHER THINGS TOO

The motor car has become an essential instrument of medical practice, and just after the end of the war the BMA established a special department to help doctors to obtain preferential delivery of new cars. A scheme was operated in conjunction with the Society of Motor Manufacturers and Traders. And at times of petrol shortage (caused, for example, by strikes in the petrol supply industry) the BMA has endeavoured to obtain priority supplies for doctors.

In 1955 the BMA fought a battle which (with the wisdom of hindsight) we may now feel was unwise. The Government announced its intention to prohibit the manufacture and use of heroin. The BMA saw this as an unwarrantable intrusion by Government in the right of doctors to prescribe whatever they considered was necessary for each particular patient, and mounted a campaign of resistance. An anonymous telephone call to BMA House from a disgruntled official in the Home Office alerted the BMA to a technical flaw in the legality of the Government's proposed action. The BMA prompted Lord Jowitt to challenge the legality of the Government's proposal in the House of Lords, and the Government retreated in confusion. The proposal was eventually abandoned.

The Association has always fought strenuously (and successfully) against the closed shop — that is, against any attempt by an employing authority to compel all its medical employees to join a trade union, not excepting the BMA itself. Notable struggles were against Willesden Borough Council in 1947, against Durham County Council in 1952 (see Chapter 9), and against the city of Stoke-on-Trent in 1968. The BMA has shown that it has no intention of allowing doctors to be dictated to by the trade union movement or anybody else. The BMA's attitude to the closed shop was well stated in 1966 in a communication to the Royal Commission on Trade Unions and Employers' Associations: "We regard the imposition of a condition of compulsory membership of a trade union as highly objectionable. The policy of compulsory membership of a trade union or professional organisation is deeply repugnant to most professional workers. The professions are profoundly attached to the principle of free association and this principle implies more than freedom to associate. It implies also freedom not to associate if the individual so chooses in the unfettered exercise of his judgment or conscience."

In 1960 the BMA published a report supporting the artificial fluoridation of public water supplies, as a measure for preventing dental caries. On behalf of preventive medicine, in 1971 the BMA published a policy on smoking and made 15 specific proposals to discourage smoking. The memorandum stated that "Members of the medical and health service professions must set an example." The BMA itself has certainly done this — for example, the standing orders of the Representative Body do not permit smoking, but a motion to suspend this standing order was regularly proposed and carried in the first hour or so at Representative Meetings in the 1940s and 1950s. Nowadays the no-smoking rule remains unchallenged throughout the meeting.

Also in 1971 the BMA published a report on *Gaps in Medical Care.* It was a sensitive and thoughtful attempt to show where medical care failed or fell short. Examples were: "The mangled motorist dying by the roadside. The friendless old lady dying alone in a cold room. The agonising toothache touring London on a Sunday. The young chronic sick condemned to a life with the old, demented, and incontinent." The report said: "The answer to these problems is not merely more money or the harassment of government departments. The national conscience — including that of many doctors — must be stirred. It is not good enough to know the facts and to assume that 'It could not happen to me,' and to pass by on the other side with averted eyes. These gaps are serious, and the profession has a duty to point them out and to see that action is taken."

Lastly, the BMA has quite frequently joined with other organisations in investigating problems. In 1961 the BMA set up a joint committee with the General Council of the Bar (as it was then called) and the Law Society to consider "the whole question of the presentation of medical evidence to courts of law and tribunals," and in due course the joint committee produced an authoritative report. It was republished in 1981. The BMA also produced several joint reports with the Magistrates' Association. In 1973 the BMA took the initiative in establishing a joint committee with the Royal Colleges, the Committee of Vice-Chancellors and Principals, and the Councils of Postgraduate Medical Education to review the existing methods of "ensuring the maintenance of the standards of continuing competence to practise and of clinical care of patients." The joint committee was chaired by Mr E A J (later Sir Anthony) Alment and produced a good report on this important but difficult subject. Since then the BMA has devoted increasing attention, albeit warily and somewhat reluctantly, to what is known as medical audit.

The tidings in this chapter are that, although the BMA's energies since 1948 have been largely and unavoidably absorbed by the problems of the National Health Service, the Association has by no means neglected its duties in those areas which were not nationalised at that time.

Chapter 7

Science and ethics

Science

Medicine is a science of uncertainty and an art of probability.
— Sir William Osler, *Aphorisms*, Chapter 5.

The Provincial Medical and Surgical Association was founded in 1832 to promote the medical and allied sciences; the original prospectus for the association described in clear and lyrical terms how this aim was to be achieved. "It is proposed to associate the Provincial Medical Practitioners of England, or at least as many as can be brought to rally round a common centre, in a comprehensive co-operating institution, which, by collecting the results of individual experience, and bringing the energies of many minds to bear on those unsettled points which have subjected medicine to the imputation of being a conjectural art, may contribute to redeem its character and to give to its operations more precision and greater certainty."

This process of scientific investigation by pooling experience was used to such good effect in the early days that by the time of the centenary year in 1932 the BMA had established for itself a reputation as an authoritative voice on medical science.

ADMINISTRATION

In 1932 the standing committee to which Council delegated preliminary consideration of major scientific matters was known as the Science Committee. Its terms of reference were to advise on those matters, not specifically referred to other committees, which related to the promotion of the medical and allied sciences, on the provision of lectures to branches and divisions, and on the library and its management. Its members were elected by the Representative Body, the Council, and the Journal Committee.

In the 1930s and 1940s the Science Committee was restricted in the amount of clinical and scientific skills available to it because it was not empowered to co-opt additional members; there was also a danger of it becoming concerned in conflicting policy decisions because it was considering and reporting on matters which had also been referred to other committees. These inherent weaknesses were corrected in 1955, when the Science Committee was given the right to co-opt up to three additional members and to appoint at least one of its own members to any ad hoc committee within the BMA which might be considering subjects with a scientific aspect.

These changes were part of a strong impetus given to scientific activities in the 1950s during the secretaryship of Dr Angus Macrae. In 1959 Council accepted a recommendation that such activities should be expanded, adding a rider to the effect that topics that the BMA investigated should not only be desirable from the purely scientific point of view, but should also have direct implications for the community at large. To reflect this wider role of the Science Committee, its name was changed in 1961 to the Committee on Medical Science, Education, and Research.

Despite these constitutional developments and the considerable amount of scientific work undertaken, a strong feeling persisted that the image of the BMA was still falling short of its founders' objective of promoting the medical and allied sciences, and that an undue amount of attention was being paid to the parallel aim of guarding the interests of the profession.

To restore the balance a memorandum was drawn up by Dr Ronald Gibson, Chairman of Council, and presented to Council in January 1968. This proposed that all the Association's scientific and medicosocial work should be concentrated under one body to be named the Board of Science and Education, the chairman of which should be a distinguished member of the medical profession. The board would be limited in size and would operate through the medium of specially appointed panels. Constitutionally, it would be under the supervision of the Representative Body and Council, but would have a measure of independence. By these means it was intended that at long last all the BMA's scientific activities should be co-ordinated under one authority, and that they should achieve the prominence in the public eye that they deserved.

The proposals in the memorandum were immediately accepted by Council and were adopted by the Representative Meeting at Eastbourne in June 1968. The former Committee on Medical Science, Education, and Research and the Annual Meetings Committee were merged into the new Board of Science and Education. The first chairman of the Board was Sir Ronald Tunbridge. Initially its membership was limited to eight, all appointed by Council, but in 1974 this number was increased to 11, three of whom were to be appointed by the Representative Body, six by Council, and two were to be junior staff elected by a process determined by Council.

The creation of the Board of Science succeeded in raising the scientific prestige of the Association. Nevertheless, the unification of all the Association's scientific activities under one semi-autonomous body, though ideal in theory, was not easy to put into practice. The fundamental weakness lay in the fact that the BMA as a whole controlled the purse-strings. This meant that if priority had to be given to other Association activities for financial or other reasons the Board of Science's resources, and thus its independence, could be endangered.

This defect was recognised by the board in the 1968 Annual Report of Council, when it emphatically stated that financing an expansive programme of scientific activities would be beyond the means of the BMA; it was, therefore, exploring the possibility of funding new projects from outside sources and it again referred to this intention in 1970. Four years later the board recommended the establishment of a charitable trust which would supply additional funds for scientific activities to augment the Association's annual allocation. In the event, and even though the recommendation had the support of the Representative Body, no such trust materialised and thus the ability of the board to carry out its remit in relation to the promotion of the medical and allied sciences had to be restricted.

In 1971 its vulnerability was clearly exposed when the Representative Body, faced with increasing medicopolitical activities and a requirement to fund these from the Association's overstrained resources, debated a motion from St Marylebone which called for an immediate investigation into the activities and accountability of the Board of Science. That motion was lost, but two from Bournemouth at the annual representative meeting of 1974 went much further; they urged that in the interests of economy both the Board of Science and the Nuffield Library should be discontinued. In support of the motions, it was argued that the BMA was a political, not a scientific, organisation, and that the Board of Science was a luxury which the Association could not afford. In reply the Chairman of Council, Mr Walpole Lewin, drew attention to the fact that the Memorandum of Association of the BMA included the provision that it should promote the medical and allied sciences, and pointed out that the Board of Science absorbed only 10% of the Association's revenue. The motions were withdrawn, but only on the understanding that an examination of scientific activities would form part of a detailed review of all the BMA's functions, finance, and staffing which had already been authorised by Council, and which was to be carried out by the General Purposes Committee.

The ensuing report of the General Purposes Committee reaffirmed that science was a primary function of the BMA, but also recommended that scientific activities should be subject to further review in the light of contemporary circumstances, and that first priority should be given to scientific work for which the Association was uniquely fitted — the preparation of reports on special subjects.

The board's status within the BMA's constitution was finally recognised and consolidated in 1978, when a working party report on the functions and priorities of the Association emphasised that scientific and ethical activities distinguished a professional from an industrial union and that such activities should not be curtailed by the BMA in order to provide additional funds for its medicopolitical work. The report recommended categorically "the continuation of the present scientific, educational, ethical and social activities of the BMA, both centrally and locally."

The scope and variety of the BMA's scientific activities

over the past 50 years are so wide-ranging as to belie any notion that the Association has become solely a medicopolitical organisation. The story can best be told by considering the various methods by which the BMA implements its scientific role.

MEETINGS

The first, and indeed only, instrument for the advancement of medical science available to the Provincial Medical and Surgical Association back in 1832 was the annual meeting, and the BMA continued to hold these important scientific events at both national and local levels.

In 1932 the annual scientific meeting was linked with the annual representative meeting, but took place on entirely separate days from the discussion of business and political matters. At the centenary meeting in that year, the scientific meeting was divided into 24 sections devoted to different medical specialties. The proceedings of each section were later summarised in the *British Medical Journal* and selected papers were published in full.

This remained the general pattern for the organisation of annual scientific meetings during the 1930s. At the Oxford annual meeting in 1936, however, there was considerable criticism of the system for publishing the proceedings. The view was expressed that papers from the scientific sections absorbed an undue amount of space in the *British Medical Journal* and that delay in publication was such that the papers might well be out of date by the time they appeared in print. The papers from the 1935 scientific sections occupied 244 pages of the journal and had been published over a period of some 25 weeks. The Editor's freedom of action in this matter was limited by a minute of Council which required him to publish the opening papers of every section. As a result of the debate at the 1936 Meeting, this restriction was lifted and the Editor and Journal Committee were given full discretion over the publication of the proceedings of the scientific sections. A further motion that the complete proceedings should be issued as a special number of the journal was rejected on the grounds of expense.

No annual scientific meetings were held between 1940 and 1947. The first to be staged after the war was at

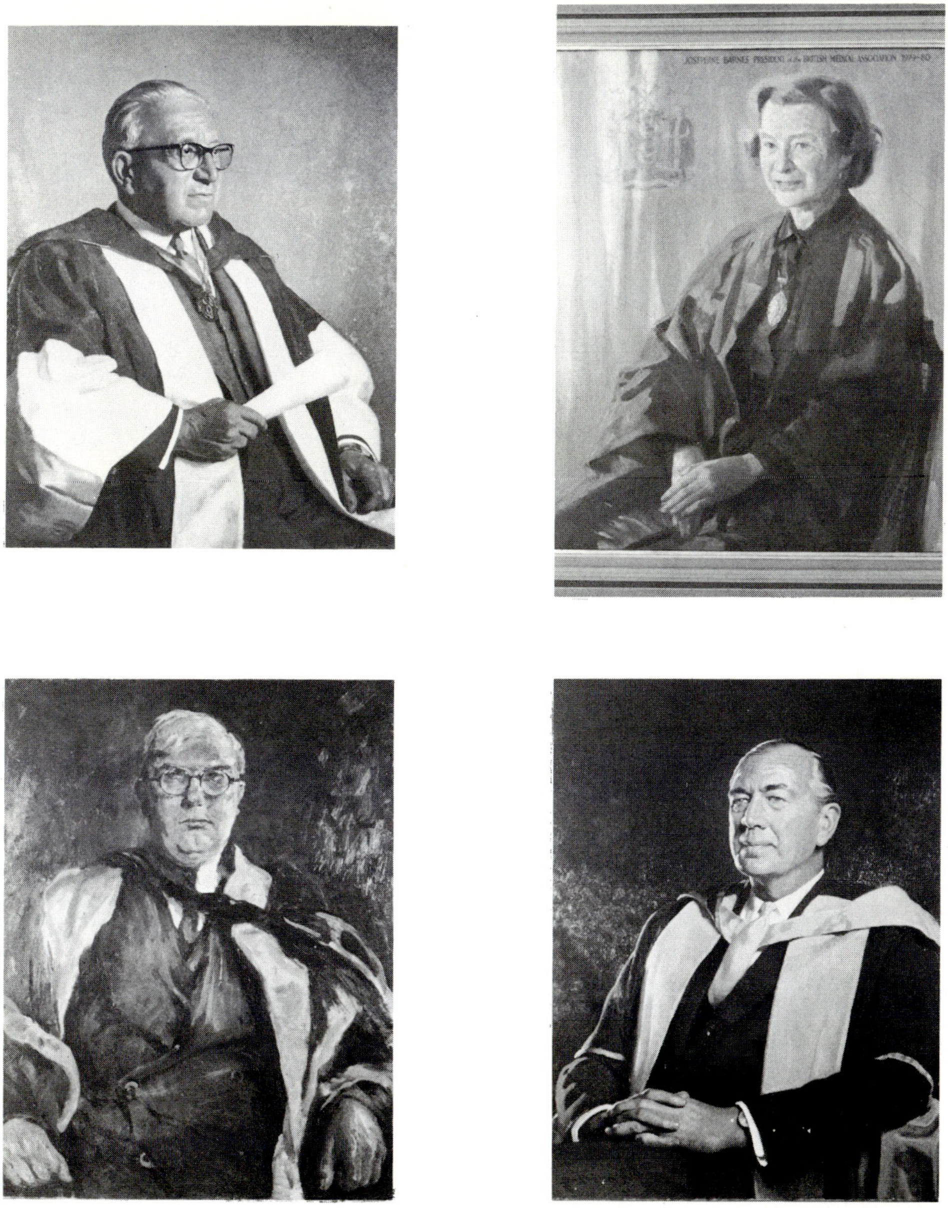

Four Portraits: Dr Solomon Wand (by Edward Halliday), Dame Josephine Barnes (by David Buchanan), Dr Charles Hill (by T C Dugdale), Dr Derek Stevenson (by Edward Halliday).

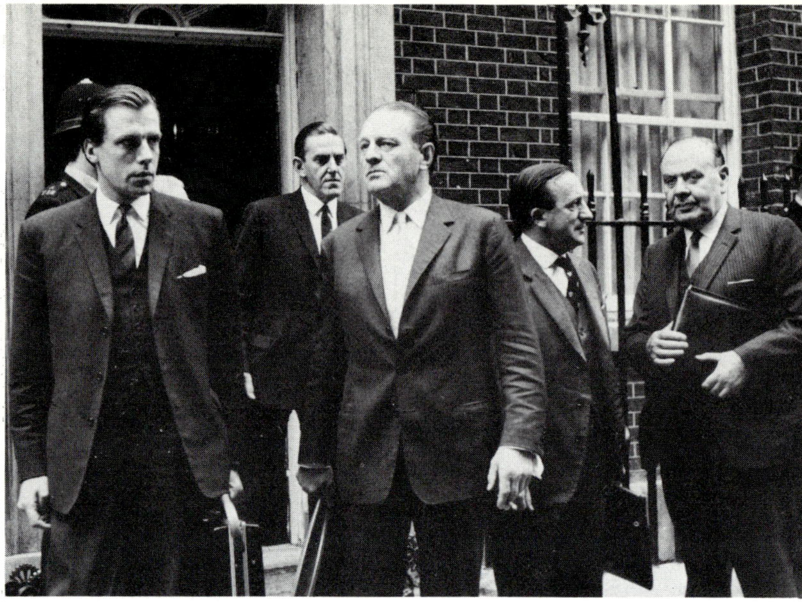

THE GREAT REVIEW BODY ROW OF 1970. BMA DELEGATION OUTSIDE NO 10 DOWNING STREET (28 MAY 1970).

L TO R: MR JULIAN ELKINGTON (CHAIRMAN, HOSPITAL JUNIOR STAFFS GROUP COUNCIL), DR RONALD GIBSON (CHAIRMAN OF COUNCIL), MR WALPOLE LEWIN (CHAIRMAN, CENTRAL COMMITTEE FOR HOSPITAL MEDICAL SERVICES), DR JAMES CAMERON (CHAIRMAN, GENERAL MEDICAL SERVICES COMMITTEE).

(*Fox Photos Ltd*)

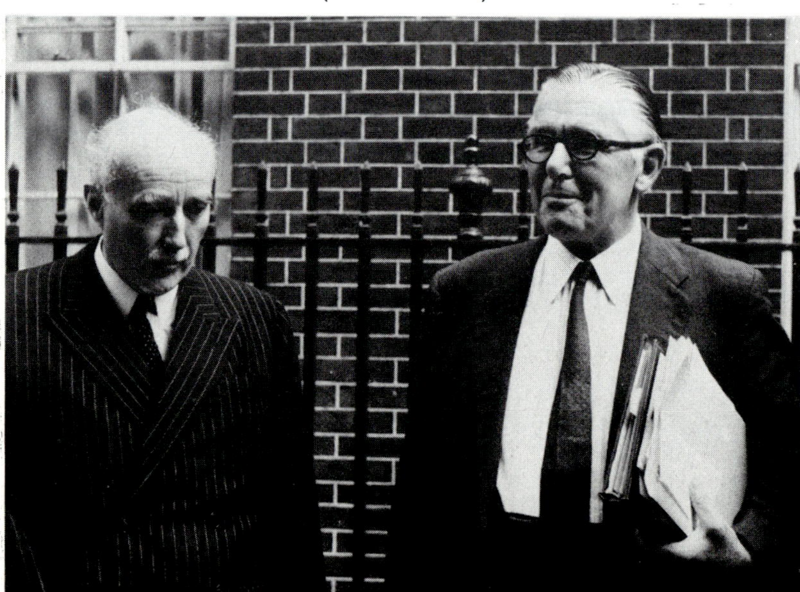

OUTSIDE NO 10: THE DEPUTY SECRETARY (DR E GREY-TURNER) AND THE SECRETARY OF STATE FOR SOCIAL SERVICES (MR R H S CROSSMAN).

(*Fox Photos Ltd*)

Cambridge in 1948 when it was decided to adopt the prewar suggestion of publishing the complete proceedings in a special volume. This appeared in print early in 1949, and in 1950 the proceedings of the 1949 Harrogate scientific meeting were also published separately. The experiment was short-lived however, and no further volumes of this nature have been published.

The shape of annual scientific meetings since 1950 has shown considerable adaptability and imagination on the part of their organisers, who have been quick to use modern ideas and technology. Dublin in 1952 saw the introduction of plenary sessions to supplement the meetings of the scientific sections. At Toronto, in 1955, round-table conferences on specific subjects were introduced. A revolutionary feature at Newcastle in 1957 was a programme of surgical operations and clinical demonstrations in the Royal Victoria Infirmary which were shown to a large audience by colour television on closed circuit. In 1960, at Torquay, came the first formal debate at a scientific meeting when a motion that "Dissemination of medical knowledge by means of television, radio, and the press does more harm than good to the health of the population" was lost by 44 votes to 43.

The scientific meeting at Manchester in 1964 was the first to have an integrated programme based on a broad theme — that of "Medicine in the 'sixties: the needs arising from a changing pattern of disease." A variation in this arrangement came at Hull in 1974 when a series of themes were chosen, all of which were covered in detail; on some occasions different aspects of the same subject were discussed simultaneously in adjacent lecture theatres.

For many years a feature of the annual scientific meeting was a museum of pathology and a trade exhibition of surgical appliances, foods, drugs, and books. At Dublin in 1952 the scope of the museum was widened by the institution of a scientific exhibition in which the subjects illustrated included the chemotherapy of tuberculosis, plastic surgery, malaria, the surgery of mitral stenosis, new contrast materials for radiography, tissue transplantation, and isotope treatment. A small historical section included documents and pamphlets from the muniment room of the Royal Army Medical College at Millbank. Certificates of merit have been awarded to the best exhibits since 1957, and every year the outstanding exhibit receives a silver cup, which was donated in 1959 by Mr Lawrence Abel who was largely responsible for the introduction of the scientific exhibition.

The scientific exhibition was an instant success and this led to a feeling that it should be made available to a wider public. In December 1960 the Science Committee proposed that as an experiment part of the scientific exhibition should be kept in being as a travelling exhibition. Council adopted this recommendation and during the months of September and November 1961 a choice of the exhibits from the scientific exhibition at Sheffield were displayed at the medical schools of Manchester, Liverpool, Leeds, and Newcastle upon Tyne. Unfortunately, although the travelling exhibition was an imaginative innovation, the expense was too great for it to be staged again after 1961.

In November 1957 a major development in BMA scientific meetings was introduced with a recommendation by the second Constitution Committee that an annual clinical meeting be held. The proposal was for a scientific function of high standard, organised on an informal basis, which would appeal to the postgraduate student. The meeting would occupy a long weekend during the winter months, and would normally be held only in those towns which could not accommodate annual meetings of the Association.

The recommendation was approved by Council and the first clinical meeting was held at Southampton in December 1958. Its organisation owed much to the fertile brain of the Deputy Secretary, Dr Walter Hedgcock. Panel discussions, general sessions, colour television, medical films, and clinical demonstrations all featured in a busy programme. Two highlights were a demonstration of a live operation for atrial septal defect, which was televised in colour from Southampton General Hospital, and a transatlantic clinical conference between a British group in Southampton and a team of United States doctors at the American Medical Association's clinical meeting in Minneapolis.

The Southampton clinical meeting was a great success. It set a pattern for the series of such meetings, which have been held regularly since 1958 and which have become more and more ambitious in their arrangements over the years.

In 1971 a further attempt was made to extend the benefits of scientific meetings to BMA members in more remote parts of the country when Council decided to establish a series of annual postgraduate meetings. The first of these was held at Inverness in September 1972, with a programme that emphasised matters of daily clinical importance to practising doctors. Further postgraduate meetings took place in Guernsey in 1973 and the Isle of Man in 1974.

In response to a growing feeling that the complexity of the different BMA scientific meetings should be rationalised, in 1977 the Board of Science recommended a policy which was adopted by the annual representative meeting at Glasgow in July. In future, one major scientific meeting would be held each year within the United Kingdom, one clinical meeting would be held additionally in the United Kingdom or overseas, and a series of symposia would be organised in London throughout the year. If desired, weekend symposia could be staged elsewhere in the United Kingdom. A fundamental change was effected by removing from Council its obligation under the Articles of the Association to hold a scientific meeting at the time of, and in the same place as, the annual general meeting. Since 1977 it has been the practice to organise one short scientific session at each annual meeting, while the main scientific meeting is held elsewhere at a different time. The first of these new-style annual scientific meetings took place at Ipswich in October 1978.

The "series of symposia," which constituted one element in this new policy, had their origins in conferences on special subjects which had been sponsored by the BMA from time to time throughout the previous 50 years. An outstanding example had occurred in April 1939, when the BMA summoned a national conference on nutrition in its widest aspects, including agricultural policy. Over a period of three days some 400 delegates from the medical profession, the farming community, government departments, and those interested in the subject from the point of view of production, distribution, social welfare, and education met in the Great Hall of BMA House. Their discussions ranged over the whole subject, from the basic food needs of the individual for the maintenance of health to the problems of increasing production of foodstuffs at home and in Europe. On the evening of the second day the discussion was extended to a wider audience in the form of a public meeting at which the Charles Hastings lecture on "Nutrition and the Public Health" was delivered by Professor V H Mottram. Three months later the proceedings of the conference were published under the same title as the lecture. The Sir Charles Hastings lecture had been instituted by the BMA in 1927 as an experiment in health education. During the 1930s it was delivered annually to a lay audience on topics of general public health interest by recognised experts in the field.

Throughout the severe economic depression of the 1930s, when the level of public nutrition was a burning question, it is to the credit of the BMA that it always treated the subject with the degree of importance that it deserved culminating in the 1939 conference. There can be no doubt that the sound food policies adopted during the war owed much to the BMA's groundwork.

In the period immediately after the war conferences on special subjects did not figure largely in BMA scientific life, but a renewed burst of activity on this front came in the 1960s when conferences on the following subjects were sponsored by the Association:

1962 acne vulgaris, and foot health;
1964 foot health (again), and safety in motoring;
1966 the teaching of first-aid; and
1967 the application of mathematical and computer methods to problems in medicine.

With the advent of the Board of Science in 1968, postgraduate seminars open to all BMA members became a specific and regular part of the BMA's scientific programme. The first of these, in March 1971, was devoted to obstetrics and gynaecology and was well attended despite a postal strike which restricted publicity. During the next two years the subjects covered included paediatrics, general medicine, addiction, geriatrics, fertility, urinary problems, and death. Initially, the seminars were one-day occasions and they were normally held during the autumn and winter. After 1974 they were called "symposia." In 1980 two symposia under the general theme of "Topics of Our Time" were staged in provincial cities: one on "road accidents and their management" at Birmingham, and the other on "hazards in the working environment" at Southampton.

To sum up this part of the story, the main change in the annual scientific meeting in the past 50 years has been the abolition of the sections. There used to be about two dozen specialty sections, each with a president and two honorary secretaries chosen for each meeting, and each with its own programme. The BMA sections played an important part in the profession: until bodies such as the Royal Society of Medicine, the Association of Surgeons, the British Paediatric Association, and the many other present-day specialist associations and faculties sprang up, it was the BMA sections which catered for the scientific interests of the proliferating specialties.

Then, in the 1950s, the BMA began to think that the specialties could be left to take care of themselves, and that it was now more important for the Association to reintegrate medicine, and also to take high-quality meetings to smaller centres. Plenary sessions, symposia, and round-table discussions therefore replaced the special sections at the BMA Meeting, and a second annual scientific meeting, on a more concentrated scale, was inaugurated to be held in smaller places.

LECTURES

Meetings organised centrally by the BMA constitute only one facet of this particular form of scientific activity. Meetings arranged by local branches and divisions of the Association for scientific, business, and social purposes have always been a vital part of BMA life. The scientific purpose has received direct encouragement by the system of BMA lectures.

In 1932 each branch and division in Great Britain and Ireland was entitled to one BMA lecture annually at the expense of the Association's central funds. During the 1930s this facility enabled local gatherings of BMA members to be addressed by eminent specialists. From 1939 to 1945 BMA lectures were suspended but they were resumed immediately the war was over.

In 1947, as a contribution to postwar reconstruction, the BMA Council set aside £1000 to provide lectures by distinguished British doctors to the medical profession in

Europe. This scheme enabled such lectures to be delivered in Czechoslovakia, Denmark, Norway, Spain, and the Netherlands.

In 1950 Council extended the system of BMA lectures to include medical student bodies. In 1956 it recorded its thanks to 96 distinguished members of the profession who had given BMA lectures during the previous year; at the same time financial caution constrained it to reject an annual meeting motion that divisions should have the option of applying for an additional lecture at the discretion of the divisional executive committee. After the advent of postgraduate medical centres in the 1960s, Council agreed in 1966 to offer BMA lectures to those centres where arrangements could be made in co-operation with the local BMA division. This was but a small contribution to the development of postgraduate centres, a movement in which the BMA, harassed by other problems, missed the opportunity to play a leading part.

The first substantial change in the system of BMA lectures came with the creation of the Board of Science in 1968. In March 1969 the board recommended to Council that the BMA lectures be available to branches and divisions only as an alternative to BMA one-day scientific symposia, that the lectures be confined to scientific subjects, that they be required to have the approval of the Scientific Programmes Panel of the board, and that travel and subsistence expenses be paid to lecturers — but no honorarium as in earlier years.

Guidelines on the conduct of scientific, educational, and clinical functions by the modern BMA division were furnished in 1977 in the report of a working party on the status of the Association. Local scientific and clinical meetings were to be of a kind not provided by postgraduate medical centres and their cost was not to exceed the division's own resources. Whenever possible social and scientific functions were to be combined.

During the period immediately after the second world war it became the custom for the Winchester Division of the BMA to arrange an annual address, in which an eminent person would speak to a mixed medical and lay audience on a theme of broad social or medical significance. In 1953 Dr Guy Dain spoke on "John Citizen and his doctor — where do we go from here?"; in 1955 Lord Beveridge took as his subject, "The problem of the aged." Through the calibre of its speakers, the Winchester address became an event of more than local quality and importance to the extent that, starting in 1958, Council made a grant to the division to help cover the expense. Speakers since that time have included Sir Keith Joseph, Lord Cohen of Birkenhead, Cardinal Heenan, Lord Goodman, Mr Edward Heath, Lord Denning, and Sir Ronald Gibson. The Winchester address developed into one of the outstanding occasions in the BMA calendar.

SCHOLARSHIPS

Since the nineteenth century the BMA has stimulated medical research by awarding scholarships and prizes, the funds for them being derived either from bequests or from special grants made by the Association itself.

In 1932 four scholarships were awarded annually to candidates qualified to undertake research into the cause, prevention, or treatment of disease. One of these was the Ernest Hart Scholarship to the value of £200, the others being ordinary scholarships of £150 each. In that year Council decided to increase the value of one of the ordinary scholarships to £200 and to name it after Professor Walter Dixon who had rendered yeoman service to the BMA over many years in administering awards and prizes. In addition to these formal scholarships, Council was prepared to make special research grants and during 1932-3 seven such grants totalling £350 were made.

Throughout the 1930s the work of BMA scholars and grantees was not allowed to go unnoticed. Reports on their investigations were made to the Science Committee and were published annually in the supplement to the *British Medical Journal.*

Early in 1939 a review of the work accomplished by scholars during previous years was undertaken to decide whether, in view of the increase in funds generally available for research purposes, the grants made by Council were being used to the best advantage. In particular, the review examined the desirability of converting the existing system of part-time scholarships to whole-time awards. The verdict of the investigation was that there was already ample provision outside the BMA for whole-time scholarships, and that the present arrangements — which had served very well — should be maintained. The one modification approved had the objective of providing the scholar with expert supervision.

No scholarships were awarded during the war and when they were again made available in 1946 as an interim measure their tenure was restricted to nine months. Experience quickly showed this period to be inadequate and from October 1947 the prewar system of awards for 12 months to coincide with the academic year was restored. The possibility of instituting full-time scholarships was rejected once more because it was felt that the smaller, part-time grants were particularly useful to younger doctors.

Several new BMA scholarships have been created since 1946. In 1948 Council established a trust fund from the sum of £5000 bequeathed to the BMA by Mr E R Insole to provide a scholarship for research into the cause and cure of venereal disease. The award is made biennially. In 1959 the Claire Wand Fund provided a travelling scholarship enabling two general practitioners to spend six to eight weeks in the United States and Canada to study the postgraduate education of general practitioners in those countries. As part of their award the two doctors concerned were able to attend the 2nd World Conference on Medical Education in Chicago. In 1970 the Edith Walsh Research Award was instituted as a result of a generous bequest "for research into cardiac and respiratory disease." The Geoffrey Holt Award is similarly offered for research into diseases of the cardiovascular system. In 1977 a bequest of nearly £48 000 was received from the estate of Mr Thomas Payten Gunton, whose career had been spent in education, and whose wife had suffered from cancer for many years. In accordance with Mr Gunton's wishes, the T P Gunton Award was created by Council for research into health education with special regard to the early diagnosis and treatment of cancer. The award is open to both medical and non-medical people. The Welsh Council administers a fund donated by the Harry and Abe Sherman Foundation, making grants to members of the Association who live and work in Wales, and who require assistance in research projects.

The tradition that the Association should make only

part-time awards was finally broken in 1967 when a BMA research fellowship was established for whole-time work. In 1970 this innovation was further extended when the T V James bequest made possible a research fellowship for whole-time investigation into the nature, cause, prevention, or treatment of bronchial asthma, open to any member of the BMA and tenable for a maximum of two years.

PRIZES

Turning from BMA scholarships and research grants to specific prizes awarded by the Association, we find that in 1932 four of the present-day prizes were already in existence — the Stewart Prize for work on epidemic disease, the Middlemore Prize for research in ophthalmic medicine and surgery, the Charles Hastings Prize for award to general practitioners, and the Katherine Bishop Harman Prize for the encouragement of research into the disorders of maternity. The BMA also offered prizes for competition by final-year students in medical schools of the British Empire; in 1929 this competition had been extended to newly qualified practitioners of not more than one year's standing.

No further prizes were instituted until 1939 when a gift of £1000 from Mr N Bishop Harman was devoted to the endowment of a biennial prize to encourage clinical research. The Nathaniel Bishop Harman Prize was to be open to hospital consultants in the United Kingdom and, as such, was designed to complement the Charles Hastings Clinical Prize for general practitioners.

After the war substantial innovations were introduced into the range of BMA prizes. In 1948 Council approved the annual award of prizes for essays written by nurses in the three categories of pupil nurses, state-registered nurses working in hospital, and state-registered nurses not working in hospital. The aim of the competition was to stimulate systematic observation by nurses. The Nurses' Prize was followed, in 1951, by the introduction of the Occupational Health Prize open to any member of the BMA who was engaged in industrial medicine. The year 1951 also saw the introduction of the Charles Oliver Hawthorne Clinical Prize. Dr C O Hawthorne, who had been Chairman of the Representative Body, left £2000 to the Association and the income from this sum was devoted to a prize for the runner-up in the Charles Hastings Prize competition.

The essay competition for medical students was reorganised in 1948 and was opened to all medical students — not just to those in their final year. Six prizes of £25 were to be awarded on a national basis, and, in addition, £150 was allocated for regional essay prizes based on the four regions of the British Medical Students' Association. By 1954 the number and quality of essays had deteriorated and Council attempted to improve matters by deciding that future subjects should have a more literary character. At the same time, a similar essay competition was established for provisionally registered practitioners, but the entries were so few that it was discontinued in 1963. The form of the Medical Students' Prize competition was again changed in 1970 when the essays were no longer written on set subjects, but the prizes were awarded for accounts of original observations on any subject of medical interest submitted either by individuals or by groups of students.

Several new prize competitions were introduced during the late 1950s and early 1960s. In 1958 a legacy from Sir Henry Brackenbury, a former Chairman of Council, was invested and the income devoted to a prize which under the terms of Sir Henry's will was to be awarded to a member of the BMA for "a study, essay, lecture, or similar contribution on a subject judged by the Council to be of immediate practical importance with regard to public health, to some medicopolitical or medicosociological problem, or to some educational question whether general, medical, or postgraduate." In 1961 a prize competition was established in memory of Walter Jobson Horne, a celebrated laryngologist, who had died in 1953. The prize is awarded annually to a member of the BMA who has advanced the science and practice of laryngology and otology, particularly in relation to general medicine. The C H Milburn Prize, first awarded in 1961, is open to any medical practitioner for research into medical jurisprudence or forensic medicine or both. Dr Charles Henry Milburn had been a member of Council from 1899 until 1918. In 1961 Dr Doris Odlum, who is a Vice-President of the BMA, endowed a prize for research in mental health. In the same year Mrs P D Holmes from Yorkshire gave a substantial sum to encourage the invention of a satisfactory appliance for incontinent women patients. The Holmes Prize was awarded in 1966.

The financing and administration of BMA scholarships and prizes came under searching review in 1960 when Council recognised that the available funds were inadequate and undertook to investigate the possibility of establishing a single trust fund into which, by deed of covenant, the Association would pay the monies normally devoted to scholarships and prizes. In 1966 a Scholarships Trust Fund was set up for the receipt of bequests for medical research. Prizes and awards, however, still posed financial problems.

In 1971 the Board of Science reported that with the exception of the nurses' competition, the number and quality of entries to the essay competitions over the previous 10 years had been extremely disappointing and the board was having difficulty in fulfilling its obligations under certain trust deeds. The advice of the Association's solicitor had been obtained, an approach was being made to the Charity Commissioners and in the meantime the prize essay competitions had been suspended.

The review by the Board of Science led to an important change of policy over prizes. Instead of their being offered for essays based on work already carried out, the Board decided to invite competition for awards to encourage prospective research and particularly pilot projects. The area of research and eligibility for an award are governed by the original trust deed of the prize competition.

SUBJECT OF THE YEAR

This imaginative proposal gave every doctor in the country an opportunity of contributing to a nationwide discussion of a chosen medicoscientific or medicosocial subject. The scheme was launched in a memorandum prepared by Dr Ronald Gibson, and submitted to the Organisation Committee in March 1959. The memorandum proposed that the chosen subject should be discussed in the first instance by "fireside groups" at home; it would then be debated by divisional meetings, which might be addressed by a speaker from a panel drawn up by the Science Committee; finally, there would be a conference at BMA House attended by representatives from all divisions. The plan was warmly endorsed by the Organisation and Science Committees and by Council and the first "Subject of the Year" chosen for debate in 1959-60 was "The Medical and Social Aspects of Adolescence."

The initial response to the project was disappointing; comparatively few divisions sent in reports of discussions and the number did not justify holding a conference. The quality of the reports received, however, was good and they were correlated in a booklet published by the BMA in 1961. Council, feeling that there was sufficient evidence to persist with the scheme, decided that the subject for 1960-1 should be health education. To provide more impetus to the project, a steering committee to advise divisions was set up under Sir Allen Daley and 43 divisions took part compared with 26 in the first year.

The "Subject of the Year" for 1961-2 was "Practical Steps in the Prevention of Chronic Disease," for 1962-3 "Health at Work," and for 1963-4 "Anxiety." The number of divisions taking part was never more than 50 and an atmosphere of increasing disillusion became apparent. The Science Committee's recommendation to Council that the "Subject of the Year" be discontinued after 1963 was not accepted, but this decision merely served to delay the inevitable. "Problems of Retirement," the subject for 1966, proved to be the last in the series.

SPECIAL SUBJECT COMMITTEES

Abstract research has never been a feature of the BMA's scientific activity. The Association has always concentrated its attention on medical problems of topical importance to the community at large. Yet no organisation is better equipped than the BMA to investigate medicosocial problems. With its large membership of doctors who have a close relationship with individual patients, the Association is naturally sensitive at an early stage to matters of concern to the general population. To inquire into those matters it can draw on a depth of medical experience not available to any other medical body.

On special subjects it has long been the practice of the BMA to set up committees of members with expert knowledge to consider the subjects in depth and report to Council and, through Council, to the annual representative meeting. In many instances, these reports have also been published. The wide range of topics covered in the past 50 years is well illustrated by the chronological list of reports by special subject committees which is annexed to this chapter (Annex 1).

EVIDENCE TO OFFICIAL INQUIRIES

The BMA has always played its full part in submitting evidence to official inquiries into matters of serious concern that have a medical aspect. Examples of such evidence are given in a list annexed to this chapter (Annex 2; see also Chapter 6).

JOINT COMMITTEES WITH OUTSIDE ORGANISATIONS

The BMA has collaborated closely with paramedical or non-medical organisations to promote scientific interests that are held in common. Two notable examples during the past 50 years have been the Association's relationships with the Pharmaceutical Society and with the Magistrates' Association.

As early as 1935 a joint conference was established between the BMA and the Pharmaceutical Society of Great Britain to consider the need for machinery to collect and disseminate information on proprietary medicines.

Between May 1935 and June 1938 10 meetings of the conference were held under the chairmanship of Sir Ewen Maclean. The final report of the conference was published in the *British Medical Journal* (1939; **i**, suppl: 209-13) and embodied an imaginative proposal for an approved list of proprietary medicines. The cost of administering such a list would, however, have been so high that the conference itself recommended delay in its implementation and the outbreak of war in the following September sealed its fate altogether.

Close contact with the Pharmaceutical Society was resumed in 1946 when the two societies conferred on problems of common interest arising from the proposed National Health Service. The conference resolved that a joint committee of the BMA and Pharmaceutical Society should be set up to compile a standard prescribers' formulary to replace the *National Formulary for National*

Insurance Purposes which had been issued by the BMA in pre-war years.

The first edition of the *National Formulary* was published in 1949 and thereafter editions appeared at intervals of about two-and-a-half years. In 1957 the title was altered to *British National Formulary*. After publication of the edition for 1976-8 it was recognised that an interval between editions of two years or more was no longer acceptable and with effect from the 1981 edition it was decided to publish more frequently, with an ultimate goal of two editions a year.

In 1946 the BMA and the Magistrates' Association set up a joint committee on psychiatry and the law. The aim of the committee was to consider all matters of common interest with special reference to observation, prevention, and treatment in relation to the medical aspects of legal offences and to make recommendations for improving and extending existing arrangements and facilitating new legislation.

The committee came to an end after 1969 but during its lifetime it was responsible for the following useful reports:

(*1*) The unstable adolescent girl. *Br Med J* 1946; **ii**: 909-12.

(*2*) Memorandum on interpretation of the definitions in the Mental Deficiency Act, 1927. *Br Med J* 1947; **i**, suppl: 101-2.

(*3*) The law relating to attempted suicide. *Br Med J* 1947; **i**, suppl: 103.

(*4*) Enuresis. *Br Med J* 1948; **i**, suppl: 143-6.

(*5*) The criminal law and sexual offenders. *Br Med J* 1949; **i**, suppl: 135-40.

(*6*) The adolescent delinquent boy. *Br Med J* 1951; **i**:1256-60.

(*7*) The law in relation to the illegitimate child. London: BMA, 1952; and summary in *Br Med J* 1952; **i**: 271.

(*8*) Cruelty to and neglect of children. London: BMA, 1956; and summary in *Br Med J* 1956; **i**, suppl: 327-8.

(*9*) The law and practice in relation to attempted suicide in England and Wales. London: BMA, 1958; and summary in *Br Med J* 1958; **i**: 1233-4.

(*10*) Memorandum on alcoholism. *Br Med J* 1961; **i**, suppl: 190-5.

SCIENTIFIC SERVICES

Apart from the investigation of specific medical subjects, since early in its history the BMA has operated certain continuing scientific services for the benefit of its members. Pre-eminent among these during the years since 1932 have been the Nuffield Library and the film library which developed into the British Life Assurance Trust (BLAT) Centre for Health and Medical Education.

NUFFIELD LIBRARY

By 1932 the library was already playing an important part in the scientific life of the BMA. Founded in 1887 to collect publications on medicine and its allied sciences, it had become one of the largest general medical libraries in the United Kingdom, second in size only to the library of the Royal Society of Medicine. The book stock of the BMA Library in 1932 amounted to some 40 000 volumes; in 1981 this figure had risen to the 100 000 mark.

The library has always received invaluable help from the *British Medical Journal* in building up its collections. Many copies of books received for review by the journal have been passed to the library, and exchange arrangements with journals published by the BMA have enabled the library to take many periodicals that it would not otherwise have obtained. This help with periodicals was greatly augmented in 1947 when the BMA started to publish *Abstracts of World Medicine* and many of the journals which had been taken by the abstracting service were in due course transferred to the library.

The number of journals received regularly by the library reached a high-water mark of over 2000 in the early 1960s. Adverse economic conditions in the 1970s resulted in a considerable reduction in this number, but in 1981 the library was still subscribing to over 1000 titles, representing a core-collection of the more important medical journals from all countries.

The rapid expansion of the library stock has naturally created problems in storage and has necessitated several changes in the buildings which have housed it over the past 50 years. In 1932 the library occupied the space in the north block of BMA House which had previously been known as the Hastings Hall. Before the end of the second world war this proved inadequate and in November 1947 the library was moved into the garden court wing, which had been built during the early part of the war. In its new home the library occupied the top two floors and the basement. The comparative seclusion of the garden court and the absence of any noise from the traffic in Tavistock Square made this an admirable site.

Even so, the need for additional storage space soon became an acute problem once more. In 1954 Council turned down a suggestion that room for the library might be found in the building to be erected on the newly acquired Burton Street site; it did recognise the importance of the library service and undertook consideration of a long-term policy for its accommodation.

Early in 1961 detailed plans were submitted to the Estates Committee for a radical reconstruction of the existing library. As the cost of this work was considered too high to be borne from BMA funds, an application was made to the trustees of the Nuffield Foundation, who generously granted the sum of £50 000 and enabled the project to proceed. The rebuilding began in January 1962 and the new Nuffield Library was opened on 2 May 1963 by the President of the BMA, Sir Ian Fraser. The library now occupied all four floors of the garden court wing with greatly improved reading-room and staff accommodation. Even more important, the equipment had been modernised in two respects: new passenger and book lifts took publications to and from the stores, and electrically operated compact shelving in the basement provided storage space for many years to come.

The creation of this extra shelf space was to prove an investment of great value in the mid-1970s with the arrival of harsh financial conditions and the necessity for tight economy. In 1975, when the call for savings was made and the future of the library was in jeopardy, the librarian vacated the upper two floors of the garden court wing and left them free for letting. With the help of the existing compact shelving and by using a large loft in BMA House as an extra store, this work of contraction was carried through by the end of 1976. A fresh source of income was thereby obtained for the Association, while the stock and services of the library were maintained at their former level.

The library exists to provide a comprehensive reference collection for those members who can visit BMA House; for those who cannot do so, the library's function is to send literature or information to them through the post. In two important respects, modern technological advances have been introduced in recent years — photocopying and computerised information retrieval.

In 1932 journal articles could be made available to members outside the library only in the form of loans, often in heavy bound volumes which were expensive to send through the post, and which might then be absent from the shelves for long periods. In 1963 photocopying articles, under the provisions of copyright law and at a minimum charge to members, was inaugurated. The service grew rapidly and proved so popular that photocopying largely replaced loans of periodicals. In 1980 7517 articles were copied.

Literature-searching for information in 1932 could be done only by manual searching through indexes by experienced library staff. During the late 1950s computerised information retrieval was introduced by the National Library of Medicine in Washington and was first used to improve the quality and speed of published indexes, such as *Index Medicus*. The system was subsequently extended to individual libraries by the installation of local computer terminals and since 1978 the Nuffield Library has made this computerised service available to members of the BMA. Initially this was done by using the terminal at the Science Reference Library, but in 1981 a terminal was installed in the Nuffield Library itself.

The full services of the Nuffield Library are available only to members of the BMA who live in the British Isles. Over the past 50 years statistics have shown a steady use of the library by some 20% of the membership every year. The BMA has also recognised a duty to make its unique collection of medical publications available to the academic world at large on strict conditions that protect the interests of its own members. In 1967 a scheme for institutional membership of the library was introduced to help the rapidly growing number of small medical libraries, particularly those in postgraduate medical centres. In 1936 a special arrangement was made that extended the facilities of the BMA Library to members of the Irish Free State

Medical Union; this service to Irish doctors remained in force until 1978. In 1959 for the first time undergraduate medical students were allowed to use the library for reference purposes on the recommendation of the dean or librarian of their medical school; this right was consolidated in 1974 when associate membership of the BMA for medical students was introduced.

The fact that the United Kingdom has no single national library to serve the medical profession has been of considerable interest since the second world war, and is further complicated by the existence of two, largely duplicated, medical library services operated by private societies — the Royal Society of Medicine and the British Medical Association. During the 1960s and 1970s several discussions between the two societies took place with a view to establishing a combined library service, but without practical result. In 1974 talks were also held between the BMA and the British Library to form a national centre for medical librarianship. These discussions also came to naught, and, in the final event, the Nuffield Library remains an independent unit under the control of the BMA and serving the individual member.

FILM LIBRARY

Eleven BMA members who went on a world tour to the annual meeting in Melbourne in 1935 brought back cinematograph films of their travels. These films were worked into a composite reel which had a special showing at BMA House in February 1936. A copy of the film was purchased by the Association and provided the first example of BMA interest in this medium.

In 1938 a show of films, mainly in colour, was given to the scientific sections at the Plymouth annual meeting and aroused considerable interest. Later that same year the *British Medical Journal* reported a suggestion that the Association should establish a central medical film library from which divisions and branches could borrow films to show at their meetings. Council gave its approval and invited donations of films by medical practitioners, but the outbreak of war in 1939 put an immediate stop to the project.

The subject was taken up again early in 1946 when

Council appointed a special committee to inquire into the scope and limitation of films for postgraduate and undergraduate medical education. The committee's report, "The Scope and Use of the Film in Medical Education," was published as Appendix II to the Annual Report of Council for 1946-7 (*Br Med J* 1947; **i**, suppl: 140-8). In accordance with its recommendations, Council proposed the establishment of a medical film bureau primarily to serve BMA divisions and branches and to act as a central office to facilitate, co-ordinate, and assist in an advisory capacity the production of medical films. Council also undertook to consider the formation of a BMA film library and the appointment of a standing committee to manage both the medical film bureau and the film library.

In 1947 the Kodak Film Library consisting of some 200 films was presented to the Association as a nucleus of its film library, and Council, after authorising the purchase of a sound projector, placed the sum of £500 at the disposal of the newly established Film Committee to acquire copies of suitable films.

In 1949 Council was able to report that the BMA Film Library was in being and that some medical films had already been shown to local divisions. It had also approved the production by the BMA of a colour film entitled "The Treatment of Infections of the Fingers and Hand," which was to prove highly successful when it became available in 1950.

A film theatre was completed in BMA House during 1950, and early in 1952 a catalogue of the stock of the BMA Film Library was published. This included technical information about each film, a synopsis of its content, and an indication of the type of audience for which it was considered suitable. The catalogue was revised and reissued in card form in 1957.

On the occasion of the First World Conference on Medical Education held in London in 1953 the Film Committee staged a successful and well-attended lunchtime showing of medical films.

In 1956 Council approved a proposal by the Film Committee that it should organise an annual competition for medical films with the award of two prizes, one for commercial and one for non-commercial producers. The choice of subject would be left to the competitors and the judges were to pay particular attention to the value of films for the BMA Film Library and the likelihood of their frequent use. Sixty-nine entries were received for the first competition in 1957.

By 1961 the stock of the Film Library amounted to 356 films, nine of which had been made directly under the aegis of the BMA. The annual borrowings from the library had risen to 1260, an increase of 471% from the first year of the library's existence.

There was a change in the administration of the Film Library in 1961. Since its inception the Film Committee had been a committee of the Association on which either the Chairman or a nominee of the Science Committee had a right to sit. In 1961 the new Committee on Medical Science, Education, and Research was created with wider terms of reference which were to include film activities. These would henceforth be administered by a Film Subcommittee of the Committee on Medical Science.

This constitutional change soon aroused considerable dissatisfaction. It was felt that the Film Library had been downgraded and that as a result film activities were failing to attract essential support from outside bodies. This criticism was so effective that the Film Committee was reconstituted in 1963 as a special committee of Council.

With the advent of tape-recordings and closed-circuit television for medical education, the work of the Film Committee became so diverse that Council came to the conclusion in 1964 that a full-time director should be appointed to manage the committee's business, to advise and discuss with film producers the problems of film-making, and to edit both films and tapes. In 1965 it was further proposed that the BMA should set up a department of audiovisual communication with responsibility for the whole field of films, tape-recordings and discs, television and video tapes. Plans were also made for establishing an educational trust to promote medical education by these means.

These plans came to fruition in 1966 when, with the support of the Life Offices Association and the Association of Scottish Life Offices, the Department of Audio-Visual Communication was established. It was supported by a trust entitled the "British Life Assurance Trust for Health Education in association with the British Medical Association." Initially the new department was administered by the Film Committee, and its first director was Mr (later Professor) Charles Engel.

BLAT CENTRE FOR HEALTH AND MEDICAL EDUCATION

The simultaneous creation of the Department of Audio-Visual Communication and of the Board of Science, which was intended to integrate all the scientific and educational activities of the BMA, led inevitably to some initial friction between the two bodies. The Film Committee held the view that as the Department of Audio-Visual Communication was financed in part by the British Life Offices Associations, and as its activities were concerned with the health education of the public, it should be allowed a degree of independence. In the end it was agreed that the Department of Audio-Visual Communication, advised by the Film Committee as a panel of the Board of Science, should be an autonomous organisation with direct access to the board. The board retained its overall responsibility.

The immediate aims of the new department were to expand the Film Library, to create an information and advisory service, to establish a reference and distribution library of audiovisual material for teaching and learning, and to help find more effective methods of teaching and learning with audiovisual media. The main purpose was of a catalytic nature geared to the improvement of education through technology.

The year 1972 marked an important stage in the development of the Department of Audio-Visual Communication. The annual income of the British Life Assurance Trust was increased from £15 000 to £50 000 and the Nuffield Foundation made a grant of £36 570 over three years to set up the Centre for Individual Learning Materials in Medical Education, which was designated by the World Health Organisation as a WHO collaborating institution. The administrative structure of the department was strengthened by the formation of an Academic Council under the chairmanship of Sir Brynmor Jones, Vice-Chancellor of the University of Hull.

In 1975 the name of the Department of Audio-Visual Communication was changed to the BLAT Centre for

Health and Medical Education to reflect the much wider nature of its work.

CONCLUSION

This, then, has been the story of the BMA's role in promoting the medical and allied sciences during the 50 years since 1932. It is a story of intense and productive activity in response to pressing medical needs throughout the community. There is no better description of this scientific achievement than the words of Sir Charles Hastings when he addressed the annual meeting of the BMA in 1862, and which he would certainly have used again on a similar occasion in 1981: "We exercise an uncertain and obscure art; but still our art is improving and the mysteries of science are every day being revealed to us . . . we stand on Mount Pisgah, like Moses of old, and look forward to the good land, where the fruit may be still more abundant, and where we may exercise our skill with still greater certainty. I think I see in this Association the promise of much future good. What has already been done fills my breast with the greatest feeling of gratification."

Ethics

> Maintenance of the honour and respectability of the profession generally . . . This means that it was recognised from the start that the profession was responsible for its own ethics. This is really the crux of any professional organisation. — HRH Prince Philip, Duke of Edinburgh, *British Medical Journal*, 1959, **ii**, 839.

The intimate relationship between doctor and patient and the degree of power given to the medical man in the consulting room and at the bedside make a code of ethical rules essential for the medical profession. When the sick are treated by all and sundry the state may step in and lay down such rules by law, as was done in the Code of Hammurabi in ancient Babylon and by the Emperor Frederick II in the Middle Ages. When medical practice reaches a more advanced stage, it is qualified doctors themselves who decide on the ethical standards of their profession and this has been a primary function of the BMA since its foundation. According to the Association's original prospectus, it set out in 1832 to maintain the honour and respectability of the profession and to promote friendly intercourse and free communication of its members and to establish the harmony and good feeling "which ought ever to characterise a liberal profession."

During its history the BMA has sought to regulate the conduct of its members towards one another and towards their patients and the non-medical public in a manner consistent with the highest standards of integrity and fair dealing. By 1932 the Association had amassed a vast store of experience in dealing with ethical matters and it was recognised as the only medical organisation in the country that was equipped to operate in these matters, apart from the General Medical Council with its statutory powers of discipline. In the words of the BMA *Handbook* for 1932-3, "The aim of the Association is to provide an experienced and impartial tribunal adapted for dealing with questions of professional conduct not so serious as to come within the purview of the GMC."

For dealing with ethical matters, well-defined machinery had been established, the core of which was the Central Ethical Committee which reported to Council and the Representative Body. Divisions and branches each had ethical committees whose procedures were governed by rules which had been framed and approved by the Representative Body. Under these rules, complaints of unethical behaviour by a member of the profession residing within the area of a division were sent to the honorary secretary of that division who would then refer the matter to BMA headquarters for guidance as to the best method of dealing with it. The ultimate sanction which the BMA possessed in ethical questions was expulsion of a guilty member. This weapon, however, had rarely been used; the role of the Association had been very much one of conciliation, not condemnation.

The ethical machinery of the BMA has been subject to little constitutional change in the 50 years since 1932, but procedures have been tightened up and clarified.

The annual meeting in 1938 conferred on Council the power of expelling a member, after due inquiry, without the necessity for a recommendation from a division or branch. Such a recommendation had previously been regarded as necessary. This change was felt necessary in those cases where a division or branch was inactive, or where a complaint had concerned conduct which had offended the Association generally rather than a local individual or BMA unit. Divisions and branches, however, still retained their right to initiate or to conduct an inquiry into any complaint arising from their area.

After this change the Central Ethical Committee set out to draft new rules of procedure under which inquiries could be initiated centrally by the BMA. This work was interrupted by the war; when it was resumed in 1946, it was thought desirable to extend the scope of the new rules to cover all ethical inquiries conducted by the Central Ethical Committee, whether initiated centrally or locally. These fresh, comprehensive rules were given the title, "Rules of the Central Ethical Committee relating to Complaints regarding Professional Conduct," and were published in the Annual Report of Council for 1946-7 (*Br Med J* 1947;**i**, suppl: 86-9). Further revisions of these rules of procedure were issued in 1950, 1965, and 1976.

In 1955 the Association's bylaws and standing orders were amended to make it clear that the Central Ethical Committee was empowered not only to inquire into cases of alleged unethical conduct but also to adjudicate on them. The only exception would be those cases in which expulsion was recommended, when Council was to have the final word. This right of adjudication by the BMA in ethical disputes where there was no contravention of the law was given legal backing by a decision of the High Court in a case brought before it in 1966.

In 1965 Council found itself unable to agree with a minute from the annual representative meeting of 1964 to the effect that all necessary administrative action over an ethical dispute should be undertaken centrally by the BMA. It remained convinced of the importance of local ethical committees.

The wide experience of ethical matters built up in BMA headquarters has been used increasingly to provide guidance to individual doctors in the form of printed matter. In 1950 a booklet entitled *Ethics and Members of the Medical Profession* was issued by the Association as a basic guide to the numerous day-to-day problems of an ethical nature which arise in medical practice. It was supplied free of charge to all newly qualified doctors. A revised edition was produced in 1953.

A complete section on medical ethics, which provided details of a code of medical conduct as well as a description of the BMA's ethical machinery, was included in the *Annual Handbook* of the Association for the first time in the edition for 1950-1. The section on ethics was given wider circulation in 1958 when it was separately published as a booklet with the title *Medical Ethics.* This procedure was repeated in 1963 and 1974.

For 30 years these successive BMA booklets provided clear and concise ethical guidance to doctors. A major revision of the 1974 edition was undertaken in 1978 by a working group of the Central Ethical Committee under the chairmanship of Mr Barry O'Donnell. A draft text produced by the working group was discussed in detail at the 1979 annual meeting and the final version was published in 1980 as *The Handbook of Medical Ethics.* This was a comprehensive publication; one chapter, headed "Ethical Dilemmas," concerned problems on which the profession had not yet reached a consensus view. A further revised edition of the handbook appeared in 1981.

Apart from publishing its own guidance on the ethics of medical conduct, the BMA has also played its part in the formulation of international codes, several of which have been drawn up by the World Medical Association. One of the first acts of that association was to produce a modern restatement of the Hippocratic Oath in September 1948, known as the Declaration of Geneva. In October of the following year the General Assembly of the World Medical Association met in London at BMA House and an International Code of Medical Ethics, based on the Declaration of Geneva, was approved. It was agreed that individual countries might vary the code according to their own practice so long as the fundamental principles were not infringed. The international code was amended by the World Medical Association at Sydney in 1968.

The World Medical Association has also issued several codes of practice on specialised ethical problems. In 1964 it drew up a code of ethics for experiments in man, which is known as the Declaration of Helsinki and which owed much to Dr Hugh Clegg, Editor of the *British Medical Journal*. A revised version of the Declaration of Helsinki was published in 1975.

The Declaration of Sydney (1968) contained a statement on the determination of the time of death. In 1970 the Declaration of Oslo provided a statement of principle on therapeutic abortion. In the Declaration of Tokyo (1975) the World Medical Association supplied guidelines for medical attitudes towards torture and other cruel, inhuman, or degrading treatment or punishment in relation to detention and imprisonment. The texts of all the World Medical Association codes may be found in the BMA's *Handbook of Medical Ethics* (1981).

The specific ethical topics with which the BMA has been concerned over the past 50 years have been so numerous and varied that it is not possible to recount them in detail. There have, however, been one or two particular subjects that have posed recurrent problems which deserve special attention.

In the conduct and etiquette of medical practice, one continual source of ethical trouble has been advertising by doctors. The BMA has been vigilant in closing those loopholes in its rules which might permit this form of unethical conduct.

In 1936 the annual meeting carried a resolution that the lay press should never be used by a practitioner to publish his change of address, to announce his movements, or to announce his surgery or consulting hours. Such information could be conveyed only in sealed letters to patients of the practice.

In 1950 the Central Ethical Committee undertook to review a statement on indirect methods of advertising which the BMA had drawn up in 1925. The aim was to provide guidance for those members of the profession who spoke or wrote for the public on medical matters. The committee, with some reason, foresaw considerable difficulty over press and radio interviews, and television appearances.

In the matter of the new medium of television, Council had already recognised that nothing could be done to conceal the identity of doctors who appeared on the screen but had decreed that nothing should be shown which would enhance their professional reputation. Fears of indirect advertising by television were not allayed, however, and the annual meeting of 1951 passed a motion that contracts for doctors to broadcast should insist on anonymity and that the BMA and the British Broadcasting Corporation should co-operate closely in the production of medical programmes. The general insistence on anonymity was in line with a resolution of the General Medical Council issued in 1934.

The revised statement on indirect advertising, which had been promised in 1950, was passed by the 1953 annual meeting as the "Report of Council on Indirect Methods of Advertising" (*Br Med J* 1953, **i**, suppl: 126-8), but it provided little help with the problems that arose. Early in 1954 it was reported to Council that the names of medical practitioners who broadcast were frequently announced, together with their qualifications. After discussions with both the General Medical Council and the British Broadcasting Corporation, the Council of the BMA reiterated in 1956 that the rule of anonymity for broadcasters should remain unaltered and this recommendation was accepted by the annual representative meeting, which also approved a revision of the 1953 "Report on Indirect Methods of Advertising" (*Br Med J* 1956, **i**, suppl: 175-7). This reassessment had been found necessary to deal with recent developments, particularly contributions by doctors to the lay press.

In spite of all the BMA's safeguards, the issue over anonymity in broadcasting deteriorated and a leading article in the *British Medical Journal* for 2 May 1959 bemoaned the way in which the ethical rules were being flouted; in the same month, Council agreed that the "Report on Indirect Methods of Advertising" should be sent to all members of the BMA in the United Kingdom, together with a statement noting with concern "the increasing frequency with which doctors' names are receiving public mention through the several media now available." In July the annual representative meeting instructed Council " to consider the present ethical rules about anonymity in broadcasting, so that no medical practitioner shall be placed in jeopardy."

In response, Council drew up a fresh "Report on Advertising and the Medical Profession" (*Br Med J* 1960; **i**, suppl: 225-8) to replace the 1956 report. In this there was the first sign of a shift from an insistence on absolute anonymity. Although this was still to be the general principle, departure from that principle would be permissible if it was (*a*) in the interests of the general public, (*b*) in the interests of the medical profession, or (*c*) an essential part of providing authoritative information for the general public. The final decision was to remain in every case with the individual doctor. These provisions were again enshrined in a further "Report on Advertising and the Medical Profession" which was approved by the annual representative meeting in July 1968 (*Br Med J* 1968; **ii**, suppl: 22-3).

Concern continued to be expressed from time to time about advertising by medical practitioners and in 1973 the Representative Body instructed the Central Ethical Committee to deal urgently with the matter. In the final event, after consulting all the standing committees, Council stood by the policy laid down in 1968 with only a few minor changes made necessary by the 1974 reorganisation of the National Health Service.

The relationship between different groups of doctors within the medical profession can give rise to disputes and complaints of unethical behaviour. In the 1930s, for example, there were frequent complaints from general practitioners about some of the activities of public health medical officers. Industrial medical officers, who treat patients at their place of work, are also at risk of trespassing on the territory of general practitioners and there have been recurrent problems in this sensitive area during the past 50 years.

In the relationship between doctor and patient, the ethical topic that has perennially come to the fore has been professional confidence. The doctor, with his privileged position in relation to the patient, has a duty to preserve secrecy on the information confided to him in the course of consultation. In the early years of the BMA the Association's policy was to regard this rule of secrecy as an absolute prohibition to disclose such information without the consent of the patient.

In 1952 Council considered that there were exceptional cases when such secrecy could involve innocent third parties in disaster. Examples, which were cited, included nursemaids suffering from venereal disease who refused to give up their work, and epileptic car drivers who continued to drive. Council put a motion to the annual representative meeting that permitted a doctor to disclose his privileged information when he regarded it as his moral duty to protect innocent persons, provided that the patient had been advised of the proper course he should take. The meeting did not support the proposal, however, and reaffirmed the existing policy of total secrecy.

In 1957 Council noted in its annual report that strong arguments were being put forward in favour of some relaxation of this policy in the public interest. In the following year the annual representative meeting passed a motion instructing Council to re-examine the possible disclosure of information to the appropriate medical authority when a doctor was aware of a disability in a public service official that might endanger life. As a result of Council's deliberations on the subject the 1959 annual representative meeting passed a motion to the effect that, due to the complications of modern life, it might be necessary on some occasions to modify the rule of absolute secrecy; any course adopted, however, must be to the benefit of the patient or protect his interest.

A lengthy debate on the subject of professional secrecy was held at the annual representative meeting in 1966; by an overwhelming majority, the meeting confirmed the policy laid down in 1959, but an important rider was added to the effect that "the death of the patient does not absolve the doctor from his obligation of secrecy. Where the patient is dead or not in a position to give consent, it is left to the discretion of the doctor to decide who, in a particular case, is the person competent to give such consent."

The amount of legislation which might endanger professional confidence began to cause increasing concern. At the annual representative meeting of 1970, the Abortion Act, the Children and Young Persons Act, and the Medicines Act were put forward as examples, and a motion from West Suffolk was passed calling on Council to resist all such encroachments on professional secrecy.

In 1971, following a survey of the whole question of professional confidence, Council revised the section in the *Members Handbook* which dealt with the subject and also published it in its annual report for 1971-2 (*Br Med J* 1972, **ii**, suppl: 117-20).

One particular aspect of professional secrecy that has caused concern in recent years is the increasing use of computers for medical records. As early as May 1971 Council promised to consider the ethical implications of computerised storage of medical information. In 1976 the BMA gave evidence to the Data Protection Committee, which had been set up by the Government to examine the possibility of establishing permanent statutory arrangements to protect personal information held in computer systems. By 1981, however, there was no sign of any immediate legislation on the subject and no intention by the Government to set up an independent data protection authority. In these circumstances, the BMA continues to scrutinise all developments for signs of infringements of medical secrecy.

The creation of the National Health Service in 1948 and the establishment of close links between the medical profession and the state gave rise to new ethical problems. As early as 1949 Council expressed its fears about the number of forms which doctors were required to complete and the possible misuse of the information contained in them. It reiterated its view that professional information, including that in official forms, could not be divulged without the consent of the patient.

Between 1951 and 1955 a thorny topic was the loan of hospital records to government departments, such as the Ministry of Pensions and Ministry of National Insurance, in connection with claims for pensions or sickness benefit. The ethical policy in this matter was finally laid down by the annual representative meeting in 1955 with provisions that such loans could be made only with the consent of or on behalf of the patient and that, wherever practical, if the disclosure of the information might have psychological effects on the patient, the practitioner who compiled the record — or, if he was not available, a nominee of the hospital authority — should be consulted on the wisdom of disclosing to the patient all the confidential information in the records.

The whole question of medical ethics in the context of a national health service was reviewed in the 1970s by a joint working party of the BMA and the conference of medical Royal Colleges and their faculties in the United Kingdom under the chairmanship of Sir Rodney (later Lord) Smith.

In 1977 the working party issued a discussion document on the ethical responsibilities of doctors practising in the National Health Service (*Br Med J* 1977; **i**: 157-9); this paper produced some hostile reaction when it was later considered by the BMA Council.

Advances in medical technology have brought with them an increasing number of ethical problems for the doctor in his relations with patients. Since the second world war the BMA has been faced with many new moral dilemmas, including those affecting therapeutic trials, experimental research in man, the transplantation of human tissue, artificial insemination by donor, and cosmetic surgery. The growth within the community of more elastic attitudes to life and death has faced the Association with intensely difficult moral questions arising from abortion, contraception, sterilisation, euthanasia, and the artificial preservation of life. The social and political environment of the times has brought to the fore such matters as non-accidental injury to children and the interrogation and artificial feeding of prisoners. The entry of the United Kingdom into the European Economic Community raised the long-term problem of harmonising the British system of medical ethics with the codes and laws of other member states. To the Central Ethical Committee of 1932 most of these issues were unknown. It is to the lasting credit of the BMA that it has not flinched from the ethical problems that have arisen since then.

Annex 1

Reports by Special Subject Committees

1933 ARTHRITIS
Causation and treatment of arthritis and allied conditions. *Br Med J* 1933: **i**: 1033-52.

1933 NUTRITION
Report of the Committee on Nutrition. *Br Med J* 1933; **ii**, supplement to 25 November, p 16.

1935 ALCOHOL AND ROAD ACCIDENTS
The relation of alcohol to road accidents: report by BMA Committee. London: BMA, 1935; and *Br Med J* 1935; **ii**, suppl: 57-9.

1935 IMMUNISATION
Report of Committee on Immunization including Vaccination. London: BMA, 1935; and *Br Med J* 1935; **i**, suppl: 282-93.

1935 NUTRITION
Family meals and catering. London: BMA, 1935.

1935 OSTEOPATHY
Theory, technique and practice of osteopathy. Memorandum by Special Committee of the British Medical Association. *Br Med J* 1935; **i**, suppl: 1-5.

1935 FRACTURES
Report of Committee on Fractures. London: BMA, 1935; and *Br Med J* 1935; **i**, suppl: 53-62.

1936 MINER'S NYSTAGMUS
Report of a Committee on Diagnosis and Certification of Miner's Nystagmus. London: BMA, 1936; and *Br Med J* 1936; **i**, suppl: 238-42.

1936 PHYSICAL EDUCATION
Report of Committee on Physical Education. London: BMA, 1936; and *Br Med J* 1936; **i**, suppl: 149-78.

1936 TRANSPORT SAFETY
Report of Committee on the Compulsory Use of Yellow Lights for Motor Cars. *Br Med J* 1936; **i**, suppl: 225-6.

1938 NUTRITION
The doctor's cookery book. London: BMA, 1938.

1939 NUTRITION
How to stock your ARP larder. One week's emergency food store chosen by the *British Medical Journal.* London: BMA, 1939.

1939 OCCUPATIONAL MEDICINE
First-aid in industry. London: BMA, 1939.

1940 NUTRITION
The doctors tell you what to eat in wartime. London: BMA, 1940.

1941 MENTAL HEALTH
Report of a Committee on Mental Health. London: BMA, 1941; and summary in *Br Med J* 1941; **ii**: 276-8.

1941 OCCUPATIONAL MEDICINE
Report of Committee on Industrial Health in Factories. London: BMA, 1941; and summary in *Br Med J* 1941; **ii**: 783-5.

1946 REHABILITATION
Report on rehabilitation by a special committee of the BMA. *Br Med J* 1946; **i**, suppl: 187-201.

1947 GERIATRICS
The care and treatment of the elderly and infirm: report of a special committee of the British Medical Association. London: BMA, 1947; and *Br Med J* 1947; **i**, suppl: 133-40.

1948 GERIATRICS
"The right patient in the right bed." First supplement to the Report (1947) of the Committee on the Care and Treatment of the Elderly and Infirm. *Br Med J* 1948; **ii**, suppl: 71-2.

1950 NUTRITION
Report of the Committee on Nutrition. London: BMA, 1950; and summary in *Br Med J* 1950; **i**: 541-4.

1950 TUBERCULOSIS
Tuberculosis and the National Health Service. Report of BMA Group Committee. *Br Med J* 1950; **ii**: 1382-5 (summary).

1951 HYDROTHERAPY
The spa in medical practice. A report of a committee of the BMA. London: BMA, 1951; and summary in *Br Med J* 1951; **i**, suppl: 173-4.

1954 ALCOHOL AND ROAD ACCIDENTS
The recognition of intoxication: report of a special committee of the British Medical Association. London: BMA, 1954; and summary in *Br Med J* 1954; **i**, 753-4.

1954 REHABILITATION
The rehabilitation and resettlement of disabled persons. London: BMA, 1954; and summary in *Br Med J* 1954, **i**: 1490.

1954 TRANSPORT SAFETY
Memorandum on medical standards for road, rail and air transport. *Br Med J* 1954; **i**, suppl: 117-22.

1955 GERIATRICS
Report of the Geriatrics Joint Subcommittee. *Br Med J* 1955; **i**, suppl: 181-90.

1955 HYPNOSIS
Medical use of hypnotism. Report of a subcommittee appointed by the Psychological Medicine Group Committee of the BMA. *Br Med J* 1955; **i**, suppl: 190-3.

1956 COAL-GAS POISONING
Report on the problem of accidental death and ill-health from coal-gas poisoning. *Br Med J* 1956; **ii**, suppl: 201-2 (summary).

1958 ALCOHOL AND ROAD ACCIDENTS
Recognition of intoxication: report of a special committee of the

British Medical Association. 2nd ed, revised. London: BMA, 1958.

1960 ALCOHOL AND ROAD ACCIDENTS
Relation of alcohol to road accidents. Report of a special committee. London: BMA, 1960; and summary in *Br Med J* 1960; **i**: 269-72.

1964 ACCIDENTS
Accidents in the home. London: BMA, 1964.

1964 GERIATRICS
Accidental hypothermia in the elderly. (A memorandum prepared for the Ministry of Health by a special committee appointed by the Committee on Medical Science, Education and Research of the BMA.) *Br Med J* 1964; **ii**: 1255-8.

1964 HYDROTHERAPY
The spa in medical practice. Revised ed. London: BMA, 1964.

1964 VENEREAL DISEASE
Venereal disease and young people: a report by a committee of the British Medical Association. London: BMA, 1964.

1965 ALCOHOL AND ROAD ACCIDENTS
The drinking driver. Report of a special committee of the British Medical Association. London: BMA, 1965.

1965 IMMIGRANTS
Report of the Working Party on the Medical Examination of Immigrants: a British Medical Association report. London: BMA, 1965.

1968 AMPHETAMINES
Report of the Working Party on Amphetamine Preparations. London: BMA, 1968 (duplicated); and summary in *Br Med J* 1968; **iv**, 572-3.

1971 EUTHANASIA
The problem of euthanasia. A report prepared by a special panel appointed by the Board of Science. London: BMA, 1971.

1971 MEDICAL CARE
Gaps in medical care — report of an inquiry by special panel appointed by the Board of Science and Education. *Br Med J* 1971; **ii**, suppl: 88-91; and *Br Med J* 1972; **ii**, suppl: 111.

1971 TOBACCO SMOKING
Memorandum on Association policy in relation to smoking. *Br Med J* 1971; **ii**, suppl: 91-2.

1972 AGE OF CONSENT
Report of the Board of Science's Working Party on the Age of Consent in Relation to Sexual Offences; summary in *Br Med J* 1972; **iii**, suppl: 180.

1972 PHARMACEUTICAL PRODUCTS
Report of the Panel on Pharmaceutical Products. *Br Med J* 1972; **ii**, suppl: 111-4.

1973 ARTIFICIAL INSEMINATION
Report of Panel on Human Artificial Insemination. *Br Med J* 1973; **ii**, suppl: 3-5.

1974 ALCOHOL AND ROAD ACCIDENTS
Alcohol, drugs and driving: a supplement to "The Drinking

Driver." Report of a Working Party of the British Medical Association. London: BMA, 1974.

1974 PRIMARY CARE
Report of the Panel on Primary Health Care Teams. London: BMA, 1974.

1975 OCCUPATIONAL MEDICINE
Report of the Working Party on the Medical Implications of Oil-Related Industry. Edinburgh: BMA Scottish Council, 1975.

1976 GERIATRICS
Report of the Working Party on Services for the Elderly. London: BMA, 1976.

1979 CHILD HEALTH
Our children's health. London: BMA, 1979.

1980 COMPUTERS
Computing in general practice: a report for the General Medical Services Committee of the British Medical Association, prepared by Paul Palmer and Cynthia Rees. London: Scicon Consultancy International Ltd., 1980.

Annex 2

Evidence to Official Inquiries

1953 INTERDEPARTMENTAL COMMITTEE ON THE ADOPTION OF CHILDREN
Memorandum of evidence submitted to Interdepartmental Committee on the Adoption of Children. *Br Med J* 1953; **i**, suppl: 240-2.

1955 ROYAL COMMISSION ON THE LAW RELATING TO MENTAL ILLNESS AND MENTAL DEFICIENCY
The law on mental illness and mental deficiency; Association's evidence to Royal Commission. *Br Med J* 1955; **i**, suppl: 211-3.

1955 DEPARTMENTAL COMMITTEE ON HOMOSEXUALITY AND PROSTITUTION
Homosexuality and prostitution. A memorandum of evidence prepared by a special committee of the Council of the British Medical Association for submission to the Departmental Committee on Homosexuality and Prostitution. London: BMA, 1955; and summary in *Br Med J* 1955; **ii**, suppl: 165-70.

1956 COMMISSION ON DIVINE HEALING
Divine healing and co-operation between doctors and clergy. Memorandum of evidence submitted by a special committee of the British Medical Association to the Archbishops' Commission on Divine Healing. London: BMA, 1956; and summary in *Br Med J* 1956; **i**, suppl: 269-73.

1959 DEPARTMENTAL COMMITTEE ON ARTIFICIAL INSEMINATION
Artificial insemination ... memorandum of evidence on the medical aspects of artificial insemination ... submitted by the British Medical Association to the Departmental Committee. *Br Med J* 1959; **i**, suppl: 289-91.

1962 GOVERNMENT COMMITTEE ON THE PROBLEM OF NOISE
Evidence to Government Committee on the Problem of Noise. *Br Med J* 1962; **i**, suppl: 194-7.

1965 ADVISORY COMMITTEE ON PESTICIDES AND OTHER TOXIC CHEMICALS
Memorandum of evidence to the Advisory Committee on Pesticides and other Toxic Chemicals. *Br Med J* 1965; **i**, suppl: 190-1.

1965 ROYAL COMMISSION ON THE PENAL SYSTEM
Interim memorandum of evidence to the Royal Commission on the Penal System. *Br Med J* 1965; **i**, suppl: 187-90.
Second memorandum of evidence to the Royal Commission on the Penal System. *Br Med J* 1966; **i**, suppl: 119-21.

1966 COMMITTEE ON THE AGE OF MAJORITY
Memorandum of evidence to the Committee on the Age of Majority. *Br Med J* 1966; **i**, suppl: 118-19.

1976 WORKING GROUP ON ORAL CONTRACEPTIVES
(Summaries of BMA evidence.) *Br Med J* 1976; **i**: 1093-4; and *Br Med J* 1977; **i**: 1101.

1978 COMMITTEE ON OBSCENITY AND FILM CENSORSHIP
(Summary of BMA evidence.) *Br Med J* 1978; **i**: 1077.

1978 WORKING GROUP ON BACK PAIN
(Summary of BMA evidence.) *Br Med J* 1978; **i**: 1082.

1978 CRIMINAL LAW REVISION COMMITTEE
(Summary of BMA view on "mercy killing".) *Br Med J* 1978; **i**: 1082.

1979 INQUIRY INTO PERINATAL AND NEONATAL MORTALITY
Br Med J 1979; 7 April, Annual Report of Council, p 14.

Chapter 8

Publications

> There is a dead medical literature and there's a live one. The dead is not all ancient, the live is not all modern. There is none, modern or ancient, which, if it has no living value for the student, will not teach him something by its autopsy. — Oliver Wendell Holmes, *Medical Essays*, "Medical Literature."

Throughout its history the BMA has been closely connected with the publication of medical information.

The development of the BMA into a medical society of national and international standing was mirrored by the growth in status of its principal publication, the *British Medical Journal*, which by 1932 had become one of the leading medical journals in the world and one of the most widely read. In 1926 the BMA had widened the scope of its periodical publishing by issuing two journals devoted to special subjects, *Archives of Disease in Childhood* and *Journal of Neurology and Psychopathology*. Monograph publications had not been neglected, since BMA reports on medical and social matters of public concern had been published on many occasions, and had come to be regarded as pronouncements of considerable authority.

By 1932, therefore, much experience of medical publishing was already at the disposal of the BMA, an experience that was to stand the Association in good stead during the 50 years that lay ahead — when swift and complex developments in medical practice, coupled with a rapidly changing social, political and economic scene, would make medical publishing a more exacting business and, at the same time, a more hazardous one.

Throughout the period of this history the overall control of most of the BMA publishing activities was in the hands of the Journal Committee, whose duties and powers were defined in 1932 as "to consider and report to the Council upon matters connected with the *British Medical Journal*." The matters referred to included the two specialist journals and all miscellaneous printing undertaken for the Association.

Executive responsibility for the *British Medical Journal* and its associated publications lies with the Editor, whose duties are described by the Articles of Association thus: "The journal shall be conducted by a paid Editor who shall be responsible for all that appears therein, except such matters as are inserted in accordance with the regulations or by-laws or by direction of the Council. The Editor shall be appointed by and be subject to the control of the Council."

In 1932 the printing and advertisement department of the *British Medical Journal* was controlled by the Financial Secretary and Business Manager of the Association, Mr Leycester Ferris-Scott.

Considerable criticism of the administration of the journal began to make itself felt in the early 1930s. It was argued that the Journal Committee, meeting as it did only three or four times a year, could hardly be capable of managing the details of such a large business concern as the *British Medical Journal* had become. It was said also that the Financial Secretary of the BMA was already too overworked to carry the extra responsibility of being Business Manager of the journal.

In 1934 the Chairman of the Journal Committee, Sir Robert Bolam, established a subcommittee to consider "methods of improving the *British Medical Journal*." Sir Robert retired in 1935, but his successor as chairman, Dr R G Gordon, was equally determined to carry out reforms and gave firm support to the subcommittee, prominent among whose members were Professor R J A Berry and Dr Guy Dain. Its secretary was Dr Hugh Clegg, Deputy Editor of the journal, to whom the Editor, Dr Gerald Horner, gave a free hand.

In considering changes to the administrative structure of the journal the subcommittee took professional advice from Fleet Street on all aspects of newspaper and periodical publication, and its deliberations bore fruit in 1936 when a new form of administration for the journal was authorised by Council. This substantially reduced the powers of the Journal Committee, which was to remain in being and was to continue to direct general policy; in addition, however, there was to be a Board of Directors for the *British Medical Journal.* This was to be appointed by the Council and was to consist of five members, elected for a term of three years, who would be paid a fee of five guineas a year. The board was to meet at least 10 times a year and any member who failed to attend a minimum of six meetings would lose his seat. The function of the board was to control the business side of the production of the journal and other BMA publications. Its chairman, if not a member of the Journal Committee, had a duty to attend meetings of that committee to give account of the board's activities. In normal circumstances the Board of Directors was expected to report through the Journal Committee, but it was given the right of direct access to Council. The first Board of Directors took office in November 1936.

Early the following year the post of Financial Secretary and Business Manager of the Association was abolished. Henceforth responsibility for the business affairs of the *British Medical Journal* was divided between a Financial Secretary to the Board of Directors and an Advertisement Manager.

The Board of Directors met at monthly intervals until 1939, and continued to function during the early years of the war. After 1943, however, it ceased to exist and the way was left clear for the Journal Committee to resume its position as the sole BMA committee responsible for the *British Medical Journal* and its associated publications.

In 1951 Council appointed a firm of business consultants to investigate the publishing methods of the British Medical Association with a view to improving efficiency and effecting economy. The consultants presented their report to Council early in 1952 and this consolidated the constitutional position of the Journal Committee by recommending that it should continue in sole control of the *British Medical Journal* and its publishing activities, with the exception of *Family Doctor.* The report went further, however, by recommending the appointment of a business manager to promote by all possible means the publications of the BMA. This recommendation was accepted and the first Business

Manager, Mr Maurice Webb, was appointed in January 1953.

Administration of the publishing department was considerably eased in 1960 when it moved into offices in the new extension to BMA House in Burton Street. Improved storage accommodation became available, which enabled orders to be dealt with more quickly, and it became possible to undertake a long overdue replacement of obsolete equipment with modern addressing and accounting machines. Through such mechanisation the advertising and subscription procedures were made much more efficient.

In 1961 Mr C W Francis, who had been Advertisement Manager since 1937, died, and in October of the same year Mr R H L Russell, the Business Manager, resigned. The loss of these key figures confronted the Journal Committee with a difficult problem. After a careful review of all the circumstances, the committee decided on a thorough reorganisation of this part of the journal's work, a process that was carried out by the new General Manager, Mr C G A Parker, who took office in December 1961 and served the *Journal* in that capacity until 1977.

The revitalisation of the business side of the BMA's publishing department in the years following the second world war led naturally to a more vigorous promotion of the *British Medical Journal* and a consequent increase in circulation figures. In the matter of circulation it must be remembered that the figures for the *British Medical Journal* are somewhat misleading from the financial point of view because a copy is sent every week, free of charge, to each member of the BMA. This fact attracts a substantial income from advertising by pharmaceutical and medical equipment firms, but if the journal is to be financially viable it is vitally important for sales to non-members of the Association to be energetically encouraged. In the case of special journals and monograph publications such a policy is even more essential.

A sales drive to promote BMA publications by advertising was vigorously pursued both at home and abroad during the 1950s. The annual reports of the *British Medical Journal* throughout that period record a growing circulation in countries outside the United Kingdom. In 1956 a special effort was made to increase the sale of BMA periodicals in North America. In 1957 the Business Manager visited Scandinavia and Holland, calling on medical booksellers, subscription agents and university libraries.

The campaign was widened in the 1960s by the adoption of various methods designed to make the *British Medical Journal* more easily obtainable by overseas readers. In 1963 subscribers in Canada and the United States were offered an "air express" delivery service; for an inclusive subscription of $50 they received their copies of the journal by air freight within two or three days of publication. The air express service was a success and, by 1966, 150 copies were being sent to North America every week by this method. In January 1967 an edition of the *British Medical Journal* was launched in Australia, where it was printed from matrices flown from London; as a result of this process Australian readers could receive their copies within days of publication instead of suffering the sea-mail delay of six to eight weeks. The text in these copies was the unabridged British version, but the advertisements were of Australian origin. In the final event this particular venture did not attract the necessary support and it was brought to an end after two years.

In March 1971, the General Manager led a trade mission of professional and learned journal publishers to the United States. This was sponsored by the Government through the agency of the British National Export Council. Visiting New York, Chicago, and San Francisco, the mission achieved much in a country that is the world's largest market for academic journals. In January 1973 a further attempt was made to break into this region by the publication in North America of a monthly *Selections from the British Medical Journal.* This was aimed at the American and Canadian doctor by culling for him from the weekly *British Medical Journal* those articles that were judged best for his purposes. Although 4000 subscriptions were received for the *Selections,* the experiment failed and came to an end after a two-year trial.

The success of this continuing promotional campaign was reflected in a substantial growth in circulation figures and in financial receipts. The circulation of the *British Medical Journal* rose from 62 000 copies in 1946 to 89 284 in 1981; of the last number, 19 380 copies were supplied to non-member subscribers. The number of non-member subscriptions increased rapidly during the 1950s; between 1953 and 1960 there was a rise of 72% in such subscriptions in the United Kingdom and 57% in those from abroad. Between 1960 and 1981 there was a further rise of 128% in non-member subscriptions.

An impressive change has taken place in the financial position of the journal department during the 50 years since 1932, and one that is of fundamental importance to the BMA as a whole. The journal accounts for 1932 showed an excess of expenditure over income of £10 916 2s 8d and this sum had to be recouped from the subscription income of the BMA. In 1938 the deficit had risen to £19 162 5s 3d. Beginning in 1943 circumstances altered radically with the journal accounts in that year showing a credit balance of nearly £6000, which was transferred to the general funds of the Association. In the years since then, with few exceptions, the *British Medical Journal* and its associated publications have made profits on a scale that have gone far to make the journal a stabilising influence on BMA finances and a major factor in keeping the subscriptions of individual members at a reasonable level. In 1978 the profit had climbed to the high peak of £213 584, part of which was devoted to increasing the journal reserves to £½m, the remainder being transferred to the current account of the Association.

Such circulation and financial achievements, however, cannot be explained solely in terms of vigorous promotion. Only the quality of the actual product can provide the real explanation and it is time to turn attention to the history of that product, the *British Medical Journal.*

BRITISH MEDICAL JOURNAL

As the official journal of the BMA, the *British Medical Journal* has to walk a difficult editorial tightrope in its discharge of the two functions of the Association — promotion of the medical and allied sciences on the one hand, and maintenance of the honour and interests of the profession on the other. In seeking to fulfil the first function, the aim must be to supply members with a weekly periodical that provides a comprehensive review of progress in the science and practice of medicine. To fulfil the second function, since 1903 the journal has included a supplement to keep members informed of the course of the Association's business and of the way in which it has performed its duties as the chief medicopolitical organisation of the profession. Much of the material to be found in the supplement is of a kind that would not normally form part of any medical journal conducted as a purely commercial undertaking. Even for members of the BMA such material can sometimes make dull reading and, in general, it is of no interest at all to non-members who may be potential subscribers to the journal.

In 1932 the supplement was contained in a separate section of the *British Medical Journal*, stitched into the centre of each issue, with its own pagination and its own half-yearly indexes. The average number of pages devoted to it each week was 12 — against 50 for the scientific text. In the same year Council agreed that greater use should be made of the supplement to publicise the activities of the BMA; this was to be brought about by making more pages available for narrative of this kind at the expense of routine entries, such as notices of division and branch meetings, and by including more reports of BMA committee meetings. The Annual Report of Council for 1933-4 records a conscious effort on the part of the editorial and medical departments to co-operate in presenting the information in the supplement in a more readable form with appropriate comment.

Following the outbreak of war in 1939 the supplement stopped being a separate insert in the *British Medical Journal* and was incorporated at the end of each issue with its own pagination. It was used to give prominence week by week to war notices issued by the Central Medical War Committee and to publish information of importance to medical practitioners in time of war, such as the protection of practices and the treatment of air-raid casualties by insurance practitioners. In 1944 it was necessary, despite the rationing of paper, to enlarge several supplements to include articles, reports, and correspondence arising from the Government's White Paper on a National Health Service. The allocation of extra pages for this particular subject continued to pose problems in succeeding years and in 1945 it was necessary to make further space available for correspondence on the demobilisation and resettlement of medical officers serving with the Forces.

The important role of the supplement and the editorial problems associated with it led to it being the subject of debate at the 1951 annual meeting. The Winchester Division proposed that the supplement should be recast as a new weekly publication, under lay editorship, to deal with medicopolitical and non-scientific matters and that it should be issued with the *British Medical Journal.* In support of the motion it was argued that such a change was essential to improve the channels of information through which BMA policy could be made known to the profession and, if necessary, to the public. The motion was passed with the deletion of the phrase, "under lay editorship." In due course Council gave the matter its consideration with the help of a memorandum by the Editor and the views of the Journal Committee, and made its report to the 1952 annual meeting. In this it emphasised the need for the supplement as an "official gazette" to publicise all BMA matters which the Articles and Bylaws required to be recorded, together with other important activities of the Association. The likelihood that such material would sometimes make dull reading was freely admitted. The report also drew attention to the fact that much information of intense interest to BMA members had to be withheld from publication because it was the subject of confidential negotiations with the Ministry of Health. Despite such difficulties, every effort was being made to make the supplement more attractive. The prewar practice of including occasional signed articles by doctors from overseas describing their medical services under social security schemes had been resumed. Further proposals under consideration were the publication of articles on the organisation and work of BMA committees, articles on subjects taken from the correspondence columns, and regular notes on current events by the Secretary. In conclusion, Council rejected the motion by the 1951 annual meeting that the supplement should be recast as a new weekly publication.

The question of the supplement was raised again at the annual meeting of 1956, which passed a motion to the effect that it should be published either separately or in the prewar form of an insert in the *British Medical Journal.* It was also suggested that the supplement might be printed on paper of a different colour. As in 1952, Council refused to take any action on these proposals, this time on the grounds that separate publication would cost an extra £6000, and that the insert method would result in an objectionable division of the scientific text into two parts.

The format of the supplement remained unchanged throughout the 1960s, and in 1970 Council was able to record that the frequency with which its reports were quoted contradicted the popular impression that it was never read. One distinguished American observer had described the supplement as "a great journal of social medicine."

Renewed efforts were made to make it more attractive to the less politically committed doctor. Features such as "Backbench Comment," tape-recorded discussions on controversial topics, and the reporting of committee meetings in a less detailed way were introduced in 1973, and more emphasis was placed on essential debates and decisions. Several topical articles were published to provide guidance on the reorganisation of the National Health Service.

In July 1974 a major change in format was made when the pagination of the supplement was made continuous with that of the scientific section. It continued to have a separate cumulative index until January 1977, when it was merged with the index to the scientific section.

Further innovations were introduced into the supplement in 1976, including the weekly personal commentary by Scrutator, a monthly socioeconomic column entitled "Commentary," and signed articles in a "Talking Point" series. An improved layout was adopted which largely abolished the small-print, three-column, committee reports; those reports were shortened and decisions were given in readily readable "boxes."

The annual report of the *British Medical Journal* for 1976 outlined its policy for the supplement as seeking to reflect accurately, but in a readable way, all shades of opinion, and explaining why and how particular decisions were taken.

Turning from the supplement to the scientific text of the *British Medical Journal,* it is clear that this section also poses considerable problems in editorial selection. With membership of the BMA drawn from all branches of the profession, the material published in the journal must cover the whole range from general practice to individual specialties. Equally, if the journal is to attract subscriptions from a scientific readership outside the BMA, its contents must be of wide interest. A study of the contents of the journal over the past 50 years quickly shows that a great degree of versatility has been employed to achieve the right balance. This task has been made that much harder by the sheer volume of original papers which the *British Medical Journal* has always attracted; in 1935 no fewer than 1008 articles were submitted to the Editor, but space for only 544 could be found in the journal. Today, over 5000 articles a year are submitted and only 20% of these are accepted.

With the outbreak of war in 1939 the shortage of paper reduced the size of the journal, but—after an initial decline—the number of papers submitted for publication rose rapidly, and the desire of doctors to put on record a wide variety of new experiences in wartime was reflected in an increase in correspondence. Editorial policy, as announced in 1940, was to select and publish those manuscripts which had topical value relating to military medicine, surgery, hygiene, and administration. The aim was to provide doctors with information and guidance that would enhance their ability to serve the country.

During one of the most critical periods of the war, on 5 October 1940, the journal still found it possible to publish a centennial number to celebrate the 100th year of its continuous publication. That the spirit of innovation was not lacking in wartime was illustrated by the introduction in February 1943 of a new feature, "Any Questions," in which a selection of inquiries from readers were answered in the columns of the journal by expert contributors. This feature has retained its popularity ever since.

The postwar years brought no diminution in the variety and topicality of the contents of the *British Medical Journal.* The issue for 22 November 1947 celebrated the 90th birthday of Sir Charles Sherrington with a series of articles on the life and work of that great physiologist and humanist. In the same year the country suffered its first big epidemic of poliomyelitis and the journal kept doctors informed of the course of events and of modern knowledge of the epidemiology and treatment of the disease by promptly publishing articles written by acknowledged experts. On 7 January 1950 a special number of the *British Medical Journal* was devoted to the commemoration of "Fifty Years of Medicine." Many distinguished doctors contributed articles on the development of medicine and surgery during the first half of the century, and a special pictorial supplement contributed towards making this an outstanding issue.

Occasionally the Editor's choice of the contents of the *British Medical Journal* has been questioned. At the annual meeting in 1953 a motion from Eastbourne asked that the composition of the journal should be altered so that a minimum of one-third of the matter should be devoted to clinical subjects of interest to general practitioners. In support of the motion it was argued that recent clinical articles had become too complex and technical to be of interest to the average reader, being more suitable for publication in specialist journals. This argument was not accepted by the meeting, which decisively rejected the motion and thereby endorsed the principle of editorial freedom.

Editorial freedom to interpret BMA policy in leading articles can also be a source of controversy. This was evident at the 1956 annual meeting when the Winchester Division moved "that this Representative Body instructs the Council to take steps to ensure that leading articles in the *British Medical Journal* reflect the policy of the Association." The background to this motion was a leading article in the *British Medical Journal* for 7 April 1956 entitled "The Gold-Headed Cane," which criticised the Royal College of Physicians of London and was considered in some quarters to have endangered joint action by the college and the BMA in difficult negotiations with the Government. The BMA Council had debated the matter and dissociated itself from the article on the grounds that it had had no prior knowledge of it, and that it was entirely the responsibility of the Editor "according to the usual practice." After a full and impressive debate the annual representative meeting in July overwhelmingly defeated the Winchester motion and gave solid support to the Editor and to the principle of freedom for editorial expression in the journal.

1958 was a year particularly rich in fresh ideas. Two new series, "Today's Drugs" and "Drug Treatment of Disease," were designed to guide the practising physician through the bewildering maze of pharmaceutical remedies. In another feature several general practitioners in different parts of the country were invited to send in up-to-date, first-hand accounts of epidemics of influenza and measles. To complement these symposia on disease in general practice, there were clinicopathological conferences which reported discussions by hospital consultants on particular cases which had come to necropsy.

Beginning with the first issue in January 1963 a major rearrangement of the various sections in the journal was effected. The leading articles and annotations were moved from the middle to the front and the first page of text was modified to provide a narrow column of "pointers" to various sections which were thought to be of special interest. "Any Questions" was brought from the back of the journal to the middle, to be grouped with "Today's Drugs" and similar matter under the general heading of "Current Practice." "Today's Drugs," which had previously been a column of news on individual drugs, became a weekly authoritative article on drugs for different conditions and diseases. Dr Hugh Clegg introduced a lighter note into a somewhat serious journal by writing, under the pseudonym of Pertinax, an occasional commentary on current events entitled "Without Prejudice," which combined wit and piquancy in an entertaining mixture.

In January 1968, during the editorship of Dr Martin Ware, Lord Platt launched a successful series, "Personal View," which remains an integral part of the *British Medical Journal* today. Contributors write about their own interests and enthusiasms, the intention being that the flavour of the articles should be that of good conversation rather than formal writing.

With the advent of the 1970s greater emphasis was placed on postgraduate education. In January 1971 a new section, "Medical Practice," was introduced which combined features from the previous "Current Practice" and "Middle Articles." It brought together the journal's main contribution — outside the leading articles — to the continuing education of doctors, and was intended to deal with the practice as much as with the science of medicine "whether in the hospital, the health centre, or the home."

"Short Reports" and "Materia Non Medica" made their first appearance in 1975. The former were original articles limited to 600 words, with one table or figure and no more than five references. They proved extremely useful for reporting single cases, side-effects of drugs, and important negative results; they enabled the *British Medical Journal* to continue to publish its traditional complement of medical articles in a much restricted space. "Materia Non Medica," short articles by doctors about their non-medical pursuits, was an answer to the criticism that apart from "Personal View" no relaxing reading could be found in the pages of the *British Medical Journal.*

An unusual and imaginative departure from the normal practice of medical journalism took place in 1975 and 1976 when the journal under the editorship of Dr Stephen Lock sponsored a series of four seminars in London, Edinburgh, Birmingham and Dublin on the subject of speaking and writing in medicine. The discussions ranged over the whole subject of medical article refereeing, subediting, presenting data, speaking and lecturing, and the MD thesis. The seminars were forerunners of a series of similar events which have been organised by the *British Medical Journal.*

In 1976 an endeavour was made to infuse a lighter note into the news pages with "Views" by Minerva, a random collection of medical facts, events, and opinions. In 1977 the book review section was radically altered to become "Medicine and Books," in which the main aims were to consider books in a wider perspective, to list every book of medical interest which had been received for review, and to ask individual writers to describe their enthusiasms.

A major change in the scientific text of the *British Medical Journal* was made in January 1981, when two separate United Kingdom editions were introduced with the object of increasing editorial content and strengthening the journal's finances. Both editions have the same content, but in the "Practice Observed" edition eight pages of "Clinical Research" articles are in miniprint; in the "Clinical Research" edition a corresponding number of "Practice Observed" articles appear in miniprint. These two specialist sections, which are devoted to general practice and to clinical research, serve to broaden the *British Medical Journal*'s coverage as a general medical journal, while preserving the usual features in ordinary-size type. The advertisements are rearranged to suit the appropriate readership.

The development of the scientific text of the *British Medical Journal* between 1932 and 1981 has shown a refreshing and inventive approach to the problems of recording the changing face of medicine and adapting to the needs of its readers. But no account has yet been given of the important contribution to the advance of medicine which has been made by articles in the journal during this period. Some prime examples of such historic papers are given in the chronological list annexed to this chapter (Annex 1).

The story of the *British Medical Journal* from 1932 to 1981 would not be complete without an account of its physical production, which is an impressive record of imaginative design and of adaptation to external difficulties.

In 1932 the composition of the journal was carried out in a printing office in the north-east wing of BMA House. The subcommittee, which had been set up by Sir Robert Bolam in 1934 to consider ways of improving the *British Medical Journal,* examined the question of design and production and this led to a major change in 1937 when the composition department was disbanded. The whole process of composition, machining, and dispatch of the journal was entrusted to Messrs Eyre and Spottiswoode on a five-year contract. The disposal of machinery and equipment freed much-needed space for the expansion of editorial office accommodation.

Simultaneously with the change in production, the typography and layout of the journal itself were radically altered, starting with the issue of 2 January 1937. The new typeface used throughout the letterpress and title page had been chosen with the advice of the eminent typographer, Mr Stanley Morison, its sole objective being to make the *British Medical Journal* easier to read. Increased legibility was achieved by using a darker type and by adopting a design, recently created for *The Times,* that was simple and free from eccentricity. A distinctive change was also made to the front cover by using grey paper instead of white and by a new design that included a scarlet device, the work of Mr Eric Gill, which embodied the staff of Aesculapius. For the first time a list of the principal contents of each issue was printed on the front cover.

Production of the *British Medical Journal* was severely affected by the second world war, when supplies of paper were restricted. As early as 1940 smaller type was being used in various sections of the journal to compensate for the fact that less space was available. In May 1941 the three printing works of Eyre and Spottiswoode off Fetter Lane in London were demolished in an air-raid; temporary arrangements ensured that issues of the *British Medical Journal* were printed and published without a break and in July 1941 the work transferred on a permanent basis to the Gainsborough Press (Fisher Knight & Co) at St Albans. This lengthened the lines of communication and that fact, coupled with a change from printing by rapid rotary to flat-bed machines, made it necessary to advance the time of going to press. From 1942 onwards paper rationing became so severe that circulation of the journal outside the membership of the BMA had to be drastically curtailed and new subscriptions were refused.

The paper ration was increased in October 1946, but the fuel crisis of February 1947 created more critical conditions than those during the war. For the weeks ending 22 February and 1 March 1947 the *British Medical Journal*, together with all other weekly periodicals, was forbidden to print at all, an event unprecedented in its history. The ban on printing arose from an agreement between the Ministry of Fuel and Power and the Periodical Trade Press and Weekly Newspaper Proprietors' Association, a body which had refused membership to the *British Medical Journal* in 1938. The BMA refused to sit down under this arbitrary ban and discovered that it did not, in fact, have any force in law. With the wholehearted co-operation of the Secretary of the Association and of staff members, two "Pemmican" issues of the journal for 22 February and 1 March were produced and circulated in duplicated form.

A new hazard to the production of the *British Medical Journal* made its appearance in the 1950s — strikes by printers and by postal workers. Early in 1956 difficulties in the printing industry caused some delay in publication. Much more serious was the printing strike of 1959, which began on 19 June and lasted seven weeks. With the help of two non-union printers, the Editor and his staff were able to produce seven 64-page issues of the *British Medical Journal.* It was a period of strenuous activity for the staff, relays of whom worked in Committee Room C of BMA House rolling individual copies of the *British Medical Journal* into wrappers. Outside the main gates of BMA House could be seen pickets of strikers. The issue of the journal for 8

August 1959, the final one of the strike series, included a full account of how publication was maintained during the strike and of the efforts which were made to impress on the trade unions concerned the vital necessity for continuing to print the journal. Much later in the period of this history, in the spring of 1980, another printing strike caused serious disruption to issues of the *British Medical Journal* published between 10 April and 31 May. Although the size of issues was reduced and their dispatch delayed, all were published in due course.

The price of paper and postage has been a perennial problem for the BMA publishing department. For a brief spell during the early 1950s the price of paper fell and contributed a measure of stability to the journal's finances. By 1957, however, substantial increases in the cost of both paper and postage were being reported and, in 1958, a suitable paper, 10% lighter than the existing one, was adopted for the *British Medical Journal* as an economy measure. The possibility of distributing the journal by other means than through the post was investigated, but no practical alternative could be found. The new paper gave rise to a considerable number of complaints from readers to the extent that, in 1961, the use of a somewhat heavier one was resumed. In 1971, however, the high cost of postage led to the adoption of another light, high-quality, paper which reduced the average weight of a copy of the journal from 12 oz to 8 oz.

A series of alterations to the design and make-up of the journal were made during the 1960s and 1970s. At the beginning of 1964 the size and shape of the page was substantially changed, making it possible to give the contents of each issue in greater detail on the cover and to print sections of the text in three columns instead of two. After consulting typographical experts, the decision was taken to change *The Times* New Roman typeface, which had been adopted in 1937, to Plantin. In 1967 an attempt was made to help medical libraries by producing the *British Medical Journal* in four volumes a year. An index was provided for each quarterly volume and in addition a cumulative annual index was made available for purchase. This succeeded in reducing the size of individual volumes, but the experiment did not prove a success and the journal reverted to two volumes a year in 1976.

In January 1968 a new cover was introduced, the design of which retained the familiar hallmarks, but which made possible a more balanced prominence to the various sections of the journal. In that year also a contract for printing the *British Medical Journal* by web-offset was signed. This process began in January 1970, and not only reduced production costs but also allowed a higher quality of reproduction, the use of better paper, and greater speed of printing.

ABSTRACTING JOURNALS

One constituent section of the *British Medical Journal* which had existed back in 1932 and which has received no mention as yet was the *Epitome of Current Medical Literature.* The *Epitome,* which first became part of the journal in 1892, consisted of abstracts of articles chosen from a wide variety of medical journals and arranged under broad subject headings. It had some six pages in each issue of the *British Medical Journal* with its own pagination and its own half-yearly index.

This attempt to provide a reasonable survey of a growing world literature within such a small compass was not really a practical proposition and it finally broke down in 1938. From 2 July of that year the name of the *Epitome* was changed to *Key to Current Medical Literature,* in which the periodicals received were arranged in two groups — general and special. Under the title of each appeared a list of appropriate articles contained in it. Only selected articles were given abstracts, and these were short and factual and were intended merely as a guide to the article itself. The *Key* had only a brief existence; it ended on the outbreak of war in 1939, the final issue being published on 26 August.

In 1946 the *British Medical Journal* reported that it hoped to resume publication of the *Key* as part of a comprehensive abstracting service. In point of fact, it was an abstracting service without the *Key* that was inaugurated in January 1947, with the publication of the first monthly issues of *Abstracts of World Medicine* and *Abstracts of World Surgery Obstetrics and Gynaecology.* The articles abstracted in both journals were selected from the principal medical periodicals published in different parts of the world. The abstracts were classified under subject headings. For the most part they were "informative" in nature to provide the reader with a clear idea of the contents of each article, but shorter, "indicative" abstracts were also included. The first editor, Dr G W M Findlay, and his assistant, Dr S S B Gilder, had at their disposal a large panel of specialist abstracters. It was confidently hoped that both journals would provide a trustworthy guide through the complicated maze of a rapidly increasing periodical literature. By 1953 about 1700 periodicals were being received by the abstracting department.

Despite satisfactory circulation figures at the outset, an early setback came in June 1952, when *Abstracts of World Surgery Obstetrics and Gynaecology* ceased publication and surgical publications were henceforth included in *Abstracts of World Medicine.* This unhappy event was attributed not only to the unfavourable economic climate of the time but also to illness among the editorial staff and, in particular, to the death of the editor of *Abstracts,* Dr Findlay.

At the request of Council in 1957 the Journal Committee prepared a report on the position and future prospects of *Abstracts of World Medicine.* Opinions were sought from subscribers all over the world, the great majority of whom affirmed that the publication of this journal was a valuable service to medicine. Circulation had risen steadily since 1947 and the 1600 periodicals which were abstracted eventually found their way to the BMA Library and made a handsome contribution to its collection. These facts satisfied the Journal Committee that there was a need for this service and that no change of policy should be recommended. Council accepted this view.

In 1968 subscriptions to *Abstracts of World Medicine* reached the record figure of 2687. Out of 104 new subscriptions from the Commonwealth, 50 were the result of a trial arrangement whereby the Commonwealth Foundation purchased copies of *Abstracts* for distribution to selected medical libraries. Nevertheless, there was a persistent background of substantial financial loss; in 1968 this amounted to £16 288. In both 1968 and 1969 there were motions to the annual representative meetings calling for *Abstracts of World Medicine* to be discontinued on financial grounds. Both motions were lost and, in an attempt to remedy the position, the Journal committee raised the annual subscription to *Abstracts* from six guineas to £10 from January 1970. This move had the effect of keeping circulation figures steady, but it served only to postpone the evil day. The committee ultimately concluded that there was no possibility of keeping losses on *Abstracts of World Medicine* within acceptable bounds and publication was brought to an end in December 1971.

For 24 years *Abstracts* had played a most useful part, particularly in the underdeveloped world, in guiding individual doctors to important reports in medical publications. The harsh fact was that it could not survive in a world of adverse economic conditions, especially in the face of competition from highly automated, comprehensive abstracting services, such as that provided by *Excerpta Medica.*

SPECIAL JOURNALS

At the start of this chapter brief mention was made of the entry of the *British Medical Journal* into the sphere of special-subject journals with the publication of *Archives of Disease in Childhood* and *Journal of Neurology and Psychopathology.* Little further development occurred during the 1930s, but in the period during and immediately following the second world war the number of titles published under the aegis of the *British Medical Journal* grew to the extent that the BMA soon owned a medical publishing business that was one of the biggest in the world. The scale of the operation is well illustrated by the list of BMA special journals that have been published during the 50 years since 1932, which is annexed to this chapter (Annex 2).

In recent years the journal department of the BMA has undertaken to act as agent for the publication of a number of specialist journals on behalf of other medical or paramedical organisations. To carry out this function it became necessary for the journal department to register with the Registry of Business Names the publishing name of "Professional and Scientific Publications." The journals published in this way include: *Annals of the Royal College of Surgeons of England*; *British Dental Journal*; *Annals of Clinical Biochemistry*; and *Transactions of the Ophthalmological Societies of the United Kingdom.*

There can be no doubt that the reputation of British medicine has been enhanced, both at home and abroad, by the special journals published by the BMA and co-sponsored, as many of them are, by the appropriate national society for the specialty concerned. The fact that 10 of the titles have developed from quarterly to monthly or bimonthly publications is a reflection of the growth in the number of papers received for publication and of the high standing of those particular journals. This high standing has been achieved not only by the scientific content of the journals, but also by the superior quality shown in their production.

MONOGRAPHS

The publications of the BMA have not been confined to those in periodical form; monographs have also played their full part. During the 1930s several series of articles on different themes, which were originally printed in the *British Medical Journal* and which proved popular, were republished in book form. The first of these, *Treatment in General Practice*, was published in four volumes between 1936 and 1940 by H K Lewis & Co. This process of reissuing useful articles proved so successful that it has been repeated at regular intervals throughout the period since the second world war and the journal department itself has undertaken publication of all the items concerned. The titles, all of which were reprints of *British Medical Journal* articles, which have been issued since 1950, are annexed to this chapter (Annex 3).

Apart from volumes of collected articles, the journal department has also published monographs on particular subjects or designed for a particular class of reader.

To guide newly qualified doctors through the complexities of medical practice in Britain the BMA published *The Medical Practitioner's Handbook* in 1954. A revised edition was issued in 1958. Administrative, business, and legal problems were all covered, and a clear account of the structure of the National Health Service was provided.

Published advice from the BMA has also been extended to those who aspire to enter the medical profession. In 1951 *The BMA Handbook of Medical Scholarships* contained detailed information on financial assistance that could be obtained towards the cost of medical education. This was followed in 1962 by the first edition of *Becoming a Doctor*, a pamphlet that dealt comprehensively with every aspect of medical education. This proved so successful that five further editions have been published.

To help doctors seeking junior hospital appointments to choose those hospitals best suited to their needs, the first edition of *The Hospital Gazetteer* was published in 1960. In this, information was immediately available on whether a particular hospital was recognised or approved for the different postgraduate diplomas, together with many other useful facts about local conditions. Further editions of *The Hospital Gazetteer* appeared in 1967, 1969, and 1972.

In August 1953 the Editor of the *British Medical Journal* undertook the work of editing and producing the Proceedings of the First World Conference on Medical Education. In September 1962 the Third International Conference on Alcohol and Road Traffic took place in BMA House and the proceedings of the conference were published by the BMA.

A serious problem that has always faced editors and publishers of medical periodicals and books has been the lack of standardisation in the form of bibliographical references and of the abbreviations of periodical titles. During the period immediately after the second world war this question was the subject of attention from the UNESCO Co-ordinating Committee on Abstracting and Indexing in the Medical and Biological Sciences, the chairman of which was Dr Hugh Clegg, Editor of the *British Medical Journal.* As a result of the committee's deliberations, an international list of medicobiological periodicals, entitled *World Medical Periodicals* was published jointly by UNESCO and WHO in 1951. This work, which was based on a document that had been used in the office of the *British Medical Journal* for several years, was compiled by Mr L T Morton, Information Officer of the journal. It provided details of all current medical journals that had been traced and of further serials that had ceased publication between 1900 and 1950. The abbreviation given for each title was based on a modification of the system in the *World List of Scientific Periodicals.* In 1957, a second, enlarged, edition was published by the World Medical Association and a third edition came out in 1961, followed by a supplement in 1968. The editorial work on all these editions was carried out in the journal department of the BMA; the compiler of the third edition and of the supplement was Mr C H A Fleurent, Intelligence Officer to the *British Medical Journal.*

Consideration of the monograph publications of the BMA cannot be ended without mentioning two recent outstanding items. In 1969 *Trends in Clinical Pathology. Essays in Honour of Gordon Signy*, published by the BMA for the Association of Clinical Pathologists, was a festschrift volume presented to Dr Signy after 25 years as Editor of the *Journal of Clinical Pathology*. The essays provide a fascinating picture of developments in clinical pathology during the previous quarter of a century.

In 1977 *Remembering Henry*, edited by Stephen Lock and Heather Windle, was published by the BMA as a tribute to the memory of Dr Henry Miller, the eminent Newcastle neurologist, who had died on 25 August 1976. Dr Miller had been director of the BMA's Planning Unit from 1967 until 1970. Contributions from a cross-section of his friends and colleagues, together with reprints of three of his own papers, made this book a fitting tribute to the man.

FAMILY DOCTOR

The BMA has always been mindful of the fact that advances in the practice of medicine by the profession must be accompanied by adequate education of the general public in health matters. During the half century of this history, the Association has played a major part in health education with the publishing activities of *Family Doctor*.

The publication of a popular health journal by the BMA had been casually discussed before the war, but the first concrete proposal came from the Science Committee in January 1948. This was referred to the Journal Committee for consideration. After a detailed examination of existing health journals and of the financial implications of a BMA publication on that subject the proposal was endorsed by the Journal Committee. Council, at its meeting on 11 May 1949, approved the recommendation and, at the annual representative meeting in July 1949, it was argued that a monthly health journal would give the profession an opportunity to give public advice on healthy living in its broadest aspect, and that such a publication was best edited by a medical organisation with lay help, rather than by a lay organisation with medical help.

In 1950 Dr Harvey Flack was appointed editor of the new

popular health journal and the first number appeared on 20 March 1951 under the title of *Family Doctor.* The magazine was put on sale at newsagents and bookstalls and an appeal was made to general practitioners to draw it to the attention of their patients. This was the first time that the BMA had issued a periodical specifically for non-medical readers. It constituted a frank recognition by the Association that medicine had ceased to be a mystery and that there was a need to supply the public with trustworthy information on the subject. It set out to provide that information in the best possible way by being entertaining.

During its first year *Family Doctor* ran into considerable difficulty. The financial deficit on the first 10 issues amounted to £65 000, considerably more than had been estimated. The marketing of a journal on sale to the general public presented the journal department with problems never before experienced. As a solution to these problems *Family Doctor* was made independent of the *British Medical Journal* and its affairs were put in the hands of a special committee, the Family Doctor Committee, which was to be directly responsible to Council. This did not prevent six different motions being put to the annual representative meeting in 1952 to the effect that the magazine should be discontinued on the grounds that it served no useful purpose, that it was a drain on the BMA's finances, and that it was not part of the Association's function to educate the public. In the event, however, the motions were defeated and the principle behind the BMA's latest entry into health education was vindicated. By 1953 *Family Doctor* was beginning to break even financially and circulation had reached the half-million mark.

At the annual representative meeting of 1953 there was some criticism from the floor that advertisements in *Family Doctor* were encouraging self-medication with proprietary medicines, and a motion from Swansea was passed to the effect that advertisements for drugs of doubtful value should not be included. During the 12 months after the meeting prompt action was taken to exclude some advertisements that had previously been regarded as acceptable.

By 1954 *Family Doctor* was already beginning to exert considerable influence. An article by the late Sir Hugh Cairns on the value of crash helmets was quickly followed by a national newspaper campaign along the same lines. A decision by the tobacco manufacturers to make available the sum of £250 000 to aid research on lung cancer followed a clear suggestion first made to them in an article in *Family Doctor*. The British Broadcasting Corporation began to make increasing use of *Family Doctor* material in its home and overseas broadcasts, and the press throughout the world started to make regular purchases of articles for reproduction.

During 1953 the first *Family Doctor* pamphlets were published, including such titles as *Feeding Your Family, Having a Baby, Infectious Diseases,* and *Feeding in the First Two Years.* These pamphlets, priced at only 3d and 6d, were distributed widely to individual readers and in bulk quantities to the profession, particularly medical officers of health. They were an immediate success. In 1956 *Family Doctor* was able to report that over 100 000 copies had been sold and that 16 different booklets were in process of publication.

As *Family Doctor* did not possess the means to invest considerable sums to advertise itself, financial stability depended very largely on sales promotion. This was pursued aggressively and with imagination. In March 1954 a stand was arranged at the Ideal Home Exhibition and was visited by 60 000 people. The venture was repeated in 1955 when the stand represented a street of shops called "Family Doctor Street for Better Living."

The year 1956 marked the first appearance of the *Family Doctor* book, *Getting Married,* which offered guidance on all aspects of marriage. The first issue of 150 000 copies was sold out within a few weeks. Another publication, *You and Your Baby,* was made available, free of charge, to every general practitioner in the country and was re-edited, at the request of many medical officers, for distribution in clinics.

By 1957 *Family Doctor* was expanding overseas. In November copies went on sale in Canada and the same month saw the publication of the first issue of *New Zealand Family Doctor,* which was produced in co-operation with the New Zealand Branch of the BMA.

The 1950s were a period of consolidation, growth, and development to a high peak of achievement for *Family Doctor.* After the initial three years when it incurred financial losses, the magazine regularly made a small profit which was transferred to the general funds of the Association. Above all, it had attained its original goal of becoming a widely accepted, authoritative, voice in health education.

Towards the end of the decade, however, an event occurred which aroused considerable controversy. The fourth edition of *Getting Married,* which was published on 2 March 1959, contained in its text material which seemed to imply approval for extramarital sexual intercourse. As *Family Doctor* was published under the imprint of the BMA, it was considered in some quarters that the Association had given its approval to the notion that chastity was outdated. The outburst of protest that came from the membership of the BMA was so strong that the Chairman of Council, Dr Solomon Wand, gave instructions on 4 March that no further copies were to be issued pending an investigation by Council. On 25 March Council confirmed his action. It expressed regret for the offence given to sections of the public and of the medical profession and instructed the Family Doctor Committee to report on the position of *Family Doctor* and its associated publications from the standpoint of both policy and finance. At the annual representative meeting in July there was a wideranging discussion of the affair. The upshot was that the meeting agreed with Council in deploring the controversial section of *Getting Married* and it supported both Council and its Chairman in their action in suspending the offending issue. There was no further general issue of *Getting Married, 1959,* but its publication was resumed in 1960 and subsequent editions have appeared regularly without adverse criticism.

When, at the end of 1959, the Family Planning Association wished to insert an advertisement in *Family Doctor,* it is hardly surprising that the *Family Doctor* Committee was hesitant and asked Council for a decision. In the face of considerable criticism, particularly from *The Times,* Council rejected the advertisement. In so doing, it reaffirmed the policy whereby *Family Doctor* accepted only those advertisements which it thought appropriate.

During 1960 and 1961 *Family Doctor* carried out a long-planned move from BMA House to Family Doctor House in nearby Chalton Street. This enabled all editorial, business, and dispatch work to be brought together. Some £16 000 had been spent on bringing working conditions in the new building up to standard and in equipping the warehouse. This cost of conversion was met entirely from *Family Doctor*'s own earnings over three years and it was still possible, at the end of 1960, to transfer a surplus of £2289 to BMA funds. *Family Doctor*'s stay in Chalton Street lasted until 1977, when it moved back to BMA House.

In 1962 ethical problems arose for *Family Doctor* when a case came before the General Medical Council. This concerned articles in *Family Doctor* and *Getting Married* between 1952 and 1958 in which the complainant felt that the author of the articles had received an unethical degree of advertisement. In its verdict the General Medical Council found the defendant not guilty of infamous conduct, but was critical of *Family Doctor* policy in the matter, which, it suggested, should be reviewed. The resulting decision by the BMA Council was that medical contributors to *Family Doctor* should henceforth be described only by name, initial, and title.

By 1963 *Family Doctor* was so well established financially that Council felt justified in setting it a five-year target to repay to the general funds of the BMA the original launching capital from 1951 to 1953, of which some £33 000 was outstanding. In addition, it was instructed to set up an adequate contingency fund as an extra safeguard for the Association's finances.

Fresh controversy hit *Family Doctor* in November 1964 with the publication of *Doctors' Orders*, a 48-page booklet designed to educate families in the elementary principles of health. The booklet was issued without prior information to the profession in order to achieve an element of surprise that would attract maximum press coverage. Unfortunately, the resulting publicity was far from favourable; a considerable amount of adverse criticism came from BMA members who felt that the membership should have been consulted. One or two divisions were highly critical of the weight of advertising in *Doctors' Orders*, particularly that relating to the food industry. After a full debate in January 1965 the BMA Council gave its approval for the publication of a new edition of *Doctors' Orders* in November 1965, but, at a further meeting in February 1965, the Council had second thoughts and decided to defer the publication date until November 1966. Several motions to the annual representative meeting in 1965 urging that publication of *Doctors' Orders* should be abandoned altogether were defeated, but this only served to postpone the inevitable. The Annual Report of Council for 1965-6 contained the bald statement that "it has not been possible to create a second edition of *Doctors' Orders.*"

The problem over *Doctors' Orders* was only one item in an increasing number of difficulties that *Family Doctor* was facing in common with most other popular magazines. One of the main causes of this change for the worse was television, which could carry health education information in a more arresting way than the printed word. Sensible medical advice was also becoming a feature in many periodicals with a larger circulation in the home, particularly in women's journals. On 8 September 1966 Dr Harvey Flack, the Editor and the moving spirit of *Family Doctor* since its inception, died. The BMA Council regretfully came to the conclusion that *Family Doctor* magazine should be brought to an end with the issue for February 1967. At the same time Council decided to continue publication of *Family Doctor* pamphlets and booklets, and, in the years since 1967, these have worthily maintained the BMA policy of playing a full part in health education.

There was a brief sequel to the story of *Family Doctor* magazine. In 1971 the *Family Doctor* group co-operated with Thomson Publications Ltd to publish a health-education journal with the title of *You.* This was not a success and publication ended after only five issues, providing melancholy confirmation that the decision to close down the original *Family Doctor* had been correct from the point of view of finance. There are, however, many members of the public whose families derived great benefit from the magazine and who still regret its loss.

BMA NEWS REVIEW

A detailed account has already been given earlier in this chapter of the supplement to the *British Medical Journal* and its role in keeping the membership informed of developments in the BMA's domestic affairs. It became apparent in the years following the second world war that the supplement was not entirely adequate for this purpose. Certain BMA news, which was classified as confidential but would also be of considerable interest to members of the Association, could not be published through the medium of the supplement, contained as it was in the *British Medical Journal* and therefore on sale to the general public. Another factor was the style of the supplement, which was necessarily factual and rather dry; with the advent of competition from popular medical publications of the newspaper and magazine type, it became increasingly important for BMA news to be presented to members in an attractive and readable manner.

The first response to this need took the form of a personal letter from the Secretary of the Association. During the 1950s Dr Angus Macrae initiated a successful series of such letters to honorary secretaries of branches and divisions under the title *Between Ourselves.* His successor, Dr Derek Stevenson, continued and extended the scope of this link between headquarters and the periphery with a monthly printed letter entitled *Lines of Communication,* the first of which was sent out in January 1959. It was marked "confidential" and circulation was restricted to members of the Council and the Organisation Committee, branch officers, divisional officers, and members of executive committees. In that first issue Dr Stevenson described *Lines of Communication* as a monthly newsletter which would contain information on matters under discussion at headquarters — partly factual, partly explanatory, and "occasionally a peep into the future so that problems can be discussed in their early stages and before they actually arise." It would not include important items of news which were not available to or published in the supplement to the journal, but the restricted circulation of the newsletter and the confidential classification of its content would allow the Secretary to provide an informal slant to the news and to give his own views on problems as they arose.

Lines of Communication was issued regularly between January 1959 and September 1966, and performed a useful function. The only matter that was the subject of some disagreement during its lifetime was the restriction on its circulation. A motion to the representative meeting of 1959, which urged that it should be sent to all members of the BMA, was referred to Council and a compromise policy was adopted of sending to the whole profession the occasional issue devoted to matters of particular importance. In 1960 the representative meeting defeated by a large majority a motion that *Lines of Communication* should be discontinued because its circulation was too limited for it to be of any use. The representative meeting of 1961 also maintained the status quo by defeating two motions, one that *Lines of Communication* should be issued in duplicated form and sent out only when important news made it necessary, the second that it should be sent to all members of the Association.

Finally, the demand for a BMA newsletter with wider circulation and with popular appeal proved irresistible. In 1966 Council authorised the replacement of *Lines of Communication* with an entirely new publication, *BMA News*, which was to be sent to the whole profession, and the cost of which was to be largely offset by advertising revenue. It was planned to appear four times a year with two further numbers to be published during the year as an when they were needed. The first issue was published in October 1966, and contained a foreword by the Chairman of Council, Dr Ronald Gibson, in which he declared that *BMA News* had been established to ensure efficient communication between the BMA Council and doctors who were working in hospitals, consulting rooms, and offices. By furnishing accurate factual information it set out to create an informed membership with confidence in its leadership.

The representative meeting in 1967 discussed a motion that *BMA News* should be developed and published regularly as a professional medical newspaper. In support of the motion it was argued that the BMA needed such a publication to provide an authoritative answer to derogatory attacks on the Association that were appearing in "fringe" medical newspapers. The response from Council was sympathetic but cautious because of the extra cost, the possibility of overlap with the *British Medical Journal*, and the problems that might arise from the division of control between a professional editor and the Secretary. No action was taken on the 1967 motion, but it foreshadowed later developments.

In 1971 *BMA News* was being issued to about 73 000 members of the profession in the United Kingdom. In 1972 Sir Paul Chambers's "Report of an Inquiry into the Association's Constitution and Organisation" (see Chapter 9) recommended that the reporting of BMA matters, which were under the control of the Secretary, should be transferred from the *British Medical Journal* to an improved

BMA News in the administration of which the Secretary should be assisted by one or two full-time expert journalists. This recommendation was not fully implemented, inasmuch as BMA domestic affairs continued to be reported by both the supplement to the *British Medical Journal* and by *BMA News*, but professional journalists were soon introduced into the production of *BMA News*.

The representative meeting of 1972 discussed a motion that "*BMA News* be published weekly and be not required to rely entirely on advertising revenue for its finance." The principle behind the motion was largely accepted by the meeting and was carried as a reference to Council for consideration of the problems of carrying it out. Council's verdict was that, while it was neither desirable nor practical to issue *BMA News* on a weekly basis, the existing interval of two months or more between issues was too long to keep the profession properly informed. It proposed the inclusion in the *British Medical Journal* of a "Secretary's Page" on a two-monthly basis timed to appear in those months when a two-monthly *BMA News* would not be published. It also concluded that to secure a radical improvement in communications it was necessary for *BMA News* to be professionally produced. A lay journalist was appointed editor in January 1974.

In May 1975 the name was changed to *BMA News Review*, it became a monthly publication, and colour printing was introduced. The size of each issue was increased to 64 pages in October 1977, and to 80 pages in April 1978. The Annual Report of Council in 1977 commented on the popularity of the Association's "modern medicopolitical magazine" which had dealt with matters affecting all branches of the profession and had focused attention on the problems of several minority groups, including radiologists, pathologists, medical teachers and research workers, medical assistants, and occupational health doctors. Progress was made in financing the publication: by 1975 the costs of production were already being met out of revenue and only postage had to be met from BMA funds; by 1980 Council was able to report that *BMA News Review* had made a profit before tax of £21 715.

Some delicate problems over editorial control were ironed out in 1977, when Council appointed a small board, responsible to Council, to advise on all matters relevant to

BMA News Review. The Chairman of Council and the Treasurer were to be ex officio members of the board.

The successful development of *BMA News Review* is reflected in the words of the 1980-1 Annual Report of Council which described it as "now an important part of the policy to disseminate information in a short, easy-to-read, style to members and to make non-members aware of the advantages of membership."

EPILOGUE

In 1932 the publishing activities of the BMA were confined to the *British Medical Journal,* two special journals, and reports on topical subjects issued at irregular intervals. By 1981 the BMA had developed its publishing business to an extent that was undreamt of in 1932. Quality has not been sacrificed to quantity — the reputation of BMA publications stands as high in 1981 as it did in 1932. Some ventures, such as *Abstracts of World Medicine* and *Family Doctor* magazine, have had to be discontinued, but they must be ranked as gallant failures for they were designed to meet definite needs felt among the medical profession and by the general public. The financial growth and scientific success of BMA publishing has taken place during 50 years that have been marked by a world war and a steady deterioration in the British economy. It is an achievement of which Sir Charles Hastings would have been proud.

Annex 1. Historic Articles in the *British Medical Journal*, 1932-1964

1932 VASO-VAGAL SYNCOPE
Lewis T. A lecture on vaso-vagal syncope and the carotid sinus mechanism. *Br Med J* 1932; **i**: 873-6.

1932 FARMER'S LUNG
Campbell J M. Acute symptoms following work with hay. *Br Med J* 1932; **ii**: 1143-4.

1935 ACHRESTIC ANAEMIA
Wilkinson J F, Israëls M C G. Achrestic anaemia. *Br Med J* 1935; **i**: 139-43; 194-7.

1935 ERGOMETRINE
Dudley H W, Moir J C. The substance responsible for the traditional clinical effect of ergot. *Br Med J* 1935; **i**: 520-3.

1938 PRAECORDIAL LEADS
Praecordial leads in electrocardiography. A joint memorandum of a committee of the Cardiac Society of Great Britain and Ireland and the committee of the American Heart Association *Br Med J* 1938; **i**: 187.

1939 ADRENALINE
Gunn J A. The pharmacological actions and therapeutic uses of some compounds related to adrenaline. *Br Med J* 1939; **ii**: 155-60; 214-9.

1941 CRUSH SYNDROME
Bywaters E G, Beall D. Crush injuries with impairment of renal function. *Br Med J* 1941; **i**: 427-32.

1944 OESTROGEN THERAPY OF MAMMARY CANCER
Haddow A. Influence of synthetic oestrogens upon advanced malignant disease. *Br Med J* 1944; **ii**: 393-8.

1945 INVERSION OF THE UTERUS
O'Sullivan J V. Acute inversion of the uterus. *Br Med J* 1945; **ii**: 282-3.

1946 HISTORY OF TUBERCULOSIS
Hart M D'A. Chemotherapy of tuberculosis. Researches during the past 100 years. *Br Med J* 1946; **ii**: 805-10; 849-55.

1948 CHEMOTHERAPY OF HEART DISEASE
Christie R V. Penicillin in subacute bacterial endocarditis. *Br Med J* 1948; **i**: 1-4.

1948 MALARIA
Shortt H E. The pre-erythrocytic stage of mammalian malaria. *Br Med J* 1948; **i**: 192-4.

1948 CARDIOVASCULAR SURGERY
Brock R C. Pulmonary valvulotomy for the relief of congenital pulmonary stenosis. Report of three cases. *Br Med J* 1948; **i**: 1121-6.

1949 PERNICIOUS ANAEMIA
Ungly C C. Vitamin B_{12} in pernicious anaemia: parenteral administration. *Br Med J* 1949; **ii**: 1370-7.

1950 CLASSIFICATION OF CONGENITAL HEART DISEASE
Wood P H. Congenital heart disease. *Br Med J* 1950; **ii**: 639-45; 693-8.

1950 SMOKING AND LUNG CANCER
Doll R, Hill A B. Smoking and carcinoma of the lung. Preliminary report. *Br Med J* 1950; **ii**: 739-48.

1952 SMOKING AND LUNG CANCER
Doll R, Hill A B. A study of the aetiology of carcinoma of the lung. *Br Med J* 1952; **ii**: 1271-86.

1954 SMOKING AS A CAUSE OF DEATH
Doll R, Hill A B. The mortality of doctors in relation to their smoking habits: a preliminary report. *Br Med J* 1954; **i**: 1451-5.

1956 SMOKING AS A CAUSE OF DEATH
Doll R, Hill A B. Lung cancer and other causes of death in relation to smoking. A second report on the mortality of British doctors. *Br Med J* 1956; **ii**: 1071-81.

1964 SMOKING AS A CAUSE OF DEATH
Doll R, Hill A B. Mortality in relation to smoking: ten years' observations of British doctors. *Br Med J* 1964; **i**: 1399-1410; 1460-7.

Annex 2. Special Journals

1926- *Archives of Disease in Childhood.* Bi-monthly, 1932 to 1937; quarterly, 1938 to 1950; bi-monthly, 1951 to 1972; monthly, 1973 to date. Initially the BMA decided to issue a journal devoted to paediatrics, but after the second world war the *Archives* became linked with the British Paediatric Association and since 1977 it has been owned jointly by the two associations.

1926- *Journal of Neurology and Psychopathology.* Quarterly, 1932 to 1973; monthly, 1974 to date. In 1938 the title was changed to *Journal of Neurology and Psychiatry* and again, in 1944, to *Journal of Neurology, Neurosurgery, and Psychiatry.*

1939- *British Heart Journal.* Quarterly, 1939 to 1959; bi-monthly, 1960 to 1971; monthly, 1974 to date. This was launched by the BMA in 1939 as the official journal of the Cardiac Society of Great Britain and Ireland, which became the British Cardiac Society in 1946. In 1977 the BMA and the British Cardiac Society became joint owners.

1944- *British Journal of Industrial Medicine.* Quarterly, 1944 to date. Publication of journal devoted to industrial medicine was first suggested by the Association of Industrial Medical Officers. The first issue of *British Journal of Industrial Medicine* was published in January 1944 as joint venture of that association and the BMA.

1944- *Annals of the Rheumatic Diseases.* Quarterly, 1945 to 1962; bi-monthly, 1963 to date. The first three volumes of the *Annals,* issued between 1939 and 1943, were published by the Empire Rheumatism Council, but at the request of the Council the BMA assumed financial responsibility for its publication in 1944. It is now the official journal of the Heberden Society.

1946-67 *British Journal of Pharmacology and Chemotherapy.* Quarterly, 1946 to 1960; bi-monthly, 1961 to 1967. First published by the BMA in March 1946 with an editorial board appointed by the British Pharmacological Society. Publication was transferred to Macmillan (Journals) Limited at the end of 1967.

1946- *Thorax.* Quarterly, 1946 to 1960; bi-monthly, 1961 to date. First published by the BMA in March 1946 at the request of the Association for the Study of Diseases of the Chest, which became the Thoracic Society in 1948. Since 1977 the journal has been owned jointly by both organisations.

1947- *British Journal of Venereal Diseases.* Quarterly, 1947 to 1968; bi-monthly, 1969 to date. After being a publication of the Medical Society for the Study of Venereal Diseases since 1925, the ownership of the journal became vested in the BMA in 1947.

1947- *British Journal of Social Medicine.* Quarterly, 1947 to date. As early as 1944 the BMA Council had adopted a Journal Committee recommendation that a *British Journal of Social Medicine* should be published, but wartime paper restrictions delayed the appearance of the first issue until January 1947. In 1953 the title was changed to *British Journal of Preventive and Social Medicine* and in 1978 to *Journal of Epidemiology and Community Health.*

1947- *Journal of Clinical Pathology.* Quarterly, 1947 to 1957; bi-monthly, 1958 to 1969; nine issues a year, 1970 to 1971; monthly, 1972 to date. First published by the BMA in November 1947 as the official journal of the Association of Clinical Pathologists, the journal has been owned jointly by both associations since 1977.

1950- *British Journal of Ophthalmology.* Monthly, 1950 to date. In 1950 the BMA took over publication of the *British Journal of Ophthalmology* which had been in existence since 1917.

1950-74 *Ophthalmic Literature.* Seven issues a year, 1950 to 1953; bi-monthly, 1954 to 1974. *Ophthalmic Literature* is an abstracting periodical, publication of which was assumed by the BMA in 1950. It had been published by the *British Journal of Ophthalmology* since 1947. In 1975 responsibility for the publication of *Ophthalmic Literature* was transferred to the Institute of Ophthalmology.

1951-74 *Medical and Biological Illustration.* Quarterly, 1951 to 1974. Launched by the BMA in 1951 to publish information on the use of visual aids. In 1969 it became the official journal of the Institute of Medical and Biological Illustration. Publication was transferred to Longman Group Ltd in 1975.

1960- *Gut.* Quarterly, 1960 to 1963; bi-monthly, 1964 to 1968; monthly, 1969 to date. Published jointly by the BMA and the British Society of Gastroenterology at the latter's request in 1959, it has been owned jointly since 1977.

1964- *Journal of Medical Genetics.* Quarterly, 1964 to 1975; bi-monthly, 1976 to date. The first periodical in English to be devoted exclusively to the medical aspects of genetics.

1967- *Cardiovascular Research.* Quarterly, 1967 to 1971; bi-monthly, 1972 to 1977; monthly, 1978 to date. Founded in 1967 under the auspices of the BMA and the British Cardiac society to be a companion journal to the *British Heart Journal.* It was to include papers on basic or laboratory work, leaving the *British Heart Journal* to concentrate on the clinical side. Since 1977 it has been owned jointly by both organisations.

1966-75 *British Journal of Medical Education.* Quarterly, 1966 to 1975. Journal of the Association for the Study of Medical Education Publication was transferred to Blackwell Scientific Publications in 1976.

1970-75 *Psychological Medicine.* Quarterly, 1970 to 1975. Launched by the BMA in 1970 to publish papers on original research in clinical psychiatry and the basic sciences related to it. Publication was transferred to Cambridge University Press in 1976.

Annex 3.
Collected Reprints

1950 *Fifty Years of Medicine.*
1951 *Any Questions?* (1st Series).
1952 *Any Questions?* (2nd Series).
1952 *Refresher Course for General Practitioners,* First Collection.
1954 *Any Questions?* (3rd Series).
1954 *Refresher Course for General Practitioners,* Second Collection.
1955 *Clinical Pathology in General Practice.*
1956 *Refresher Course for General Practitioners,* Third Collection.
1957 *Emergencies in General Practice.*
1964 *Today's Drugs.*
1966 *Charles Hastings and Worcester, 1794-1866.*
1966 *Child Care.*
1966 *Health Centres and Group Practices.*
1966 *Obstetrics in General Practice.*
1967 *Is there an Alternative?*
1967 *Treatment of Common Skin Diseases.*
1968 *The New General Practice.*
1968 *Porphyria — a Royal Malady.*
1969 *Diseases of the Digestive System.*
1969 *Practical Psychiatry.*
1970 *Road Accidents and the Family Doctor.*
1970 *Joints and their Diseases.*
1970 *The New General Practice — II.*
1970 *Today's Drugs/1.*
1971 *Today's Drugs/2.*
1971 *Urinary Tract Disease.*
1972 *Gynaecology in General Practice.*
1972 *Problems of the Newborn.*
1972 *Progress Reports from Gut.*
1973 *Clinical Endocrinology.*
1973 *Emotional Problems in Childhood and Adolescence.*
1973 *Today's Drugs/3.*
1974 *Medicine in Old Age.*
1974 *Progress Reports from Gut.* Series 2.
1974 *A New Look at Infectious Diseases.*
1975 *Personal View: an Anthology.*
1975 *Surgery of Violence.*
1976 *Aspects of Sexual Medicine.*
1976 *Problems of Childhood.*
1976 *Statistics at Square One.*
1976 *Today's Treatment/1.*
1977 *Bone and Joint Diseases.*
1977 *Today's Treatment/2.*

1978 *Today's Treatment/3.*
1979 *ABC of Ophthalmology.*
1979 *Epidemiology for the Uninitiated.*
1979 *How to do it.*
1980 *The First Year of Life.*
1980 *Marital Pathology.*
1981 *ABC of Ear Nose and Throat.*
1981 *ABC of Hypertension.*
1981 *Procedurees in Practice.*

Chapter 9

Constitution

In any case, no one has ever claimed that the democratic process produces the *right* answer. It only claims to produce an answer acceptable to most people. — HRH Prince Philip, at BMA House on 28 October 1959.

The centenary history of the Association, by Ernest Muirhead Little, described the adoption of a new constitution in 1902, in which the Representative Body was created as the supreme policy-making organ of the Association. New local units were created — the divisions, so called because they approximated to the Parliamentary constituencies. The divisions elected the Representatives, while the branches (which still existed, and generally covered several divisions), elected most members of the Council. Thus the Association had two-chamber government, the two houses being elected (as in many federal constitutions, such as those of Australia and the USA) by different geographical constituencies of the same electorate. Sidney and Beatrice Webb described this as a complicated constitution but said that it included "all the devices of advanced democracy." By 1932 the Council included a large block of members (about one-third of the Council) elected by the Representative Body. Michael Foot called the BMA constitution "a democratic machine seemingly constructed by Dr Strabismus."*

The centenary history also described how in 1913 the BMA called the first annual conference of representatives of the local medical (and panel) committees, which had been set up by law to help administer the new Lloyd George scheme for national health insurance. The history also

* *Aneurin Bevan* by Michael Foot, Volume Two (Davis-Poynter, 1973).

described how the conference adopted the Insurance Acts Committee of the BMA as its executive, and how that committee was thenceforward representative both of the BMA and of the local medical committees, which were mainly composed of general practitioners participating in the Lloyd George scheme — not necessarily all of them being members of the BMA. Thus was born the curious concept of a BMA committee officially recognised as representing non-members of the Association as well as members, and enjoying some consequential autonomy.

In 1934 the Council became concerned about the position of consultants and specialists within the representative machinery of the Association, and decided to form a consultants and specialists group for England and Wales, another for Scotland, and a third for Ireland. Each group had a committee, and an annual meeting of group members was held in each hospital region, to which non-members could also be invited. The hospital regions were much the same regions as those later adopted for the National Health Service.

In 1947, in anticipation of the advent of the regional hospital boards under the National Health Service Act, the Council began to think of creating regional councils of the BMA. This idea was destined to be mooted again and again, but it never really caught on — except in those regions where there had always been a well-established branch of the BMA, such as the Northern Region. Here the North of England Branch had always been strong and active since its formation in 1864.

Back to the 1930s. In 1938 the Ophthalmic Group of the BMA was formed: perhaps the most important of all the special groups, because its committee has always been recognised by the Government as the negotiating body for the ophthalmic branch of the profession. In 1945 the Ophthalmic Group put forward a scheme for a national eye service. Other important groups — for example, the Psychological Medicine Group — were also formed in the 1930s.

REGIONALISATION

The first Scottish Secretary was appointed in 1919. In 1936 the Representative Body asked the Council to consider appointing a Welsh Secretary but the Council appointed instead a medical secretary for the Metropolitan Counties Branch, as a pilot scheme for strengthening the Association's peripheral organisation generally.

The Council stated in 1937 that it would "probably be necessary in the near future to develop a system of regional secretarial organisation to implement and stimulate the medicopolitical and other activities of the Association in the divisions and branches." Even so, 40 years were to elapse before this idea came to full fruition. In 1943 the Representative Body asked for full-time regional secretaries to be appointed as soon as possible after the war, and in 1945 the Council prepared to do this. Alarmed at the cost, however, the Council decided instead to enlarge the Head Office staff and to require the assistant secretaries at Head Office to spend about a third of their time in the regions — an arrangement which came to be known as the "parish priest" system.

In 1945 the Northern Ireland Committee was formed, and in due course became the Northern Ireland Council, like the Scottish Council (formed in 1957 from the much older Scottish Committee) and the Welsh Council (formed in 1968 from the Welsh Committee). Assistant secretaries were appointed for Northern Ireland in 1960 and for Wales in 1967.

Although the Council had jibbed at the suggestion of having regional medical secretaries throughout the UK, regional offices were soon established in each of the regions of the National Health Service in England — except for the metropolitan regions, which were served by Head Office. There had long been a fine Scottish office in Edinburgh, and this was supplemented by one in Glasgow. The Welsh House was opened in Cardiff in 1951, and the Northern Ireland House in Belfast in 1961. The national offices in Belfast, Cardiff, and Edinburgh carried a wide range of responsibilities, while the regional offices were mainly intended to provide a typing, duplicating, and circularising service for the honorary secretaries of BMA divisions and branches, and for the regional consultants and specialists committees. Each regional office was in the charge of a high-quality clerical officer (sometimes shared with the Medical Insurance Agency) who was entitled the regional officer. In 1949 a conference of regional officers was held at

BMA House, London, and this then became an annual event.

Not until 1977 did the Association finally decide to create a network of provincial medical secretaries and industrial relations officers throughout the country. This development was actuated by the report of a working party under the Chairman of the Representative Body (Dr A A Clark) which envisaged the appointment of "field organisers" who would be "immediately on the spot when trouble occurred and ... would be an immediate and ready source of help and advice on personal professional problems" to the individual member. This network is costly, but it is in a sense the BMA's equivalent of the breakdown service by AA patrols, which is undoubtedly the principal inducement to join the Automobile Association.

THE SEARCH FOR A JOINT PROFESSIONAL ORGANISATION

An important development in 1949 was the formation (on the initiative of the BMA) of a joint consultative committee of professional bodies. Those originally included were the BMA, the British Dental Association, the Law Society, the Bar Council, the Institute of Chartered Accountants in England and Wales, the Royal Institute of British Architects, and the Royal Institution of Chartered Surveyors. During the first postwar Labour Government, with its overwhelming Parliamentary majority, there was a feeling in the BMA that to face the massive rise in the power of organised labour and the growing influence of the Trades Union Congress, it would be wise for the professions to draw together and to create some joint organisation that could formulate and express the professional point of view on national questions. Professional workers tend to be individualists, however, and the professional societies and organisations had difficulty in finding enough common ground to make the formation of a joint professional body worth while. Nevertheless, this first effort by the BMA became a permanent fixture, but only in a very informal way: the secretaries of the participating organisations have continued to meet informally at regular intervals to discuss common problems and to dine together. In 1979, for example, they discussed radio and television programmes about the professions, incomes policy and the professions, collaboration between the professions in the countries of the EEC, and the question of professional judgment being brought under the scrutiny of the Ombudsman.

A second attempt was made by the BMA in 1952. A joint emergency committee of the professions was hastily formed to fight a determined attempt by the Durham County Council to impose a closed shop — compulsory union membership — on all its employees, including its doctors, nurses, and other professional staffs. The emergency committee was formed by the BMA with the British Dental Association, Engineers Guild, National Union of Teachers (whose General Secretary, Sir Ronald Gould, played a leading part), Royal College of Midwives, and Royal College of Nursing. After a long fight, ending in arbitration by the Industrial Court, the professions won their battle with Durham, but an attempt by the BMA to establish the joint committee on a permanent and wider basis came to nothing.

In 1960, following a motion on the subject at the ARM the previous year, the BMA convened a conference at BMA House to consider a proposal to form a confederation of professional associations. Of the professional organisations 25 were represented and some distinguished persons were present. After thorough debate, however, it became clear that there was no consensus in favour of a professional confederation, though everyone was in favour of ad hoc consultation between professions when the occasion arose, as had previously happened on the closed shop, on the question of securing tax relief on professional subscriptions, and on certain other matters. This attitude was disappointing to the BMA leaders, but the conference highlighted the great diversity of interests of the professional associations. They had different structures, some being qualification-granting, others learned societies, and others having protective functions; and also there were substantial differences in the distribution of the members of the professions between various types of employment — Government, local authority, industry, and private practice.

In later years further attempts were made by others — Sir Frederick Catherwood, for example, when he was Chairman of the British Institute of Management, and Sir David Napley, former President of the Law Society — to promote some kind of joint professional organisation, and the BMA has been invited to take part in all these enterprises. But at the moment of writing the formation of a joint professional body, as a counterpart to the Trades Union Congress and the Confederation of British Industry, still seems to be far away. Perhaps the best prospect lies in a body formed in 1978 — the Managerial, Professional and Staffs Liaison Group, in which the present BMA Secretary, Dr John Havard, has played a leading part. This body has recently obtained Government recognition as the federation representing politically independent, professional, and managerial trade unions.

ANXIETIES ABOUT THE BMA'S CONSTITUTION

Soon after the inauguration of the National Health Service dissatisfaction with the Council of the BMA erupted and the criticism was made that it was out of touch with the membership. There was also criticism of the conduct of business at representative meetings. In August 1948 the Winchester Division, activated by some young doctors who were destined to reach great positions in the Association, such as Dr (later Sir) Ronald Gibson and Mr H H Langston, circulated a memorandum that caused a considerable stir. The nub of the argument was that the Council had eventually led the profession into the NHS because it was out of touch with the feelings of the membership at large. The Council considered these complaints and reported that "many of the existing electoral areas are too extensive to allow members of Council to have effective contact with their constituents, and that what is needed is the division of the country into more compact electoral areas. . . ." So the number of members of Council directly elected by the membership at large in the United Kingdom was nearly doubled (from 22 to 40), and the number of members of Council elected by the Representative Body was nearly halved (from 20 to 13). There were some other smaller changes, and the size of the Council was increased from 66 to 77.

Dissatisfaction with the Council was not the only problem, however. At the special representative meeting which made these changes, in March 1950, the Winchester Division moved: "That the Representative Body is dis-

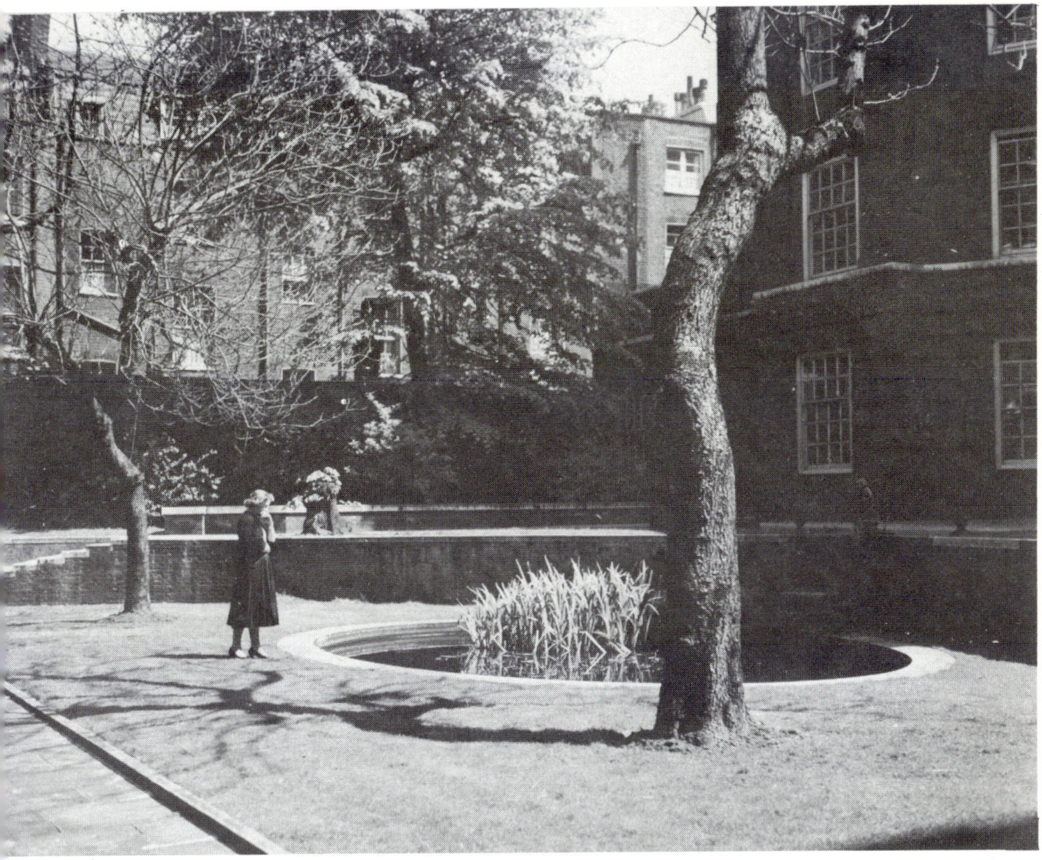

NCE CHARLES DICKENS'S GARDEN: THE GARDEN COURT AT BMA HOUSE WITH THE NUFFIELD LIBRARY ON THE RIGHT.

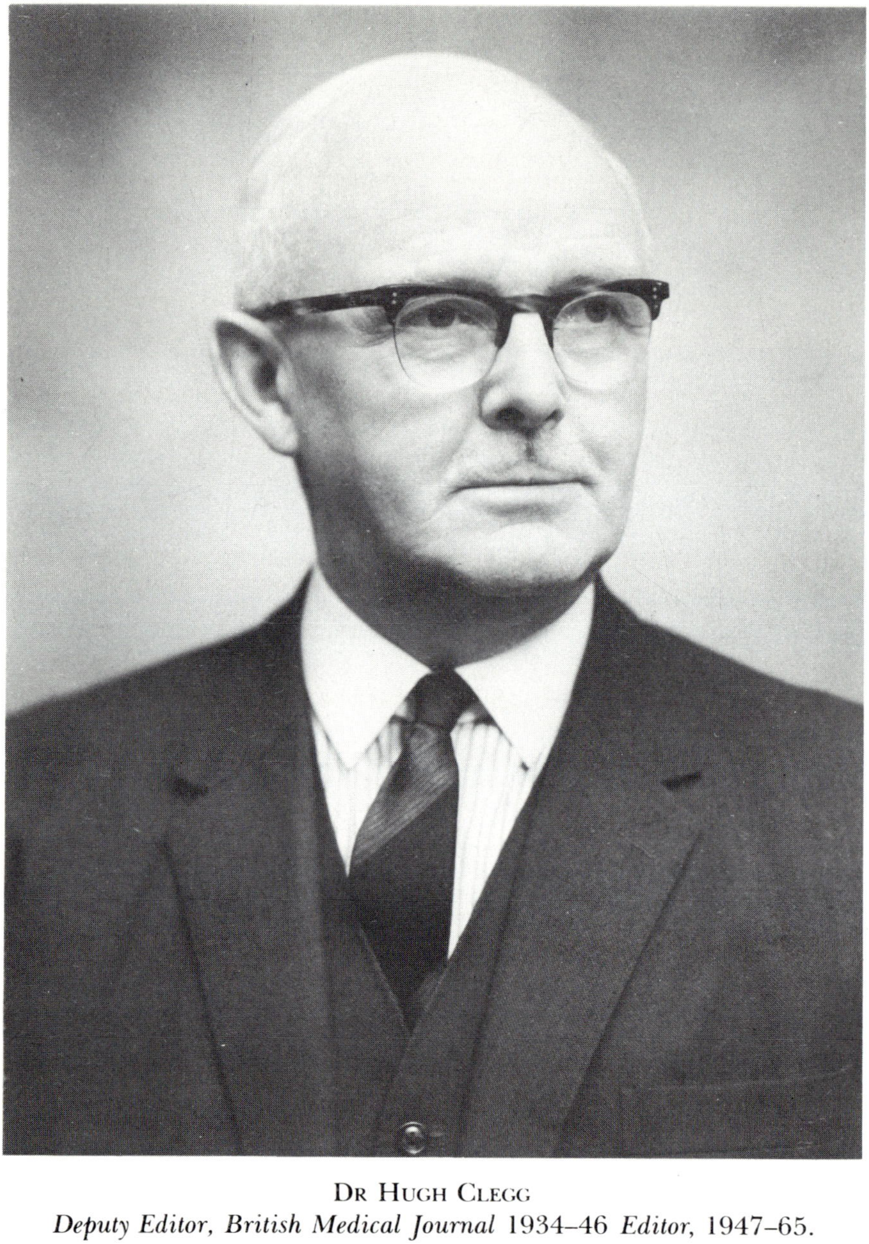

Dr Hugh Clegg
Deputy Editor, British Medical Journal 1934–46 *Editor*, 1947–65.
(*Bassano and Van Dyk*)

satisfied with the present indefinite relationship of the Autonomous Bodies to the Association and instructs Council to prepare a statement for presentation to the next ARM defining its relationship to these bodies." This was evidence of disquiet which was felt in more quarters than just the Winchester Division. The "autonomous bodies" were the General Medical Services Committee (successor to the Insurance Acts Committee) and the Central Consultants and Specialists Committee, which had full powers to determine policy and action within their own fields (general practice and hospital practice) and were not subject, within those fields, to approval by the Council or by the Representative Body. Lord Horder said that the existence of autonomous bodies had been viewed by many Representatives with considerable anxiety. Both the profession and the public looked to the Association — not to any committee of the Association — to represent the considered views of doctors in the United Kingdom.

The Chairman of Council (Dr E A Gregg) and the Chairman of the General Medical Services Committee (Dr S Wand) made a spirited defence of "autonomy," explaining that it was a device, conceived by Sir Henry Brackenbury, by which a BMA committee (the old Insurance Acts Committee) had been recognised by the authorities as representing all panel practitioners, even though some of them were not members of the BMA. In the end the meeting omitted the first part of the Winchester motion and passed the second, asking Council to define its relationship to the autonomous bodies. The Council appointed a special committee, but meanwhile the ARM 1950 laid down that the autonomous powers of these bodies should require to be specifically renewed each year.

The Representative Body continued to campaign against autonomy, resolving in 1951 "that in the light of recent events, the obvious disadvantages which have accrued from the autonomy of certain Standing Committees of the Association have created situations which are detrimental to the interests of the profession. . . ." But the Council did not agree. In April 1952 it reported: "In spite of any dangers which may be inherent in an arrangement of the kind now in operation, the effect of this arrangement has been to secure a measure of unity within the profession in putting forward its view which could not have been achieved under any rigid constitutional position. . . . In the view of the Council the advantages of the present arrangement far outweigh any disadvantages."

The agitation against "autonomy" grumbled on. The autonomous powers of the General Medical Services Committee and of the Central Consultants and Specialists Committee were renewed annually by the ARM, and the renewal resolution always stated that "the Representative Body looks to these Committees to ensure (*1*) that no action is taken by either which may prejudice the interests of another part of the profession without full prior consultation with the appropriate interests, and (*2*) that their autonomous powers will be used so as to expedite and not to delay the work of the Association." But many thought that this was an empty formula. In May 1953 Dr Ronald Gibson of Winchester wrote a long and important letter to the *BMJ* calling for the appointment of a constitution committee, primarily to reform and strengthen the Representative Body vis-à-vis the autonomous bodies. In a later letter, Dr R Hale-White of St Marylebone wrote: "It is a most regrettable fact that the RB is no longer the parliament of the Association. . . . Autonomous bodies and unity cannot exist together. The first step therefore will be to devise a form of Representative Body that will render autonomy of committees as unnecessary as it is undesirable."

THE SECOND CONSTITUTION COMMITTEE

And so, exactly 51 years after the great reconstitution of 1902, the ARM 1953 decided that a constitution committee should be appointed, composed half of Council members and half of others. The Chairman was Mr H H Langston of Winchester. Its terms of reference were: "To examine and report on the present structure and constitution of the Association with special reference to the reorganisation of the Representative Body." The committee was invited to "review the changes which have occurred during the last 50 years and the problems created by the enormous increase in the membership of the Association and the great increase in the association of the State with the provision of medical services for the community."

The report of the Constitution Committee filled 20 pages of the *BMJ* of 23 February 1957. The committee said that it had been impressed "by the essential soundness of a structure which, designed half a century ago, has served its purpose well and has withstood two major political crises affecting the basic principles of medical practice; the disruptive effect of two world wars; and the less dramatic but equally important gradual extension of the State's responsibility for health and welfare." This was certainly no mean achievement, and was a great tribute to the first Constitution Committee which devised the constitution of 1902.

The main conclusions of the second Constitution Committee were as follows.

(*a*) That the division should remain the basic unit of the Association's constitution.

(*b*) That the second tier unit — the branch — should be realigned with NHS regions — that is, branch areas should as far as possible be conterminous with those of the regional hospital boards; and that the branch council should be the representative organ of the profession in the region.

(*c*) That the Representative Body should be reduced in size ("in order to secure maximum efficiency in the conduct of business") from 500 to 350 members, by imposing restrictions on the number of Representatives that the larger divisions could appoint. No change was proposed in the existing system that the divisions were the constituencies for the election of the Representatives, except for small special representation of Public Health Service members; but it was recommended that four Representatives should be added from the Central Consultants and Specialists Committee.

(*d*) That the ARM Agenda Committee should be given power to "composite" motions, and to select motions for priority debate.

(*e*) That the Association should hold a second annual scientific meeting — short, concentrated, and of high professional standing — in smaller centres.

(*f*) That as regards the Council, the existing (post-1949) constitution was satisfactory.

(*g*) That the Scottish Committee (created in 1903) be renamed the Scottish Council, to increase the prestige of the Association in Scotland.

(*h*) That existing practice, under which the autonomy of the General Medical Services Committee and the Central Consultants and Specialists Committee was subject to annual renewal by the Representative Body, provided a sufficient safeguard against divided counsels and disunity in matters of policy in the profession, and should be continued.

(*i*) That the partnership between the Royal Colleges and the Association in joint negotiating machinery in respect of the hospital services (the Joint Consultants Committee) should continue.

The Constitution Committee did not recommend the creation of any new committee to represent the younger members of the profession, but before long the Registrars Group was reconstituted in order to represent all grades of hospital junior staff up to and including senior registrars, and was renamed the Hospital Junior Staffs Group. The regional registrars groups were renamed hospital junior staffs regional groups. And in 1958 the Junior Members Forum was created, an annual meeting of young (unestablished) doctors, which was also attended by the leaders of the Association. This became a permanent feature of the BMA constitution and in 1961 its chairman was made a member *ex officio* of the Council.

The ARM 1957 accepted most of the recommendations of the Constitution Committee, but rejected two of the most important. It rejected the proposed realignment of branches to fit NHS regions, with the conferment of regional functions on the branch councils. This rejection illustrated two strong traits in the BMA character: firstly, a strong attachment to the old branch structure dating from the earliest infancy of the Association (the first branch was formed in 1835); and, secondly, a deep suspicion of the idea of the BMA conducting medicopolitical functions at regional level. This suspicion probably arose from a feeling that any medicopolitical activities at regional level might be dominated by hospital interests, and this would not be congenial to the other branches of the profession.

The second main proposal of the Constitution Committee which was rejected by the RB was that its own size should be reduced. Here again is another strong thread in the BMA's history: a marked reluctance by the supreme decision-making organ — the Representative Body — to undergo any slimming cure. Part of the explanation of this is probably the crude one — that most Representatives enjoy a week away from home, with some exciting debates and agreeable entertainments, and with part of their expenses paid. But the real explanation lies deeper, in a strong feeling that the Representative Body should be a true "parliament of the Association" with room for the representation of all areas and all sections of the profession.

In the first Council debate on the Constitution Committee's report, Dr O C Carter of Bournemouth put it thus: "The most grievous thing of all is the suggestion to cut down the size of the Representative Body. I am sure such a measure would discourage interest and many people would feel that the Representative Body would be composed of a caucus and new people would not come in."

In 1961, in one of its recurrent economy campaigns, the Council created an important new committee, the General Purposes Committee. This took the place of seven committees (the Office, Staffing, Financial Advisory, Estates, Catering, Legal Actions, and Parliamentary Elections committees). The General Purposes Committee immediately became one of the most influential committees of the Association.

Complaints increased about the conduct of business at the ARM. So many criticisms were received after the ARM at Sheffield in 1961 that the Organisation Committee decided to make a "searching inquiry into the causes of the growing frustration at this and earlier meetings and to suggest possible remedies." The report of this inquiry was published in April 1962. Mindful of the fate of the Constitution Committee's proposal in 1957, the report said that "the Council has not seen fit to recommend that the size of the Representative Body should be reduced." The Council also reported that: "Divisions should retain the right to submit to the Representative Body motions on any matters which they consider of sufficient importance for debate." Having thus tied its hands with two ropes, the Council could make only relatively minor proposals for streamlining the conduct of the ARM. They introduced the system of "accepted motions." These were motions which reaffirmed existing policy or were self-evident or otherwise non-controversial; they were marked "A" in the agenda, and were not normally debated. The Council also gave encouragement to the Agenda Committee to make much more use of the "priority motion" procedure. Such motions were marked "P" in the agenda and were given preferential positions in the timetable. Thirdly, the Council proposed to alter the timing of the publication of its annual report, to avoid the necessity for a supplementary report. Fourthly, it was decided to hold the ARM within the span of one week (instead of extending over a weekend). These changes, though relatively minor, have stood the test of time and have certainly helped to make the ARM more manageable.

Anxiety about the Association's constitution kept rising to the surface. In its annual report in 1964, Council said: "In 1957 the Constitution Committee made suggestions for reform to the Representative Body, but some of its major recommendations were not adopted. The Council is convinced that there must now be a searching re-examination of the whole structure of the Association, and it has appointed a small committee to do this." The report was appended to the Annual Report of Council published in May 1966, and was discussed and amended by the ARM that year. The Council then instructed the Organisation Committee to revise the report, adding some further suggestions of its own.

The revised report on the constitution of the British Medical Association was published on 26 November 1966. It was a complicated document, but contained some important general statements.

> During the past few years, there has been growing unrest both about the unwieldy constitution of the Association and the increasing difficulty of co-ordinating the work of different sections of the profession.
>
> The Association's structure was reviewed by a special Committee in 1953-7, but the radical proposals of the Committee received little support. There has therefore been no essential change in the constitution of the Association itself, which apart from a few minor amendments has remained unaltered since 1903.
>
> The Representative Body, though democratically elected, is not numerically representative of the various branches of the profession.
>
> The Representative Body must remain the governing body of the Association, and the problem therefore is to resolve the apparent conflict between the sovereignty of the Representative Body and the independence of the autonomous bodies.
>
> The criterion which decides the size of the Representative Body was laid down more than 60 years ago. . . . The growth of the Association's membership has resulted in a steady upward progression in the size of the Representative Body.
>
> A new Representative Body should, we believe, satisfy two criteria: (*a*) fair geographical representation; (*b*) fair proportionate representation as between the sections of the profession. In meeting these criteria it is, we believe, essential to achieve some reduction in the size of the Representative Body.

And, with regard to the Council:

> Basically, many of the problems arise from the fact that it has never been clear whether the Council is acting as an executive body administering the affairs of the Association according to the instructions of the Representative Body, or whether it is a second debating assembly.

The ARM 1967 debated (and rejected) a motion that an independent firm of management consultants should be engaged to examine the structure of the BMA. The meeting also debated (and rejected) a motion that the published report on the constitution of the British Medical Association should be referred back to the Council. This was moved by the East Yorkshire Branch which (like the Winchester Division in 1948) had made a special study of the subject and had produced a rival set of proposals. Although the reference back was defeated, the ARM agreed that the East Yorkshire memorandum should be referred to Council "for consideration and report back at the ARM 1968."

In its next annual report, the Council put forward yet another set of proposals for amendment of the constitution of the Association. This time the Council recommended a much smaller Council (not more than 50), mostly elected by the Representative Body. The Council also recommended that all committees should be appointed by the Council. Finally, the Council recommended a reduction in the size of the Representative Body to 300.

These proposals were discussed at the ARM in 1968 at Eastbourne. In a series of tangled debates, several of the Council's proposals were torn to shreds by the Representative Body. The meeting decided that the Council should not be the executive of the RB, but should continue to be elected largely by the members of the Association, grouped in geographical constituencies. The ARM also rejected the proposal that all the members of the standing committees should be appointed by the Council, and finally rejected the proposal that the size of the RB should be reduced.

In one of the debates Dr Harry Fidler (of Bradford) remarked that the constitution was now changed every year. If the pattern of the preceding years was followed there would be four constitutions in four years. It was indeed becoming clear to all that the repeated reviews of the constitution in the years 1953-68, with the plethora of widely different proposals for amendment and the constant power struggle between the Representative Body, the Council, and the autonomous committees, were signs of a deep-seated malaise. The BMA leaders began to think that a consultant should be called in — from outside the profession.

But not all was gloom: 1967 saw a great increase in the representation of hospital junior staff, partly in response to agitation by a militant pressure group, the Junior Hospital Doctors Association (see Chapter 10). The Hospital Junior Staffs Group Council was enlarged to include 50 representatives from the regions, and participation in the affairs of the group was made open to all hospital junior staff, whether members of the BMA or not. For the first time, the Representative Body in 1968 reflected the composition of the profession, and it was noted that the big block of hospital doctors had taken a prominent part in the debates.

THE CHAMBERS SAGA

In 1970 the General Purposes Committee considered the possibility of a working group to deal with the "relationship between the members, the Representative Body, and the Council," but came to the conclusion that whoever served on such a group would look at the matter subjectively, since they would be members of the Association. So the Chairman of Council (Dr Ronald Gibson) told the Council on 1 April 1970 that the General Purposes Committee thought it would be better, as a first step, "to consult an expert in the matter." In due course the Representative Body endorsed this idea, and after considering a number of possible candidates for the job, Sir Paul Chambers was approached and accepted the invitation to undertake an independent review of the Association's constitution.

Sir Paul Chambers was Chairman of the Royal Insurance Group of companies, and had been Chairman of Britain's biggest manufacturing company, Imperial Chemical Industries. He was 67, and had had a brilliant career in high finance (he was the inventor of the PAYE system of taxation) and in big business. Here indeed was a highly intelligent and completely independent pair of eyes to put the BMA constitution under the microscope.

Sir Paul Chambers studied the earlier reviews of the

BMA constitution, but came to the conclusion that they were not very relevant to his inquiry. (This may have been his first mistake.) He attended meetings of the Representative Body, the Council, the autonomous bodies, and other committees. He had discussions with chairmen, and with rank-and-file members of the profession, including non-members of the BMA. He studied the constitutions of other bodies, such as the Royal Colleges, the Law Society, and the Institute of Chartered Accountants (but not any of the great trade unions). He conducted his inquiry alone, but he requested and received from the staff of the Association what he described as "an endless stream of facts and figures."

Sir Paul Chambers completed his report in 1972, and it occupied 23 pages of the *BMJ* of 6 May 1972. It was destined to cause a cataclysm within the BMA: three special working parties, eight Council meetings, four representative meetings, and three years of heated controversy. At the end of the battle, some of its most important recommendations were rejected.

Sir Paul's diagnosis of the faults of the existing BMA constitution was brilliant: but his recommended treatment was so drastic that many sincere observers feared it would lead to the death of the patient before effecting a cure.

Here are some of the salient passages in the Chambers Report*:

> The weaknesses in the organisation arise from the desire to have a democratic constitution and . . . members as a whole prefer to live with the weaknesses in order to retain democratic control. In my view the most serious faults can be attributed not to the maintenance of democratic control but to the deviation from the principles of simple democratic control with adequate delegation of powers to subordinate bodies.
>
> The reasons for the vesting of quite explicit *and detailed control* in the Representative Body of the BMA are historical. The Council was originally the body to which members delegated powers to act on behalf of the Association. Unfortunately, members became very dissatisfied with the Council's performance towards the end of the nineteenth century and were determined to put things right. In my judgment the action they took then was wrong and this is one of the factors which have bedevilled the organisation and the efficiency of the BMA ever since. Instead of making a radical

* Wherever italics are used, they were used by Sir Paul Chambers.

change in membership of the Council itself and giving the new Council fresh and clear policy directives, it vested detailed and overriding powers in a new body, the Representative Body, *without effective rules for delegation of any of those powers to the Council, and it retained the Council as a body democratically elected by the members instead of leaving it to be appointed by the Representative Body as its (the Representative Body's) executive instrument*.... Thus, because of actions taken many years ago, the BMA now has *two* bodies, the Representative Body and the Council, with conflicting and overlapping functions, and both of these bodies are for the most part directly elected democratically ... what is at fault is the present form of duplicated democratic control, without proper delegation of executive action, which has been developed over many years.

Under the BMA's system the membership as a whole appoints members to a large Representative Body and *also* elects members of a large Council so that the latter (the Council) is in one sense the executive body of the Representative Body but in another sense, as it is not elected by the Representative Body, it is not the instrument *chosen by the Representative Body* to carry out its wishes but is another democratically elected debating chamber responsible also to those who elected it. This system is peculiar to the BMA and is a further cause of confusion preventing the necessary delegation of powers to decide and to act without reference back where the matter is both urgent and important.

Thus Chambers had correctly detected that the BMA had an elected House of Commons (the RB) and an elected upper House (the Council), but no Cabinet. He also drew attention to the curious attitude of the BMA to non-members.

The Law Society which has a membership of about 80% of the solicitors of the country is not only recognised as speaking for all solicitors — non-members as well as members — but also has certain rights of discipline over non-members as well as over members and rights to agree certain fee scales with the authorities concerned which are binding on non-members as well as members. Yet the Law Society does not allow non-members to play any part in its organisation, in its election to committees, or in its decision-making. There is thus no good reason for the BMA practice of giving doctors who choose not to join the BMA the right to take part in the election of members of BMA committees.

Sir Paul Chambers enunciated some general principles, two of which were not to everyone's taste.

> Then there must be an assumption that the Association intends to co-operate wholeheartedly with the Government in the task of making the National Health Service successful.
>
> A principle which is evident from the election arrangements proposed is that junior doctors throughout the profession are given equality not only of voting rights but also of representation throughout the organisation.

When he came to his proposed remedies, Chambers suggested that the boundaries of the BMA's local units should be aligned with those of the NHS districts, areas, and regions. He suggested a BMA area council in each area, and a regional co-ordinating committee of the BMA in each region. He also proposed to abolish the existing branch system. So far so good: all this had been proposed before.

With regard to the central machinery, however, he was much more iconoclastic.

> As a second democratically elected body subordinated to, but not technically an executive arm of, the Representative Body, the Council is an anomaly and it is proposed that this should be replaced by a relatively small *Central Executive*. ...
>
> The two *autonomous committees* will cease to exist. ... The two autonomous committees will disappear under these proposals.

This was the fuse that lit the powder magazine.

Chambers proposed no alteration in the size of the Representative Body but recommended that half the Representatives should be elected on a craft basis and half through the divisions. He proposed that all committees (including the Central Executive) should consist of Representatives and be elected by the Representative Body. He also proposed that every committee should be composed half of senior doctors and half of juniors.

Thus Chambers accurately diagnosed the causes of the perpetual tug-of-war in the BMA constitution between the Council and the Representative Body, and the constant rivalry between these two controlling (though competing) authorities and the autonomous bodies. He formed the view that this amounted to much more than a constitutional system of checks and balances, and he proposed: (*a*) that the Representative Body should be made fully representative of all areas, crafts, and age groups; (*b*) that the Council and all standing committees should be clearly subordinated to the reconstituted Representative Body; and (*c*) that the BMA should stop trying to speak for non-members.

The second of these proposals amounted to the abolition of the existing Council, General Medical Services Committee, and Central Committee for Hospital Medical Services. Sir Paul's second mistake was to express this revolutionary proposal in short, sharp terms, not wrapped in sugar-coating of any kind. Not unnaturally, the proposal sparked off an explosion of anger and resentment in the Council and in the two committees that he had earmarked for summary execution.

On 26 April 1972 Sir Paul Chambers presented his report to the Council and pulled no punches. The Council received his presentation with restraint and even with respect, but fired the opening shots in what was to be a long campaign. The Council decided to hold a special representative meeting in November 1972 to debate the report.

On 5 July 1972 the Council held a special meeting (which, incidentally, was Dr Solomon Wand's last attendance after 37 years on Council) and agreed an interim report to the SRM. But the Council reserved the most contentious issue, the proposed abolition of the autonomous committees, for further study by a special working party.

The Council's interim report accepted Chambers's proposal that BMA local boundaries should be redrawn to conform with NHS boundaries, accepted in principle his proposals for the reconstitution of the RB, and even accepted his proposal that the Council be reconstituted as a small central executive. But the real gristle of the Chambers Report was remitted to the special working party.

The Council met again on 30 August 1972 to receive the report of the special working party, which was in the form of a draft supplementary report of Council to the forthcoming special representative meeting. The draft was described by one member of Council as "an ingenious scheme to keep virtually intact the existing Conference of Representatives of Local Medical Committees and GMS Committee structure." Another said that "the draft report offered autonomous status to the other standing committees, so that there would be more tails wagging the dog." A third remarked that it was doubtful "whether the BMA membership as a whole would accept something which was an attempt to be all things to all men." Despite these pointed and well-founded criticisms, the Council adopted the draft with little change and its supplementary report to the SRM was published in the *BMJ* of 16 September 1972.

The report made no bones about the Council's desire to reject Sir Paul Chambers's advice on the autonomous committees. The Council said: "So far as the central negotiating committees of the crafts are concerned — the two present autonomous bodies and the Public Health Committee — the whole purport of this [the Council's] report is that they should continue in the redesigned organisation to carry out their existing functions." The Council also envisaged quite plainly that there would continue to be national craft conferences for general practitioners, hospital medical staff, and community physicians, and proposed an arrangement (which was eventually adopted) by which a joint agenda committee would channel motions to whatever annual meeting (representative meeting or craft conference) was considered appropriate to debate them. With regard to the composition of the RB, the Council frankly admitted "that its present proposals relating to the composition of the Representative Body differ fundamentally from those advanced by Sir Paul Chambers," and withdrew the views it had expressed in its interim report. Finally, the Council said: "The Council acknowledges that in many respects the proposals are lacking in detail, but it considers that it would be a profitless exercise to fill in the detail until it knows whether — or to what extent — the general principles outlined are acceptable to the Representative Body."

The Council did not have long to wait for an answer. The special representative meeting on 15 November 1972 was in an excited and angry mood. Sir Paul Chambers was invited to address it, and did so forcefully: "There should be working committees and not democratically elected debating societies. . . . All committees should be committees of members of the Association. In any other professional body this would be so obvious that it would have been absurd even to say it. It happened to be necessary at BMA House. Those who chose not to join the Association should not take part in the determination of its policy and should not be made the excuse for maintaining a cumbersome and inefficient system in which certain committees were given autonomy, which, in effect, meant freedom from the ultimate control of the Representative Body." (Applause.)

Sir Paul Chambers was accorded a vote of thanks by acclamation, and received a standing ovation. Dr G D H Shephard of Gloucestershire then moved: "That this meeting believes the BMA should accept the Chambers Report in its entirety." He said he felt that the Council's proposals were totally unacceptable. They did not imply change. They implied compromise in an attempt to maintain the old order in a new guise. After a two-hour debate, in which emotions ran high, the Gloucestershire motion was carried — by 153 votes to 149.

But this was not the two-thirds majority which was necessary for a policy decision by the RB, so the meeting then discussed a motion from Somerset to accept the Chambers Report "in principle." This was carried by 217 votes to 92. The Council then held an emergency meeting, after which its chairman (Mr Walpole Lewin) made a statement. He said: "... The fundamental principles of Chambers are to be adhered to. That is taken to include the abolition of autonomy and the fact that a voice in the affairs of the Association in the future will be limited to its members." On behalf of the Council, Mr Lewin undertook to prepare a further report in the light of the decision by the Representative Body that the Chambers Report should be accepted in principle.

The Council set up another special working party (which met six times) and held a two-day meeting in March 1973 to produce proposals for implementing "Chambers in principle." The working party's report was a faithful reflection of the Chambers proposals, following them as closely as was practicable, and giving cross-references to the Chambers Report at all relevant points. It was a masterpiece of draftsmanship, containing 16 "propositions" (a word deliberately chosen by the draftsmen, in case the Council might wish to disown any of them in its recommendations). But the report was, of course, anathema to the autonomous committees. At the two-day meeting of the Council, the Chairman of the GMS Committee (Dr James Cameron) conveyed a formal request to the Association on behalf of the Conference of Representatives of Local Medical Committees, "to maintain the LMC/Conference/GMSC structure within its constitution": the implication being that if the Association refused this request, that structure would separate itself from the BMA and continue to represent general practitioners independently. Dr Cameron had already written to the Chairman of Council saying: "All members of the Association . . . are faced with a situation which must cause every one of us the greatest concern . . . A conflict, an open breach within our ranks will produce a situation from which nobody can win; everyone will be the loser." Dr Cameron said he was prepared to compromise, but the one thing his committee could not compromise on was the principle of the LMC/Conference/GMS Committee structure. The Chairman of the Central Committee for Hospital Medical Services (Dr C E Astley) was even more emphatic. He said that if Chambers was to be effected unilaterally by a "madcap group" in the Representative Body, it would be going back on all the promises and authority that the BMA had given to the political wing of the hospital side.

Despite these strident objections, the "Chambers in principle" report was included in the Annual Report of Council for discussion by the divisions and by the Representative Body. But the Council said: "It is, in the Council's view, tragic that at a time when all should be concentrating upon the problems of NHS reorganisation and the United Kingdom's entry into the EEC — to name but two issues — the Association should find itself divided on the best way of ordering its own affairs." And the Council went on to recommend "that no decision be taken at this stage" on four unpalatable propositions of the Chambers working party. These were their proposals for the reconstitution of the standing committees (including the autonomous committees), their propositions that only BMA members should be eligible to serve on standing committees, that the Junior Members Forum and the Hospital Junior Staffs Group should be abolished, and that Council should be reconstituted with a membership of only 19 (plus eight non-voting members).

More than a whole day of the ARM at Folkestone in June 1973 was devoted to discussion of the constitution. The Chairman of Council moved: "That this meeting, in the light of the view held and conclusions reached by various standing committees in respect of the acceptance of 'Chambers in principle' by the SRM last November, is of the opinion that a new situation now exists which must be examined very closely in view of the risk of fragmentation of the profession, and because the whole package of 'Chambers in principle' may no longer be acceptable, the individual recommendations of the Council on the Propositions of the working party must be discussed in detail."

Out of courtesy to the host division, Dr L P Ribet of Folkestone was called to speak first and said "The abolition of longstanding machinery for collecting the views of all GPs and representing their interests should not be implemented. So strong has been the feeling on that score that a special meeting of LMCs has agreed, if necessary, to set up an independent organisation of family doctors directly answerable to LMCs and through them to all GPs. There is no doubt that in the eyes of the GPs, pre-eminent among the functions of the Association is its continuing role as the voice of all doctors and not merely BMA members."

This speech by a loyal BMA Representative, and host to the meeting, set the tone of the debate. But the radical reformers did not go down without a fight. Dr H L Leaming of Council said that if the motion were passed it would be interpreted in the world outside and throughout the membership of the Association as rescinding the decisions made in November. That would be a disaster and, because of the antics of its two autonomous committees, the BMA would lose any vestige of credibility that remained.

The reaction against "Chambers in principle" had now set in, however, and the Chairman of Council's motion was eventually carried by a large majority. The next day, the issue of autonomy was tackled head-on. Dr J H Marks of Council moved: "That no reorganisation of the BMA can be effective which does not take into consideration the LMC/Conference/GMSC structure and the parallel machinery of regional committees for hospital medical services/Hospital Medical Staffs Conference/CCHMS, and which does not confer delegated authority upon the GMSC, the CCHMS, and any other committee of similar stature." After a long and tense debate, and after adding to the motion the words "for example, the Hospital Junior Staffs Group Council," a vote was taken by roll call (an unusual event) and the motion was carried by 246 votes to 86.

The leading article in the *BMJ* of 16 June 1973 summed up in these words: "So a federalist rather than a unitary structure is seen at present as a more suitable framework for representing doctors in facing their near-monopoly

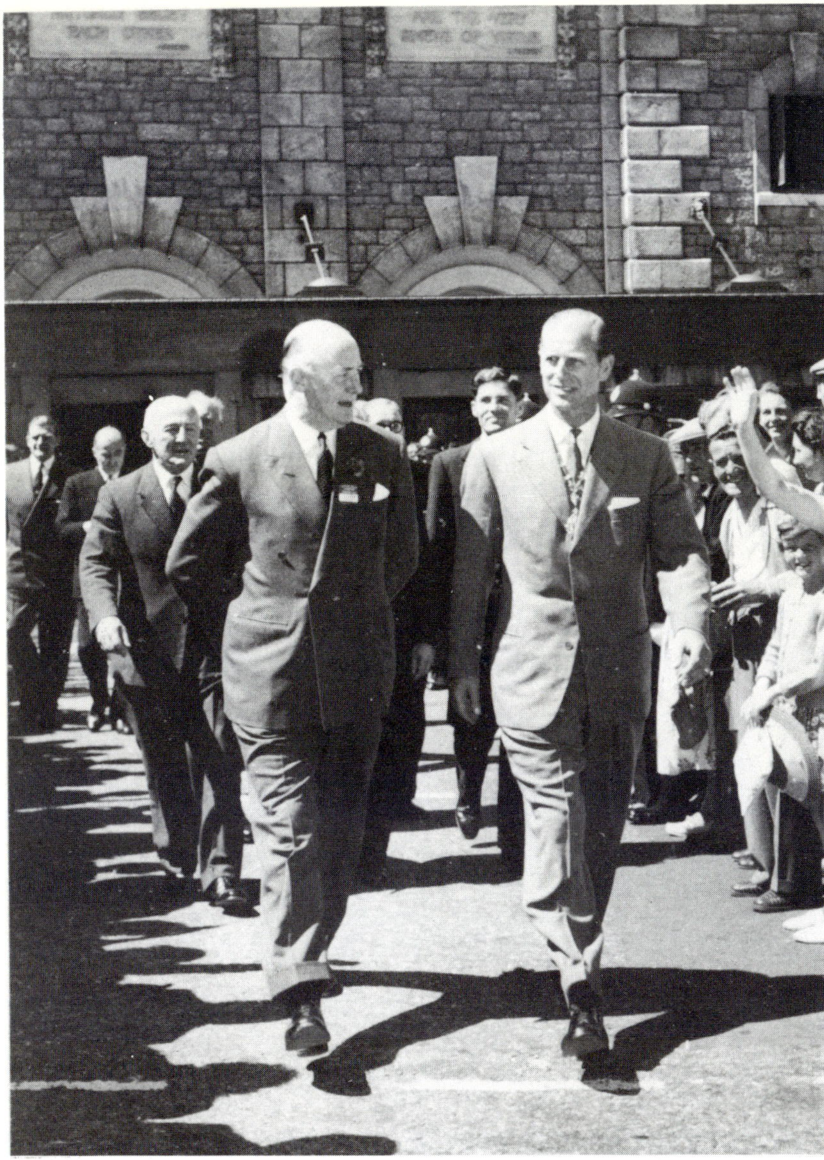

Prince Philip at the Annual Meeting (Torquay, 20 June 1960). L to R: Sir Arthur Thomson (Deputy President), Sir Arthur Porritt (President-Elect), HRH the Duke of Edinburgh (President).

(*Sean Hickey*)

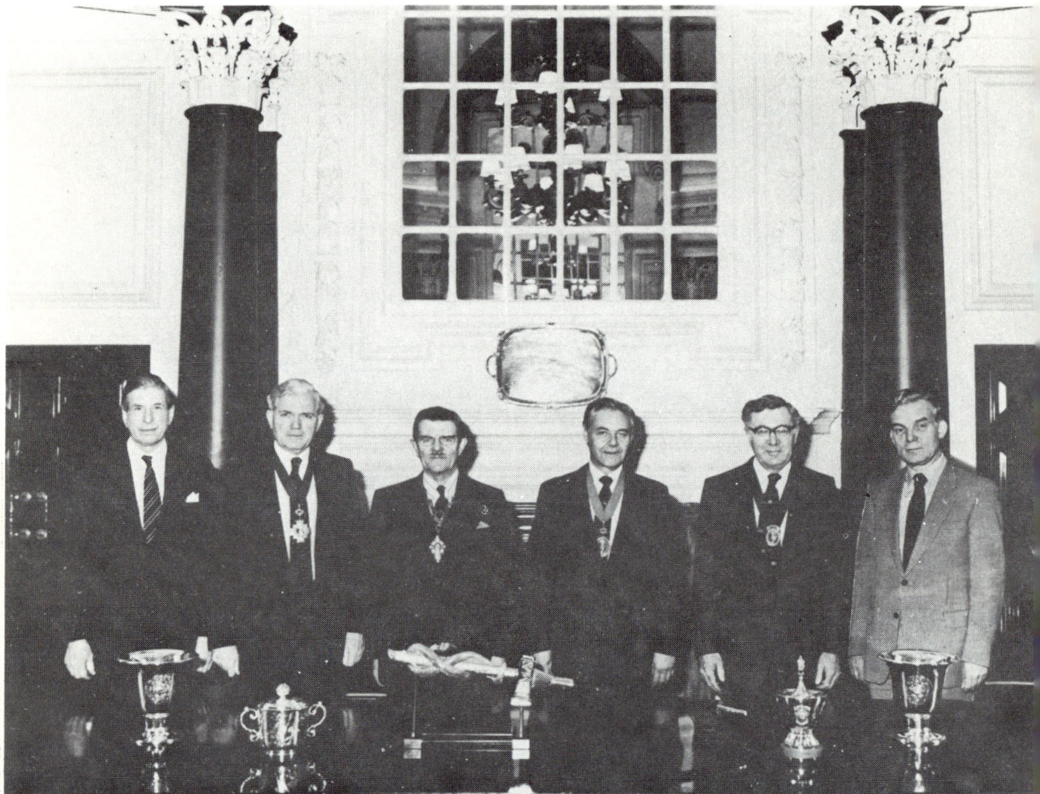

THE LEADERSHIP, 1981–2.

L TO R: DR JOHN HAVARD (SECRETARY), MR ANTHONY GRABHAM (CHAIRMAN OF COUNCIL), JOHN WALTON (PRESIDENT), DR JOHN MARKS (CHAIRMAN OF REPRESENTATIVE BODY), DR T[illegible] KEABLE-ELLIOTT (TREASURER), DR STEPHEN LOCK (EDITOR).

employer — the National Health Service. . . . Nevertheless, an appreciable minority of doctors will still regret that throughout the Chambers saga compromise seems to have been the objective in preference to radical change. . . . Moreover, some very useful parts of Chambers emerged relatively unscathed from the scrupulous attentions of the Council's working party, the Council and the RB: strengthening of the peripheral structure of the BMA to match the new Health Service; the firm establishment of the juniors' position; a new-style Representative Body dealing with major policy matters, and probably considerable reduction in the size of the Council itself."

We are now approaching the end of the Chambers story. After the Folkestone ARM the Council appointed yet another special working party to draft yet another report on the constitution, in accordance with the decisions made by the Representative Body at Folkestone. The special working party's report was debated twice by the Council, and discussed by all the standing committees. The final text, as settled by the Council, was published in the annual report on 27 April 1974.

The rock on which all the previous attempts had foundered was circumnavigated with these carefully chosen words about the autonomous committees: "As standing committees of the Association these craft committees are subject to the authority of the Representative Body. Moreover, the committees themselves have no corporate status and, indeed, apart from the BMA have no status so far as the Companies Acts and the Industrial Relations Act are concerned. Nevertheless, without the structures on which these craft committees rest the Association cannot substantiate its claim to represent *all* doctors in the NHS. Therefore, in order to ensure the integrity of the Association as the mouthpiece of all doctors these craft bodies must operate *within the Association,* and it follows that in matters affecting the interests of doctors engaged in the NHS it is necessary that policies should be formulated and implemented with the full agreement of both the RB and the craft committees."

These words indicated that there was to be a condominium between the Representative Body and the autonomous bodies. The Council's report went on to recommend:

(*1*) that "delegated authority" (the emotive word "autonomy" was quietly dropped) should be conferred by the Articles and By-laws upon the CCHMS, the GMS Committee, the new Central Committee for Community Medicine, and the Hospital Junior Staffs Committee;

(*2*) that slightly narrower "delegated authority" should be conferred upon the other four negotiating committees (Armed Forces, Full-time Medical Teachers and Research Workers, Occupational Health, and Private Practice);

(*3*) that the Representative Body should be reconstituted on a half geographical and half "craft" basis, with a total membership of about 600;

(*4*) that the RB and the craft conferences should meet in the same week and that there should be a joint agenda committee;

(*5*) that the Council should be reconstituted with five members *ex officio*, 20 elected by the standing committees, 12 elected by the RB but from the standing committees, and 17 elected by the RB on a geographical basis (in other words, the Council was to be the executive of the RB);

(*6*) that the standing committees should be reconstituted, and two of them abolished; but that two important new special committees be created: the Executive Committee of Council (concerned mainly with medicopolitical issues) and the Finance and General Purposes Committee (concerned mainly with the domestic business of the Association).

A leading article in the same issue of the *BMJ* said: "Those who have been closely involved in working out the reforms hope that they have found the right mixture at last. They certainly know how much time and effort it has taken."

The last SRM on this topic was held on 27 February 1975, and the Council's proposals were accepted without demur. The whole Chambers saga had convulsed the Association for three years, and it was tragic that so much time, energy, and heat were expended by the leaders and senior staff of the BMA on a purely introspective task. Sir Paul Chambers was once asked why he had chosen to make his most explosive recommendation ("The two autonomous committees will cease to exist") in such provocative terms. He replied that he thought the medical profession should be sufficiently intelligent and mature to receive advice in plain and unambiguous language, and he was clearly scornful of the way in which his report had been treated. Perhaps, however, Sir Paul was guilty of an error of judgment. The good doctor takes infinite pains to convey unpalatable news to a patient in a gentle and diplomatic manner, and it would have been prudent to approach the BMA in a similar way.

Let us end this part of the BMA's story by quoting some words spoken in 1980 by the Rt Hon James Callaghan, then Leader of the Labour Party: "The Party may discuss its internal conditions to such an extent that it disgusts all those with whom it comes into contact. . . . Comrades, for the time being we have had enough of discussion."

THE SEARCH FOR AN EFFECTIVE SANCTION

The widespread resentment within the BMA at the fact that the Council and the Representative Body, albeit after a titanic struggle, eventually took the medical profession into the National Health Service in 1948 led to a feeling that the BMA would have fought more successfully if it had been a trade union. Everyone was aware that the trade unions had massively increased their power and prestige in the nation, especially since the advent of the Labour Government of 1945, and the suggestion was made that the BMA should convert itself into a trade union. Nobody liked the suggestion. Doctors are individualists, not collectivists, and there are many features of trade unionism that are anathema to them: the political levy, the closed shop, the strike (in the true sense of complete withholding of labour), and picketing. But there was still a feeling in some quarters that, now that most of the practice of medicine had been nationalised, the medical profession might be wise to unionise itself, while endeavouring to avoid the more unattractive features of trade unionism.

The Council sought legal advice on this question and a detailed report was published in February 1949. The lawyers showed that the matter was not a simple one. Straightforward conversion of the BMA into a trade union would not be practicable, because of company law; and in any case a trade union of doctors would not enjoy the powers and immunities of a trade union of workmen because (in the opinion of eminent Counsel) doctors did not fall within the definition of "workmen" in the Trade Union Acts 1871 to 1913, or in the Trade Disputes Act 1906.

The lawyers recommended, however, that the BMA could acquire many of the additional powers which it sought by a device which would be entitled the British

Medical Guild. This would not, in fact, be a guild of members, but a trust fund administered by a board of trustees. The guild would be independent of the BMA, but the trustees of the guild would be the members of the BMA Council. These trustees could lawfully invite doctors to take collective action in a dispute with their employers, and could make payments to any doctors suffering financial hardship as a result of loyalty to the collective policy. The trustees of the guild could do many other things which the BMA Council was prevented from doing because of the legal status of the BMA as a registered company, limited by guarantee, and because of the restrictions imposed by its Memorandum of Association. In other words, the British Medical Guild would be a kind of trade union shadow of the BMA.

This ingenious scheme was adopted by a special representative meeting on the 30 March 1949, but not without some questioning. The British Medical Guild was inaugurated by a donation from the National Insurance Defence Trust, a fund which the general practitioners had had the foresight to create in 1919. The general practitioners now formed a second trust fund, the General Medical Services Defence Trust, with wider terms of reference, and the Central Consultants and Specialists Committee and the Public Health Committee followed suit by establishing similar defence trusts for their branches of the profession. The GMS Defence Trust was fed by deductions from the remuneration of NHS general practitioners (the system which trade unions call the "check off"), while the other two trusts had to rely on voluntary contributions from doctors, with the inevitable consequence that they did not accumulate the large funds which the general practitioners had at their disposal (and which they used generously in defence of the whole profession whenever crises arose). The British Medical Guild was financed by contributions from the four defence trusts.

Hitherto, almost the only sanction available to the BMA had been to refuse to publish advertisements for a particular employer in the *British Medical Journal*, and to name his employment in the "Important Notice" (or "BMA blacklist") in the journal. Henceforward, when the BMA Council wished to organise collective action to protect the interests of the profession they adjourned their meeting and immediately reconvened as the trustees of the British Medical Guild. In the great remuneration dispute of 1957 (see Chapter 5), the BMA Council interrupted their meeting on 27 March to hold a meeting of the trustees of the guild, who approved the terms of a first-rate message to every member of the profession, and ordered preparations to be made to organise the "phased" or "progressive" withdrawal of general practitioners from the NHS. Under this scheme the general practitioners in certain areas would be invited to resign their contracts. They would be subsidised by practitioners in other areas, and also by hospital doctors who were to be asked to contribute 5% of their remuneration to a special fund for helping the general practitioners in their action.

The threat of collective resignation from the State service had been used once before, in 1923, when the Insurance Acts Committee had collected the resignations of 97% of panel practitioners. In 1957 the resignations were not actually collected, because the BMA decided to co-operate with the Pilkington Royal Commission. There was, however, a good deal of criticism of the plan for "phased withdrawal": the general feeling seemed to be that all general practitioners should be invited to resign together, or not at all. And there were those who expressed doubts about the practicability of organising withdrawal. A correspondent in the *BMJ* wrote: "Furthermore, most doctors' personal economy is geared to their quarterly cheques, for living and practice expenses, house and motor-car repayments, and, by no means least, school fees. How many can possibly afford to throw this overboard for some ethereal 'strike pay' or collection of mythical private fees, and how many would want to?"

Such doubts prompted the GMS Committee to set up a special subcommittee to examine as a matter of urgency all aspects of the problem of preparing an alternative medical service in the event of the profession ultimately withdrawing from the National Health Service. After a time the subcommittee recommended that its task should be remitted to an independent investigator "of recognised eminence and authority." The person chosen was Sir Frank Newsam, a retired Permanent Under Secretary of State of the Home Office.

The Newsam Report was published in the *BMJ* on 17

January 1959 and covered 10 pages. Sir Frank's terms of reference had been widened: "To investigate any deficiencies in, and frustrations arising from, the present scheme for providing family doctors' services in the National Health Service, and to suggest practical modifications or alternative schemes." Unfortunately, his first and principal conclusion did not endear him to his readers. He wrote: "The National Health Service is here to stay. It is an essential feature of the welfare state. The welfare state is a continuation in peacetime of the spirit which won the war. It is unrealistic of doctors to think of withdrawing from the National Health Service. The inevitable result would be the formation of a fully salaried service." The Newsam Report was promptly disowned by the Council of the Association.

The Council proceeded to publish a statement that: "In the event of any future unresolved disputes with the Government ... it believes that total withdrawal of service would be the most effective and quickest way of securing a just solution, but that this would only be possible if the profession was united and resolved to make a stand on principles rather than on a matter of remuneration. During the period of withdrawal there would have to be reliance predominantly on private practice."

At the same time the Council published a detailed report by a new subcommittee of the GMS Committee which, after the disappointment of the Newsam Report, had tackled the problem afresh. They discussed total withdrawal, either to a contributory medical service or to private practice; partial withdrawal (as in the recent scheme for "phased withdrawal"); and other possible sanctions, such as reduction of lists, withdrawal from the administration of the NHS, and withdrawal of certification (which they admitted would be a breach of contract). It was all set out in great detail. At the same time attention was drawn to an action recently taken by the medical profession in Austria, when for two days surgeries were closed and family doctors dealt only with emergencies, while hospital doctors provided only a Sunday service.

Some of the urgency of the search for an effective sanction was removed when the Pilkington Royal Commission created the Review Body system which, it was hoped, would provide a means of regularly settling medical remuneration without serious dispute. Meanwhile, however, the Amending Acts Committee had been beavering away at schemes for an alternative medical service (that is, alternative to the NHS), and in 1961 they produced two such schemes which had been worked out in great detail. One was for a fully alternative service to replace the NHS, and the other was for a service designed to operate alongside the NHS (the "side by side" scheme). These two schemes were approved by the Representative Body and filed "for future reference should the necessity arise."

It has already been related (in Chapter 5) that early in 1965, in the explosion of wrath that followed the Fifth Report of the Review Body, the trustees of the British Medical Guild collected the undated resignations of over 17 000 general practitioners and held them for months as a threat hanging over the head of the Minister of Health. It was widely understood that the British Medical Guild was merely a front organisation for the BMA and it must be recorded that this collective and coercive action by the BMA was profoundly shocking and repugnant to many doctors, including some leading figures in the profession. This impelled the BMA to continue its search for a sanction that would embarrass and put pressure on the Government, without damaging the interests of patients, without affronting public opinion, and without causing ethical or moral reservations among doctors themselves. This was indeed a tall order. Moreover, the sanction of resignation from the NHS and a return to private practice, however difficult it might be for most general practitioners, was practically impossible for hospital doctors because the hospitals were (with very few exceptions) owned and managed by the NHS.

When the outgoing Labour Government in May 1970 refused to publish the Twelfth Report of the Review Body until after the General Election, the staff drew up a list of 11 possible sanctions, and steps were taken to activate the central and local machinery of the British Medical Guild and to mobilise professional and public opinion. As a result, the Government agreed to publish the Review Body's report on 4 June.

The great dispute which then broke out has been described in Chapter 5. Briefly, the Government decided to pay only half the Review Body's award to general practitioners and consultants, and to refer the question of the other half to another tribunal, the National Board for Prices and Incomes. The Kindersley Review Body promptly resigned in disgust. The object here is to relate that two days after the Government's announcement, a printed "Message No 1" was issued by the trustees of the British Medical Guild to all general practitioners and hospital doctors in the NHS. It called on them to embark on the following sanctions.

> (*1*) To cease to co-operate in the administration of the NHS, that is to withdraw from all negotiating, advisory, and administrative bodies, both central and local.
>
> (*2*) To cease to issue certificates of incapacity for work. In this connection the message stated: "It is appreciated that failure to supply National Insurance certificates is a breach of the terms of service of NHS doctors; nevertheless, the trustees are in no mood to be deterred from advising the profession to proceed. The situation is so serious that direct action of this kind is fully justified." The message also said: "The steps recommended here will not interfere with the treatment of patients, which will continue as usual."

A poster was issued for display in doctors' surgeries, headed "Why I cannot sign your medical certificate." Whole-page advertisements were placed in the national newspapers, headed: "The bitter pill doctors are being asked to swallow." The BMA demonstrated with the utmost vigour that the medical profession was not prepared to allow itself to be trampled on.

Not all doctors approved of these militant tactics, and there were loud criticisms of the BMA's actions. The majority, however, approved. Between 4 and 25 June 1970, 1603 messages were received at BMA Headquarters, and of these 84% supported the BMA's actions and 16% opposed them. One of the approvers wrote: "It would be futile and wrong to say that I have always agreed with BMA policy and decisions, indeed sometimes I was driven to near despair. But I am glad and proud to be a member of the BMA now."

On 12 June 1970 the British Medical Guild issued Message No 2. It included some "Notes on the Independent Review Body," and brief details of contingency plans for possible withdrawal from the NHS. In addition, a ballot card was enclosed, on which every doctor was invited to answer the question: "Are you prepared to withdraw from the National Health Service if the Government will not assure the continued existence of the independent Review

Body, and the honouring of its awards in the terms defined by the Royal Commission, without reference to any other tribunal?" The ballot card was returned by 57% of doctors: of these, 70% answered yes to the question.

Meanwhile, the staff at headquarters were carefully preparing a second phase of sanctions, but on 19 June there was a change of Government and the dispute was settled (Chapter 5).

In the course of this vehement struggle the Deputy Secretary had minuted the Secretary in these terms: "I cannot help feeling that both the GMS Committee and the CCHMS ought to set up a small sanctions subcommittee consisting of a very small number of people not committed to other work who should be told to get down to really detailed planning about a programme of sanctions and a scheme for an alternative medical service, so that we can continue this war, or embark upon a fresh war in the future, with very detailed plans all ready on the spot." After the settlement of the dispute this was done. Quietly and without publicity, a sanctions working party was established which in due course drafted a "Sanctions Plan for Emergency." (It was later published in the *BMJ* of 9 November 1974.)

The plan made clear that the steps recommended were designed to affect administration rather than clinical care. The plan was originally prepared in successive phases: firstly, withdrawal of goodwill — for example, refusal to participate in the administration of the NHS — then withdrawal of non-contractual services, such as voluntary out-of-hours work, and, finally, withdrawal from the NHS and return to private practice. The plan was kept constantly under review and modification, and was later changed into a series of options, any one of which could be chosen as the appropriate measure in any particular dispute.

An important development came in 1970. The new Conservative Government introduced an Industrial Relations Bill which was designed to regulate the activities of trade unions. The BMA, the British Dental Association, the Royal College of Nursing, and the Royal College of Midwives together represented to Ministers that professional negotiating bodies should be excluded from the scope of the Bill, but the Government made it clear that the Bill was intended to cover the professions, including all branches of the medical profession. Yet the Bill was drafted in such a way as to make it impossible for the BMA to register in its existing form as an "organisation of workers" and to continue to perform its traditional functions within the framework of the new law, because registration under the Bill and registration under the Companies Act were to be made mutually exclusive.

The BMA therefore found itself faced with the following alternatives: (*a*) to wind up the Company of the BMA, distribute the assets and start again from scratch, founding a new BMA as a trade union registered under the new law; (*b*) to abandon its negotiating (medicopolitical) role and to become purely a scientific and social body; (*c*) to found a parallel organisation, linked in some way with the BMA and registered as a trade union under the new law.

Each of these courses would have led to the virtual extinction of the BMA as we know it, because even (*c*) would have stimulated an irresistible demand from a large slice of the BMA's membership to be allowed to join only the parallel trade union and not to pay the additional subscription which would be required for full membership of the BMA.

Prolonged discussion with Ministers and officials produced no solution to this problem and it appeared likely that the BMA would have no alternative but to adopt course (*c*) as the least objectionable of the three possibilities. The Association (and the other professional negotiating bodies) was in an exceedingly serious predicament. Then in November 1970 the Deputy Secretary of the BMA made a suggestion to the Department of Employment to the effect that a provision should be inserted in the Bill whereby recognised professional negotiating bodies with their status and constitutions as existing on 5 October 1970 (the date of publication of the Government's proposals) should be registrable as "staff organisations" in a special section of the register of trade unions. The Department extended a cautious welcome to this suggestion and in due course, after further negotiation, the Special Register was created by sections 84-86 of the Industrial Relations Act 1971. The BMA was duly entered in the Special Register, and thus acquired all the privileges and responsibilities of a trade union registered under the Act without any change in its constitution.

Subsequently this Act was repealed by the next Labour

Government and the BMA again found itself threatened, but in the end the protected position of bodies in the Special Register was preserved by the Trade Union and Labour Relations Act 1974. Thus, 25 years after the BMA had first seriously contemplated becoming a trade union, the Association was registered as a trade union under the law, but without giving up its status as a company registered under the Companies Act. Since then the BMA has enjoyed dual status: it carries on all its traditional functions as a professional association which is a company limited by guarantee, and it also has the status and protection of a trade union listed under the current legislation.

While the Conservative Industrial Relations Act was in force, an important declaration was obtained from the Government. The BMA requested the Government to recognise the Association as the "sole bargaining agent" under the Act for general practitioners and hospital doctors. The Permanent Under Secretary of State at the DHSS replied: "The Department has conducted . . . negotiations exclusively with the Central Committee for Hospital Medical Services in respect of all NHS hospital doctors, and with the General Medical Services Committee in respect of all general practitioners; it would appear that these two groups of doctors have in effect constituted bargaining units and the committees have been in effect sole bargaining agents. . . . The Department has no proposals for change. . . ."

In 1975, when the Secretary of State for Social Services (Mrs Barbara Castle) made it clear that the Government was determined to proceed with legislation to enforce the separation of private practice from NHS hospitals, the consultants embarked on a campaign of collective resistance. Their sanction did not follow exactly the carefully worked out Sanctions Plan for Emergency — which illustrates the difficulty of getting doctors to conform to any agreed collective policy. The Central Committee for Hospital Medical Services urged all consultants to limit their work to the treatment of emergencies and other urgent cases, and to the continuing care of patients already in their wards. At about the same time, the hospital junior staff embarked upon a programme of sanctions because of dissatisfaction with the progress of negotiations on a new junior staff contract. The Hospital Junior Staff Committee advised junior doctors to keep to a 40-hour week, "worked flexibly according to local needs," and to deal with new emergencies only. This, again, was not consistent with the BMA's Sanctions Plan, but the junior doctors' sanctions caused grave embarrassment to the NHS authorities.

It must not be supposed that the conferment by Parliament of trade union status on the BMA, and the use by the BMA from time to time of collective sanctions, were universally popular among either doctors or the general public. Far from it. Headlines such as "Hospital consultants call for one-day strike as pay protest" (which appeared in *The Times* of 20 July 1977 during the ARM at Glasgow) were profoundly shocking to many BMA members as well as to public opinion. The whole aura of trade unionism and collective pressure, especially when (as was often unavoidable) the interests of patients were indirectly disadvantaged, was deeply repugnant to many doctors. The BMA leaders decided to put their dilemma fairly and squarely to the Royal Commission on the National Health Service. The Association's memorandum of evidence (1977) said: "On one notorious occasion (in 1970) the Government decided not merely to halve the award to certain doctors and dentists but also to refer the report of the Review Body to another tribunal for a second opinion. This made a mockery of the independence of the Doctors' and Dentists' Review Body, which promptly resigned. The question that this poses is: What is the medical profession to do in circumstances such as these? Is it to acquiesce in gross interference by the Government in the independence of action of the profession's Review Body, without anything more than protests? Or are doctors to adopt the measures of protest and self-defence which have been used for generations by the labour unions, of taking so-called industrial action? And is there a risk that the medical profession will one day be forced into the highly regrettable position of having to withdraw its labour — that is, to go on strike, which is the weapon which is used (and accepted by the public — the so-called "right to strike") by most of the trade union movement?"

The Royal Commission offered no direct answers to these questions, perhaps mistakenly regarding them as rhetorical. But in a section headed "Avoidance of Industrial Action," the Royal Commission said: "Those who work in the NHS have special responsibilities towards patients, and it is clear that the great majority are conscious of this. It is essential that they should be, but it is equally important that the Government should not take advantage, or seem to take advantage, of the obligation health workers feel towards patients. . . . There are no magic wands to be waved in this field."

We can all say Amen to that.

Chapter 10

Miscellany

Sainte-Beuve, as he grew older, came to regard all experience as a single great book, in which to study for a few years ere we go hence; and it seemed all one to him whether you should read in Chapter XX, which is the differential calculus, or in Chapter XXXIX, which is hearing the band play in the gardens. — Robert Louis Stevenson.

FINANCE AND ESTATES

Almost the whole of the 50 years covered by this book were a time of mounting financial difficulty, both for our country and for our Association. The fall in the value of money, and the vast expansion of the membership and work of the BMA, have combined to produce the remarkable change in the finances of the Association which is shown in the following table. The figures are derived from the BMA's financial statements for 1932 and for 1980.

	1932	1980
	£	£
Income	157 785	9 578 809
Expenditure	157 676	9 970 755
Surplus/(Deficit)	109	(391 946)
Net Assets	264 339	3 001 893

The feverish activity undertaken by the Association in the months leading up to the introduction of the National Health Service necessitated heavy expenditure, and the income and expenditure account for 1948 showed a deficit for the first time for 20 years. In 1949, therefore, the ordinary subscription was raised from three guineas to four guineas: the first increase since 1923. Ten years later, in

1959, the BMA successfully applied to the Inland Revenue for tax relief to be granted on the BMA subscription under Section 16 of the Finance Act 1958.

The building of the north and south wings of Tavistock House, which was begun in 1938 but was interrupted by the war and impeded by bomb damage, was completed in 1950. This marked the completion of those plans for the development of the BMA's site in Tavistock Square which had been approved by the Council in 1926. Further plans evolved and in due course the Burton Street wing was added. In 1951 work was in progress on the members' dining room and the Hastings lounge, in which was incorporated the lovely mahogany panelling originally made for BMA House at 429 Strand.

In 1962 the BMA took a momentous step: the Association bought the freehold of Tavistock House from the Bedford Estate for £120 000. BMA House in Edinburgh had been extensively reconstructed and ceremonially reopened in 1957. Since the second world war the BMA has also acquired offices in Cardiff, Belfast, and ten regional centres. The total amount of real estate owned by the BMA is now probably worth about £30 million.

A steep rise in the cost of paper in 1951 (due to stockpiling of timber by the Americans because of the Korean war) caused a serious and unexpected deficit in the Association's publishing activities and an overall deficit in the BMA's accounts of £131 000. A special Finance Inquiry Committee was set up which organised an economy campaign (the first of many), and a firm of management consultants was engaged to review the business management of the Association's publications and the administration of the Association generally.

The Great Hall at BMA House was redecorated in 1964, but the Council decided that the Association could not afford the heavy cost of completing the coffered ceiling in accordance with Sir Edward Lutyens's original design. The ceiling remains unfinished to the present day.

In 1969, after another economy campaign, the BMA Council decided that there must be another rise in subscription rates, and publicly acknowledged the help of the Medical Insurance Agency in limiting the impact of the increase on the younger member. In addition, constant efforts were made by the permanent staff to run the

Association as efficiently and as economically as possible. The Council reported in 1969:

> ... Staff economies would be difficult to achieve without cutting work load. This is an extremely difficult problem to tackle. It is easy to start new projects, but exceedingly painful to discontinue them. Every project has its enthusiastic supporters, who vigorously resist any suggestion that it has served its purpose and should be brought to an end. ...
>
> An Administrative Working Party meets every month to keep our office methods and machinery under continuous review. Modern developments in mechanisation are constantly examined and adopted whenever it is economical and advantageous to do so. The Council has decided, after a thorough study of what is acknowledged to be a most difficult subject, to computerise a proportion of the subscription and membership records, on an exploratory basis. If the experiment proves successful, the whole of the subscription and membership records will be computerised.
>
> Training courses have been introduced for newly appointed Officials and Committee Executive Officers, and an introductory course has been held for the Assistant Regional Officers.

In 1971 the Secretary published a six-page review of the Association's finance and administration, in which he examined in detail the possibilities of moving BMA Headquarters from London to a provincial centre, or of partial decentralisation — that is, moving certain departments out of London. The review also discussed the pros and cons of carrying further a policy adopted in 1968 of filling the assistant secretary grade with lay officials rather than medical, and mentioned the possibility of reducing the senior staff (both medical and lay) by some accelerated retirements. The trouble with all these successive economy campaigns, however, was that when it came to the crunch both the Council and the Representative Body were invariably unwilling to agree to any reduction in the manifold activities of the Association.

The fact is, of course, that the medical profession needs a strong and active representative association. The BMA Council's annual report for 1976-7 ended with the words: "It is impossible in a report of modest length to give anything like a complete picture of the gigantic task which is involved in speaking, and fighting, for the medical profession in the economic, political, and social climate of this country at the present time."

It was frequently pointed out that the BMA's recurrent financial shortages would not be so great if all, or nearly all, doctors became members. The BMA is firmly committed to the principle of voluntary membership, but has always been disappointed that a quarter or even a third of the profession are not members. In April 1978 the Council stated: "Bearing in mind the BMA's record of service to the profession since 1832 and its elaborate structure for democratic representation of all views, it is a matter of great regret to the Council that there are many doctors who choose to remain outside the membership of the Association." A survey in 1979 showed that 91% of BMA members thought that national negotiations on pay and conditions of service were the BMA's most important function. Non-members benefit from these negotiations as much as members, and loyal BMA members consider it surprising and shabby that many doctors are prepared to accept the fruits of BMA negotiations while declining to contribute to the cost of them.

In 1951 the membership comprised 77% of the profession in the United Kingdom, and 85% of the working profession (that is, not including retired doctors). BMA membership reached the highest figure ever at the end of 1961 — 76 673 — but the next day the Australian branches became the independent Australian Medical Association and the BMA membership figure fell correspondingly. At the end of 1980 there were 65 650 BMA members, including nearly 9000 overseas. The membership in the UK represented about two-thirds of the profession. In addition, there were over 5000 associate members, a new category created in 1974 for medical students.

One thing which the BMA is proud to provide for the whole profession — regardless of membership or non-membership — is charitable or benevolent aid in distress. The BMA administers several charitable funds that help doctors, their widows, and their families when disaster strikes. The total sum paid out in such grants since 1932 amounts to at least £1 million. When disaster struck the coasts of Lincolnshire and East Anglia in 1953, and the sea flooded over the land, the BMA helped the stricken doctors both in cash and in kind: an assistant secretary was sent up with a stock of new medical instruments to visit the doctors and to replace the instruments that they had lost.

In 1932 the Treasurer of the Association was Mr Nathaniel Bishop Harman FRCS, who held the office with great distinction from 1924 to 1939. He designed and presented the lovely ceremonial staff (or mace) of the Association, and also gave the Treasurer's Golf Cup. The responsibilities and anxieties falling on the shoulders of the Treasurer have increased immeasurably in the past 50 years, and the Association owes a great debt of gratitude to all its distinguished line of Treasurers, but perhaps most of all to the man who is Treasurer when these lines are being written, Dr J E Miller. No Treasurer in recent times has displayed greater mastery of his exacting office.

RELATIONS WITH THE PRESS

One of the most important developments in the past 50 years has been the enormous growth of the interest shown by the press and radio, followed by television, in medical science and the medical profession. The BMA has responded to this by establishing its Press and Information Department, which has become one of the most important parts of its machinery. Indeed, it would not be too much to say that the BMA Press Office has become the public relations department of the entire medical profession.

In 1938 the Council reported: "It has been evident to the Council for some time that there is need to educate public opinion on behalf of the Association and to secure a wider appreciation of the views of the profession on medico-sociological problems. ... The Council has appointed a Public Relations Officer to the British Medical Association (Mr A W Haslett). . . ." In 1943 the Council also appointed a part-time adviser in public relations, Mr Colin Hurry, who was to help the BMA for many years and (partly because of his distinctive Edwardian style of dress) present a striking figure in the background at many important meetings. In 1954 a part-time press officer was appointed to the BMA in Scotland.

The BMA's first objective has been to provide for journalists an information service on medical matters, and the large corps of medical journalists (greatly expanded in recent years by the creation of "paramedical" newspapers, many of which are circulated free-of-charge to members of the medical profession) are the first to acknowledge that the

BMA gives them a first-rate service. The second objective of the Press and Information Department has been to explain carefully to the media the BMA's point of view on any medical matter. At times of controversy this has excited great activity. In the 1957 remuneration dispute, for example, the BMA's case was brought to the notice of the public by press statements, press conferences, spokesmen on radio and television, whole-page advertisements in national newspapers, and posters in doctors' waiting rooms. In addition, a document setting out the profession's case was sent to Members of both Houses of Parliament.

Since 1937 the BMA has employed a parliamentary agent to identify and examine all Bills and parliamentary papers that might affect the interests of the medical profession, and daily information about parliamentary affairs is circulated to the staff at BMA House by the Press and Information Department. In recent times this parliamentary work has been considerably augmented.

Throughout its existence the Press and Information Department has also been responsible for dealing with requests for information from the lay public, many of whom seem to regard the BMA as the fount of all knowledge in medical matters. By 1967 the department was dealing with 18 000 inquiries a year from journalists and members of the public.

An increasingly important function of the BMA has been to make representations to the media about the way in which medical topics are handled. In 1951 the BMA Council noted with concern "the laudatory references sometimes made to medical practitioners in announcements regarding forthcoming television programmes and also in the actual performances" and decided to discuss the problem with the General Medical Council. In 1954 a BMA deputation met the Director-General of the BBC to discuss various matters in relation to radio and television programmes on medical themes. In 1955 longstanding differences between doctors working in hospitals and the press came to a head with complaints of press behaviour in connection with an operation to separate Siamese twins at the British Postgraduate Medical School at Hammersmith. The Chairman of the BMA's Public Relations Committee called a conference of all the interested parties. The press warmly welcomed this initiative, and all the main press organisations — representing proprietors, editors, and working journalists — as well as the BBC, agreed to attend. The Ministry of Health sent an observer. As a result a committee was appointed, with Dr Guy Dain as chairman and Sir Linton Andrews (Chairman of the Press Council) as deputy chairman, to examine the subject in detail. After much discussion a statement on "Routine Procedure at Hospitals" was drafted, together with an explanatory memorandum, but the BMA Council prudently remarked: "Neither the doctors nor the journalists who took part in these meetings are under any illusion that the problem of establishing a harmonious and mutually acceptable relationship between the medical profession and the press has now been solved."

There have been some further instances of unwarranted intrusion into the doctor-patient relationship, especially concerning new and startling medical discoveries; and there have been some radio and television programmes whose treatment of highly technical and complex subjects has been superficial and unbalanced. In these cases the BMA has made strong representations in the appropriate quarters. In general, however, the BMA has been fortunate in the quality of the journalists who have covered medical matters. We have seldom, if ever, encountered the unacceptable face of journalism — the nauseous voyeurism of some photographers, the reckless trivialisation of profoundly serious issues, and "cheque book journalism." In 1955, one of the distinguished Soviet doctors visiting Britain as a guest of the BMA expressed his astonishment and distaste at the manner in which one of our national newspapers had presented a particular news story (it was not a political item) and he expatiated on the advantages of press censorship. Now, after a quarter of a century, there are signs that the great profession of journalism, with all its immense power for good or evil, has something to learn from the medical profession in the matter of self-regulation.

OTHER NEW DEPARTMENTS

When medicine was nationalised in 1948, the BMA took over a well-known medical agency located in BMA House, the British Medical Bureau, and expanded it into the BMA's own medical employment agency. At first it was entitled the Medical Practices Advisory Bureau, but later this name was changed to the Personal Services Bureau. Both these titles indicate that the agency is more than merely an employment agency: it provides advice on a variety of practice and employment problems, such as partnership agreements and the terms of contracts of service.

In 1963 the coming into operation of the Review Body system prompted the formation of a statistical department at BMA House, and in 1976 this was converted into the Economic Research Unit.

In recent years the complexities of modern employment legislation (which concerns general practitioners as employers, and hospital doctors, and other doctors, as employees) have necessitated the formation of a legal department. The BMA now also has a recruitment (of members) department, a professional relations unit which provides rapid two-way communication between headquarters and the periphery, and a personnel department to manage the BMA's own staff.

The older departments already in existence in 1932, such as the library and the filing registry, now provide greatly expanded services. There has been much elaborate mechanisation, particularly in the typing and print room, in the secretarial centre (which provides pooled secretarial services), and in the personal records of members and non-members. The volume of traffic in the post room has grown enormously in the past 50 years, and some new problems have arisen. The staff have been instructed in precautions against letter bombs. In the postal strike of 1971 the BMA organised its own "pony express," using members of committees as couriers from BMA House to the regional offices, which then arranged onward distribution of urgent letters and documents. A priority circulation of the *British Medical Journal* to all BMA offices, to division secretaries, and to hospitals, postgraduate centres, and other places where doctors congregate, was also organised. Problems have arisen from other strikes too. In strikes of public transport workers key members of the Head Office staff have slept on camp beds at BMA House or stayed overnight in nearby hotels. Emergency supplies of lamps and candles were used during strikes in the electricity supply industry.

THE PLANNING UNIT

In 1966 the Representative Body expressed the wish that a "forward planning committee" should be set up. The Council sensibly decided that such a "think tank" should consist of eminent people not already immersed in BMA committee work, and that it should not be tied down to the formality of committee procedure. So a planning unit was established, with Professor Henry Miller, Dean of Medicine and later Vice-Chancellor at Newcastle upon Tyne, as its director and with a distinguished team of members. The unit quickly published a remarkable series of reports, prepared by expert panels which included non-medical members, on intensive care, aids for the disabled, computers in medicine, and primary medical care, as well as a guide to research funds. Although the reports made it clear that they did not purport to be statements of BMA policy, the chief medicopolitical committees nevertheless looked askance at the planning unit's activities and when Professor Henry Miller completed his promised term as director the unit was allowed to lapse.

Another valuable department of the BMA which was axed in one of its economy campaigns was the Career Service: an advisory service to young doctors, students, and schoolchildren about careers in medicine. In 1969 the BMA Career Service received 700 new inquiries. The medical director visited 14 medical schools, and a "careers convention" at Glasgow was attended by about 500 students. The Career Service was initiated in 1967 and discontinued in 1975.

RELATIONS WITH OTHER BODIES

Other medical bodies, which are legion, may be divided into two categories: those which are friendly to the BMA, and those which are hostile. Of those which are friendly, the first to be mentioned is the Conference of Representatives of Local Medical Committees, which is almost a part of the BMA machinery. There have been occasions when the views of the BMA and the conference have diverged on particular issues, but the leaders of the two bodies have always gone to great lengths to avoid any open clash and to arrive at some mutually acceptable compromise. The most obvious example in recent years was when the Representative Body of the BMA voted to adopt "Chambers in principle" (see Chapter 9).

For most of the time the BMA enjoys friendly and mutually respectful relations with the Royal Colleges. There have certainly been occasions, described in this book, when the Presidents of the Royal Colleges have done or said something which embarrassed or irritated the BMA, and there have also been occasions when the BMA embarrassed or even shocked the Royal Colleges. But the estrangement has always been short-lived, and the BMA's joint committee with the Royal Colleges — the Joint Consultants Committee — has worked smoothly and prestigiously. The BMA fully acknowledges the high professional standing of the colleges, and for their part they have come to recognise more and more that the BMA plays an essential and sometimes thankless role on behalf of the medical profession.

The BMA enjoys close and cordial relations with the British Dental Association, which is represented on several BMA committees. The BMA has or has had joint committees with the Royal College of Nursing, the Pharmaceutical Society, the Magistrates' Association, the British Veterinary Association, and the Trades Union Congress. Relations with the TUC have been friendly and mutually respectful, mainly because divisive issues have been avoided, but the BMA has resented the fact that successive governments have punctiliously consulted the TUC and the Confederation of British Industry about such things as pay policy and have neglected to consult the professions. The BMA has publicly pointed out that neither the TUC nor the CBI can claim to speak for the professions, a point that was at last conceded by the Government in 1976.

The BMA has always been on good terms with the Society of Medical Officers of Health (now the Society of Community Medicine), the Medical Women's Federation, the Society of Occupational Medicine, and the Royal Society of Medicine. The BMA has also enjoyed close and mutually helpful relations with the medical defence societies (the Medical Defence Union, the Medical Protection Society, and the Medical and Dental Defence Union of Scotland), though the smooth water was ruffled in 1977 when the BMA seriously considered the possibility of launching its own scheme of medical defence and indemnity, in collaboration with a well-known firm of insurance brokers. But the plan was abandoned.

The Medical Insurance Agency is independent of the BMA, but it was founded on the initiative of the BMA, has its head office in BMA House, shares some regional offices with the BMA, and now also shares a computer with the BMA. So the two organisations have worked closely together. A notable example of collaboration was the highly successful personal accident insurance scheme for BMA members which was launched by the MIA in 1958.

Now a brief word about an organisation that is ambivalent in its attitude to the BMA, neither consistently friendly nor consistently hostile: the Overseas Doctors Association. It is of recent origin and the BMA was indulgent towards its formation, but its philosophy differs fundamentally from that of the BMA towards the immigrant doctor. The traditional attitude of the BMA is that an overseas-qualified doctor, once registered in the UK, is to be treated exactly the same as any other registered medical practitioner. There should be no discrimination of any kind against him, and no discrimination in his favour. He should be completely integrated with the rest of the medical profession in the UK, and the BMA deeply regrets that the EEC Directives infringe this principle by drawing a distinction between doctors who have qualified within the European Community and doctors who have qualified outside it. The Overseas Doctors Association, on the other hand, seems to consider that overseas-qualified doctors are a distinct group that should be treated differently, even in some respects preferentially, from the rest of the profession.

The hostile organisations were set up in opposition to the BMA by groups of doctors dissatisfied with some aspects of the BMA's policy or performance. Originally the Medical Practitioners' Union was an organisation of diehards implacably opposed to the National Insurance Act of 1911 and angry with the BMA for capitulating to it. Many years ago, however, it moved politically to the left, and in 1968 it was swallowed up by the Association of Scientific, Technical and Managerial Staffs, a left-wing trade union. The General Practitioners Association had a brief existence in the "winter of discontent" of general practice in the early 1960s. The Junior Hospital Doctors Association was set up as the Hospital Junior Staff Action Group in September

1965, just two months *after* the BMA had published proposals for dramatic improvements in the pay and terms of service of hospital junior staff. Probably the young militants who formed it were not even aware of the effort which the BMA had already launched on their behalf.

It is fashionable to say that splinter groups serve a useful purpose by keeping the BMA on its toes. There is some truth in this, but it can also be argued that they divert the effort of the BMA into unproductive squabbles and fragment the profession's united front. On 7 June 1970, when the BMA was fighting vehemently against the Government's decision to halve the award of the Review Body and destroy its independence, the Secretary of State (Mr Richard Crossman) wrote in his diary*: "The BMA has met and decided on a partial strike but fortunately for us the junior hospital doctors' breakaway union had come out on our side, and so had the Medical Practitioners' Union. We have at least succeeded in splitting them that much." And on 5 December 1975, when the BMA was in furious argument with Mrs Barbara Castle about the "pricing" of the new junior staff contract she noted in her diary: "The break-away JHDA is trying to horn in on the act."

The most hostile of the splinter groups has been the Hospital Consultants and Specialists Association. A long-established and respected Regional Consultants and Specialists Association was taken over in 1970 by a small group of militant consultants who felt that they had been badly let down by the BMA and the Royal Colleges. They proceeded to wage war against the BMA. In 1974 they invited their members to resign from the BMA — an unkind cut — and 850 did so. Despite behind-the-scenes efforts by some of their leaders to bring to an end their unproductive feud with the BMA, the HCSA continued to explore every avenue to obtain separate negotiating rights, appealing to the Government, the National Industrial Relations Court, the Commission on Industrial Relations, and the Advisory Conciliation and Arbitration Service. All these moves were unsuccessful, but the BMA turned the other cheek and offered the Hospital Consultants and Specialists Association (they had dropped the prefix

* *The Diaries of a Cabinet Minister,* Vol III, by Richard Crossman (Hamish Hamilton and Jonathan Cape, 1977).

"Regional") reserved seats on the CCHMS, on the Negotiating Subcommittee, on the General Purposes Subcommittee and on the Central Manpower Committee. These magnanimous offers were rejected by the HCSA, who continued their hostile campaign. Notwithstanding these moves the BMA has persisted patiently in its efforts to reach an accommodation with the HCSA.

FAITHFUL UNTO DEATH

On 6 February 1952 the public relations officer went round the offices at BMA House with grievous news. That evening an assistant secretary (EG-T) wrote in his diary: "At about 11 am John Pringle put his head into my room and announced that the King was dead. We were all completely stunned. . . . All our hearts go out to the Queen and Queen Mary, but above all to the new Sovereign, poor Queen Elizabeth II — a charming shy girl of 25, mother of two young children, called to the Throne at a time of appalling international tension and economic crisis at home. . . . May her reign, as someone said at lunch, turn out to be 'sixty glorious years'." On the following Monday the staff filled the office windows and, in respectful silence, watched the coffin of King George VI borne on a gun carriage past BMA House on its way from Sandringham to Westminster Hall — just as the staff had watched the coffin of King George V make the same melancholy journey in 1936.

On 17 April 1962 the Chairman of Council, Dr Ian D Grant, died in his sleep in the Secretary's flat at BMA House. In June 1964 Dr J T McCutcheon died of a massive heart attack, a few weeks after taking office as Scottish Secretary. In January 1980 the Welsh Secretary, Dr M L Cattell, died in the train on his way from London to Cardiff after a Council meeting.

On 26 February 1966 Sir Guy Dain died at the age of 95. The Council publicly regretted "the passing of one of the most outstanding members of the profession in the twentieth century." He had been Chairman of Council from 1943 to 1949, the whole of the stormy period covering the introduction of the National Health Service. He was diminutive in height, but great in stature: a pocket battleship.

In 1936 Lord Nuffield was elected an honorary member of the Association "in view of the great benefits he has bestowed upon the community and upon medicine by his gifts to hospitals and medical research." He gave something like £30 million, mostly to medicine, in his lifetime. The BMA library is named the Nuffield Library in his honour.

In 1951 the first Council Dinner since 1938 was held in the Great Hall at BMA House. The traditional toast was to "the common health," and on this occasion the Minister of Health responded to the toast. The BMA Council dinners were brilliant occasions at which the guests included Ministers of the Crown, Ambassadors and High Commissioners, and Presidents of the Royal Colleges and of other national institutions such as the Royal Society and the Royal Academy. In 1954 the guest of honour was HRH Prince Philip, Duke of Edinburgh, who proposed "the common health," and again it was the Minister of Health who responded. In 1973 the Prime Minister (the Rt Hon Edward Heath) responded to the customary toast, the other guests including the Archbishop of York, three Secretaries of State, and the Lord Chief Justice.

In 1954 the BMA Council, stimulated by Dr S F Logan Dahne who was an expert in heraldry, took steps to acquire the grant of a coat of arms. The design contained an allusion to the founder of the Association in the form of the "maunche" of the Hastings family. The lion in the original design proved unacceptable to the Lord Lyon King of Arms, whose heraldic rule is absolute in Scotland where it was proposed also to have the arms registered. It was therefore replaced by a blue lion passant. For a motto the words "With head and heart and hand" were taken from Sir Charles Hastings's inaugural address to the Association in 1832, words which had been used by Sir Tudor Thomas as the title of his presidential address in 1953. The armorial bearings were finally granted to the Association in 1956.

Also in 1956 the Book of Valour was instituted, in which heroic deeds by members of the medical profession are recorded in a book which is permanently on display at BMA House. And in the same year the Fellowship of the British Medical Association was created, to recognise outstanding service given by members of the Association to their local divisions or branches.

The British and Canadian Medical Associations arranged to hold a joint meeting in 1959 in Edinburgh, and HRH the Duke of Edinburgh graciously accepted the invitation of both Associations to be their President for the year 1959-60. The *BMJ* commented: "The occasion will be a landmark in the history of the two organisations, for this is the first time that a member of the Royal Family has paid so signal an honour to either." Prince Philip was installed as President of the BMA on 28 October 1959, in the Great Hall at BMA House, having first been received by the Officers in the Centre Room — which Lutyens had placed directly over the Great Gate. Since then the room has been named "The Prince's Room."

Prince Philip was no mere figurehead as President. In his Presidential address he said: "Different people will think different things about the British Medical Association. To me it is one of those things which entirely justify our idea of freedom and democracy: freedom because the essence of freedom is self-control as opposed to some form of outside direction, and democracy because the people who exercise the control are ordinary members of the profession." During the year he frequently requested information and comment from BMA House on a wide variety of topics, and altogether kept the senior staff on their toes. In 1960 he flew by helicopter to Torquay to hand over the Presidency to Sir Arthur Porritt, and fulfilled a busy day of engagements — presiding briskly and wittily over the annual general meeting, touring the scientific and pharmaceutical exhibitions, taking the chair at a grand Presidential Luncheon, and officiating at the adjourned annual general meeting, which was held (in baking sunshine) in the covered tennis courts of the Palace Hotel.

Other brilliant annual meetings were held in Bournemouth in 1934, Belfast in 1962, and Oxford in 1963. The Annual Dinner at Belfast was attended by the Prime Minister of Northern Ireland (Viscount Brookeborough), the Speaker of the Northern Ireland House of Commons (Sir Norman Stronge, assassinated in 1981), the Duke of Abercorn, the General Officer Commanding (Lt General Sir John Hackett), and the Lord Mayor of Belfast. At the Oxford Meeting of 1963 the Archbishop of Canterbury preached the sermon at the official religious service at Christ Church Cathedral, the Presidential reception was held at Blenheim Palace, and the Prime Minister (the Rt Hon Harold Macmillan) proposed the toast of the Association at the Annual Dinner, in his role as Chancellor of the University. He said that in the past 15 years there had developed between the government of the day and the medical profession a partnership that was unique. There was no parallel, so far as he knew, with any other profession in the country, or in any other country with the profession. It jogged along rather like a marriage. But on the whole it had proved a success. The President, Sir George Pickering, said it was difficult to make an objective assessment, but were he an ordinary citizen who had the misfortune to be seriously ill he would be as well taken care of in this country as in any other. He was proud to be at the head of the British Medical Association because it was the only body which united all doctors, whether they were what transatlantic friends called pill doctors, cutting doctors, sleeping doctors, or talking doctors.

In 1966 a Hastings Centenary Clinical Meeting was held at Worcester to commemorate the death in 1866 of Sir Charles Hastings, the founder. A service was held at Hastings's grave, and a reception in the room at the Royal Infirmary where Hastings founded the Association. A memorial address was delivered by Lord Cohen of Birkenhead, President of the General Medical Council and Past President of the BMA. It is through the generosity of Lord Cohen that each President of the BMA is presented with a Past President's badge on his retirement from office.

Let us end this chapter by paying tribute to some of the BMA members who in the past 50 years have attained high office or great distinction outside medicine. The list includes five Cabinet Ministers: Colonel Walter Elliott (1932-40); Viscount Addison KG (1945-51), who was the first Minister of Health from 1919 to 1921 and was again in the Cabinet from 1930 to 1931; Baroness Summerskill (1950-1); Lord Hill of Luton (1957-62), a former Secretary of the BMA, who also became Chairman of the Governors of the BBC from 1967 to 1972; and Dr David Owen (1977-9), the first medically qualified Foreign Secretary.

Viscount Malvern was Prime Minister of Rhodesia from 1933 to 1956. Sir Earle Page was Prime Minister of

Australia from 1939 to 1940. Sir Milton Margai was Prime Minister of Sierra Leone from 1960 to 1964. Sir Seewoosagur Ramgoolam has been Prime Minister of Mauritius since 1965. Dr Hastings Banda was Prime Minister of Malawi from 1963 to 1966, and has been President of Malawi since 1966. Dr B H Sheares was President of Singapore from 1971 to 1981.

Sir Selwyn Selwyn-Clarke was Governor of the Seychelles from 1947 to 1951; Lt General Sir Alexander Hood was Governor of Bermuda from 1949 to 1955; and Lord Porritt was Governor General of New Zealand from 1967 to 1972.

Among others who have held high non-medical offices since 1932 are Lord Adrian OM, who was Chancellor of the University of Cambridge from 1968 to 1975, Lord Cohen of Birkenhead who was Chancellor of the University of Hull from 1970 to 1973, and Lord Pitt of Hampstead, who was Chairman of the Greater London Council in 1974-5. Sir Donald Pollock Bt was a captain of industry, being Chairman of Metal Industries Ltd (1924-51) and of the British Oxygen Company Ltd (1934-7).

Among those who achieved fame as authors are Somerset Maugham, James Bridie (O H Mavor), A J Cronin, and Richard Gordon (G W Ostlere, once an assistant editor of the *BMJ*). Dr Louis Boyd Neel forsook medicine for music and became a world-famous conductor. Among many famous medical athletes is Sir Roger Bannister, the first man to run a mile in under four minutes.

The medical profession can boast a long line of Fellows of the Royal Society, and a proud group of winners of the Victoria Cross. Only one person has ever achieved both of these immense distinctions, and he was a doctor. Brigadier J A Sinton, a Belfast graduate, was awarded the VC in 1916 for conspicuous bravery and devotion to duty during an action in Mesopotamia. Thirty years later he was elected FRS for his work on malaria and kala-azar.

Only one doctor has won the George Cross. Captain J R O Thompson RAMC was posthumously awarded the GC in 1944 for outstanding heroism when the hospital ship *St David* was dive-bombed off Anzio. The ship was sinking rapidly and Captain Thompson organised parties to carry the seriously wounded to safety in the boats, inspiring all by his coolness and resource. When the ship was about to founder and all were ordered to save themselves, he returned alone in a last effort to save one remaining patient who was still trapped below. Captain Thompson went down with the ship.

A SECOND ROYAL PRESIDENT

Finally, it is a great pleasure to record that in 1979 HRH the Prince of Wales graciously accepted honorary membership of the Association, and in 1980 the Representative Body unanimously elected Prince Charles to be President of the Association in its 150th year, 1982-3.

Chapter 11

The shock troops of the middle classes*

Cet animal est très méchant, Quand on l'attaque il se défend.
— La Ménagerie, by Théodore P K, 1868.

The half-century covered by this book has been a turbulent period of medical history. The medical profession has gone through three revolutions: social, scientific, and organisational. The social revolution was mainly brought about by the war, or rather by the two world wars which, in retrospect, were really one great war with a 20-year armistice in the middle. The first world war destroyed the power of the landed aristocracy. The second levelled the professions and the mercantile masters, and transferred power to the labouring classes and their unions. Mr Anthony Wedgwood Benn has said that "the power of the trade unions is as great as that of the old landowners."

The 1930s were still gracious times. At BMA House, the immediate past Chairman of the Representative Body, Dr C O Hawthorne, always wore a grey topper on Council days. A Welbeck Street physician used to travel to consultations in the country in his chauffeur-driven Rolls Royce, dressed in top hat and tails. Years later, a much-respected general practitioner remarked that his patients had been very willing to pay a guinea a mile for *that.* A Glasgow professor of surgery took a taxi from London to Windsor, dressed in grey morning tails and an elegant panama hat — the weather was hot. The social revolution put an end to all this.

The revolution in medical science has been almost incredible. Since 1932 we have witnessed the arrival of

* I do not claim authorship of this title. I think this description was applied to the BMA in a newspaper, but I have failed to trace the reference and can only express my thanks to whoever may have invented it. EG-T.

chemotherapy, antibiotics, psychotropic drugs, elaborate endocrinology, high energy radiation and postirradiation surgery in oncology, the iron lung, the heart-lung machine, kidney dialysis, and organ transplantation. We have seen the acceptance of the concept of multidisciplinary teams of specialists and the introduction of intensive-care units for neonates, postoperative patients, and acute medical emergencies. We have recently seen fertilisation of the human ovum in vitro, with the subsequent birth of a healthy infant, and genetic engineering. In diagnosis, the past half-century has witnessed the introduction of angiography and other precision radiological techniques, wonderful developments in endoscopy, the invention of ultrasonics, nuclear scanning, and computed tomography. This long list is by no means exhaustive.

High technology medicine is enormously expensive. Increasing specialisation with escalating cost was the chief (though not the only) reason for the nationalisation of the hospitals in 1948. Even before the damage and destruction of the second world war the voluntary hospitals were verging on bankruptcy. Sir Harry Platt has written: "It was clear to anyone that after the war in which we had wasted millions of our national assets, the voluntary hospitals would need to be supported financially from central government funds." The municipal hospitals were already supported from *local* government funds, but these also were insufficient. Professor Harry Eckstein has referred* to "the inability of the old major sources of finance (private payments for services rendered, philanthropy, and local taxation) to foot the bill for a really modern system of services."

The introduction of the National Health Service was a watershed for the medical profession, and hence for the BMA. For 116 years it had been a professional society of doctors, almost a private club — like many other "literary and philosophical" societies founded in the nineteenth century. True, it had always performed a medicopolitical function. The Association established a Medical Reform Committee in 1837, a Parliamentary Bills Committee in 1863, and a Medico-Political Committee in 1903. But after 1948 this role grew far more important, and the BMA

* *The English Health Service* by Harry Eckstein, Harvard University Press, 1964.

became the belligerent defender of the political and economic status of the medical profession. Indeed, with its resources and determination, it found itself carrying the torch for the whole of the middle class, which was under siege in the postwar world from fiscal policies, egalitarianism, and collectivism.

It was natural, but not inevitable, that the nationalisation of medicine should lead the BMA to become increasingly preoccupied with medicopolitical matters, especially the negotiation of pay and conditions of service of doctors. There were trade unions (and other bodies too) that were ready and willing to take over the representation of the medical profession, such as the Medical Practitioners Union, the Confederation of Health Service Employees, and the National Association of Local Government Officers. But in such unions the interests of doctors would have been subordinated to those of the "big battalions" of non-medical members. And so, although many doctors disliked it, the BMA organised and armed itself for political and economic warfare.

How successful has the BMA been in this expanded role? Is it "the strongest trade union in the world"? Or a paper tiger? The answer lies somewhere in between. One of the curious features of the BMA is that its standing is far higher outside the medical profession — among the general public, the media, and other professions — than within it. Sir Paul Chambers noted that most criticism came to him from members who themselves did a great deal of work for the BMA. Perhaps this is a healthy sign, but it does not make life easy for BMA leaders. Barbara Castle referred in her diary to "The horrible job of having to speak to two audiences: the one in front, and the one behind." The BMA leaders usually have to address three audiences simultaneously: the Department of Health (or whoever is the other party to the negotiation or dispute), public opinion, and their own very demanding and critical army behind them.

BMA members, all of whom have had a university education and most of whom are individualists, are much less likely to obey instructions from the leadership and "follow the party line" than members of labour unions. In addition, the old-established trade unions impose discipline on their members by methods which are deeply repugnant to the BMA, such as the closed shop and picketing, but these are the measures which enable the unions to use their ultimate weapon — the strike, or total stoppage of work — with so much effect.

The BMA fully recognises that this weapon is not available to the medical profession. It can be argued that in the last quarter of the twentieth century the strike weapon is an anachronism which should no longer be tolerated at all. The hardship inflicted by some strikes on innocent and defenceless bystanders is uncivilised. But so long as society regards the right to strike as an essential democratic freedom — and (in 1981) applauds the Poles for claiming it — who can blame the BMA for searching long and hard for some kind of sanction that the nationalised medical profession could legitimately use in defence of its vital interests? So far the search has been in vain, though the BMA has found some surprisingly effective ways of exerting collective pressure. At the time when the choice of a suitable crest for the BMA's coat of arms was being discussed, the then public relations officer suggested a boa constrictor.

Pari passu with the increasing involvement of the BMA in politics and in economic argument (though not necessarily or entirely because of it), there has been a decline in the esteem of the medical profession. The same process has occurred elsewhere. W S Lawson, in his centenary history of the South Australian Branch of the Australian Medical Association (1979) wrote:

> These changes marked the end of a more gracious era. Perhaps the turning point occurred when the National Health Scheme . . . was introduced in 1952. Nothing would ever be the same again no matter how desirable some of the benefits accruing to society as a whole may have been. The health, and particularly the medical expectations of the population were heightened immensely by an increased demand for tangible treatment with measurable outcomes regardless of cost. Inevitably doctors became greatly concerned with the financial rewards available to them for every aspect of their work. Some would say this influence led to a decrease in the quality of personal attention which the patient received. One of the effects was a reduction in the respect previously shown to doctors and a lowering of the esteem in which the profession was held in the public eye. During the 1970s there was a trend for people in all westernised communities to demand greater accountability by all professions and simultaneously to become highly

critical of their standards of performance in meeting their professional commitments.

These words might just as well have been written about the United Kingdom.

Perhaps as a reaction to these trends, the BMA has tenaciously persevered with its scientific, educational, and ethical functions. In recent years some critics have urged that these activities should be left to other bodies — such as the Royal Colleges and specialist societies, and the General Medical Council — so that the BMA could concentrate all its energies and resources on its protective role for the medical profession. But the BMA has adamantly refused to do this, and in the past 50 years its scientific and ethical activities, especially its scientific publications, have grown in scope and stature.

Although the world is entirely different from that into which the BMA was launched, the Association has retained some of its original characteristics. It is still dominated by the provinces, rather than by London.* It is still deeply attached to the voluntary principle, to the extent of being quixotically considerate to non-members. At the annual meeting, although such typically Victorian features as the whole-day excursion, and the annual dinner (in white tie and tails) have now disappeared, the meeting still goes ceremonially to church in academic dress and listens with a discerning ear to the sermon.

Long before 1932 the BMA ceased to discriminate in any way against women doctors. The first woman to be elected to the Council was Dr Christine Murrell, in 1924. The first woman President was Dame Josephine Barnes, in 1979. The BMA is also completely multiracial. The Association has a great many non-European members, and they have held office in local divisions and branches, in the Council and committees, and in the Presidency.

In the past 33 years the BMA has spent much time agonising over its own constitution. This is yet another consequence of the socialisation of medicine. When so much in their professional lives has to be negotiated with a near-monopoly employer, all categories of doctors are determined to be adequately represented in the negotiating

*The most influential element in the Representative Body is probably the so-called "northern block" of Representatives from the Midlands and the North.

body; and along with all this democratic machinery they *also* expect the BMA to be capable of acting quickly and incisively on their behalf. It is not easy to find a constitution that fulfils both these requirements.

And yet, despite all the pressures of modern times, the BMA remains very much a club, even a family. The wives and daughters — and husbands and sons — of BMA members have played an increasing part in the activities of the Association. For the most part the staff display a degree of loyalty to their employer that is characteristic of a family firm. Mr John Huish and Mr George Perkins retired in 1973 after 44 years and 48 years on the staff. Mr John Randall retired in 1979 after 47 years. In 1981 Mr Christopher Prosser retired after 51 years of service. Many other examples of devoted service could be cited. A lay official who left for another post in 1975 wrote: "I have enjoyed myself immensely during the ten years at BMA House where urbane and civilised company has made the roughest going more than bearable. My memories will be of a place where people smiled more readily than they scowled and where, even in times of crisis, laughter was heard more than angry voices."

The past 50 years have seen the BMA move from a gracious, bygone age, through the consuming fires of war, and through withdrawal from Empire, into a harsh, collectivist world where the Association has had to fight and fight and fight again for the profession which it loves. The BMA has a fine motto: With head, and heart, and hand. An alternative might be:

Nemo me impune lacessit.

Appendix A

A Selected Chronology 1932-81

1932 Publication of *History of the British Medical Association 1832-1932.*
Centenary dinner at the Albert Hall. HRH the Prince of Wales proposed Toast to "The British Medical Association" (28 July).
BMA membership 35 070.

1933 Hitler became German Chancellor.
Government published Warren Fisher Report on the shortage of officers and nurses in the medical and dental branches of the Armed Forces.
BMA published report of Committee on Nutrition.

1934 Incorporation of Federal Council of the BMA in Australia.
Report by BMA Committee on Medical Education.
BMA formed Consultants and Specialists Groups.

1935 Memorandum by BMA on the Theory, Technique, and Practice of Osteopathy.
Domagk reported the effect of prontosil on streptococci.
Report of BMA Committee on the Relation of Alcohol to Road Accidents.

1936 BMA founded Board of Registration of Medical Auxiliaries.
Report of BMA Committee on Medical Aspects of Abortion.
Lord Nuffield elected honorary member of the BMA.

1937 BMA accepted invitation from Trades Union Congress to form a joint standing committee.
BMA compiled register of doctors willing to render service in the event of national emergency.

1938 Publication of revised version of BMA report on *A General Medical Service for the Nation.*
The Munich crisis.
BMA membership 38 030.

1939 Central Emergency Committee reconstituted and other arrangements made to organise the medical profession for a national emergency.
BMA published memorandum on hospital policy.
Outbreak of second world war.

1940 Medical Planning Commission appointed.
Annual representative meeting and annual scientific meeting cancelled.

1941 BMA House bombed.
BMA set up Industrial Health Committee.

1942 BMA published draft interim report of Medical Planning Commission.
Government published Beveridge Report.

1943 Representative Committee of the profession appointed, for discussions with Minister of Health on proposed National Health Service.
Mass miniature radiography service inaugurated.

1944 Captain J R O Thompson RAMC won George Cross.
Publication of Government White Paper on a national health service.
BMA questionary on the White Paper.

1945 Special representative meeting on Government's proposals for a national health service.
End of second world war.
Election of Labour Government.
BMA membership 51 508.

1946 Government introduced National Health Service Bill.
Special representative meeting to consider the terms of the Bill.
World Medical Association founded at BMA House, London.
National Health Service Act obtained Royal Assent.
First BMA plebiscite on the Act.

1947 Presidents of the Royal Colleges wrote to the Minister of Health (Mr Aneurin Bevan).
Special representative meeting decided to enter into discussions with the Minister.
Negotiating Committee published result of discussions.
BMA formed Film Library.

1948 Special representative meeting to settle form of second plebiscite.
Second BMA plebiscite: 90% disapproval of the National Health Service Act.
Special representative meeting on the Act.
Minister of Health (Mr Aneurin Bevan) undertook to amend the Act.
Third BMA plebiscite: 52% against accepting service under the Act (and the Scottish Act).
BMA Council decided to recommend co-operation in the new service (5 May).
Special representative meeting advised the profession to co-operate in the National Health Service (28 May).
Inauguration of National Health Service (5 July).
British Commonwealth Medical Conference held at BMA House, London.

1949 BMA and Pharmaceutical Society published new *National Formulary*.
Special representative meeting on remuneration of general practitioners (29 March).
Separate special representative meeting, on BMA constitution, decided to found British Medical Guild (30 March).
Third General Assembly of World Medical Association held at BMA House, London.

1950 BMA formed Registrars' Group.
BMA issued booklet *Ethics and Members of the Medical Profession.*
Special representative meeting changed the constitution of the Council.
Outbreak of Korean war.
North and south wings of BMA House completed.
First article by Doll and Bradford Hill in *BMJ* on link between smoking and cancer of the lung.

1951 BMA launched *Family Doctor* magazine.
First Council dinner since 1938.
BMA founded Caribbean Council.
Special representative meeting on reform of the National Health Service.

1952 Danckwerts Award.
Inauguration of scientific exhibition at the annual meeting.

1953 Hastings Room opened at BMA House, London.
First World Conference on Medical Education, London, organised by BMA.
Council of World Medical Association met at BMA House, London.

1954 BMA asked Government to set up inquiry into medical manpower.
Dedication of BMA war memorial.

1955 BMA published Strachan Report on hospital staffing structure.
Visit of six Soviet doctors as guests of BMA.

1956 Government published Guillebaud Report on the cost of the NHS.
Collective resignation of Government doctors in Malta.
Remuneration claim submitted on behalf of general practitioners and hospital doctors.
First national conference of consultants and specialists.
Six representatives of BMA visited USSR.
Hungarian uprising, and Suez emergency.

1957 Report of Second Constitution Committee.
Royal Commission on Remuneration of Doctors and Dentists in the NHS appointed.
Special representative meeting on whether to co-operate with the royal commission (1 May). No decision.
Second special representative meeting decided to submit evidence to the royal commission (12 June).
Demonstrations on closed circuit television at the annual meeting.
Government published Willink Report on medical manpower.

1958 Medical Services Review Committee (the Porritt committee) appointed.
BMA inaugurated Junior Members' Forum.
First annual clinical meeting.

1959 BMA published Abel-Lewin report on hospital building.
Fifth British Commonwealth Medical Conference held at BMA House, London.
HRH Prince Philip installed as President.

1960 Report of Royal Commission on Remuneration of Doctors and Dentists in the NHS.
Special representative meeting on Royal Commission report (19 May).
Second special representative meeting accepted the Minister's offer to implement the recommendations of the Royal Commission "as a whole as they stand" (28 September).
End of conscription for National Service.

1961 Government published Platt Report on medical staffing structure in the hospital service.
Leading article in *BMJ* on the "First Spaceman" (22 April).
BMA membership 76 673.

1962 Joint Review Body Evidence Committee established.
First discussion with Ministry of Health about medical implications of UK joining the European Economic Community.
"New Deal" for Forces doctors.
Porritt Report published.
First national conference of public health medical officers.
Commonwealth Medical Association founded.

1963 First Report of the Review Body.
Reconstructed Nuffield Library opened.
Annual representative meeting supported the setting up of area health boards "as this would increase co-ordination and co-operation between the three parts of the service."
Special representative meeting criticised the "pool" system of remunerating general practitioners.
Annual meeting attended by Archbishop of Canterbury and Prime Minister.

1964 Special representative meeting approved special case to the Review Body on behalf of general practitioners.
Second meeting of Council of Commonwealth Medical Association held at BMA House, London.

1965 Fifth Report of the Review Body on the special case for general practitioners. Great dissatisfaction.
British Medical Guild collected undated resignations of general practitioners.

BMA published *A Charter for the Family Doctor Service.*
Special representative meeting (24 March) held in conjunction with special Conference of Representatives of Local Medical Committees. Decided to pursue negotiations with the Minister on the charter, and meanwhile to hold the resignations.
Second special representative meeting (23 June) decided that negotiations on the charter should continue but that the undated resignations would continue to be held.
BMA published *An appraisal of the Hospital Service.*
Hospital Junior Staff Action Group formed.
19th General Assembly of World Medical Association held at BMA House, London.

1966 Hastings centenary meeting at Worcester.
Seventh Report of the Review Body (4 May).
Special representative meeting (21 June) decided that the Review Body's award be accepted and that the undated resignations be "withdrawn."
Government imposed pay standstill (20 July).
Responsibility for negotiations on the remuneration and terms of service of hospital doctors transferred from Joint Consultants Committee to Central Committee for Hospital Medical Services.
BMA News launched.
Report of Council on constitution of the BMA.
BMA established department of audio-visual communication, with support of British Life Assurance Trust.

1967 Memorandum on the Current Problems of Hospital Medical Staff (the "hospital doctors' charter") submitted to Minister of Health.
BMA "blacklisted" all medical vacancies under local authorities.
BMJ published article on "Medicine and the Treaty of Rome" by N G C Hendry (13 May).

1968 Final joint report of negotiations with health departments on the hospital doctors' charter.
Report of Royal Commission on Medical Education (Todd Report) published (4 April).
Ministry of Health merged with Ministry of Social

Security under new Secretary of State for Social Services (Mr Richard Crossman) (5 April).
BMA established the Board of Science and Education.
Government published Green Papers on the administrative structure of the National Health Service in England and Wales (July) and in Scotland (December), proposing unification under area boards.

1969 Special representative meeting criticised Green Paper proposals.
BMA published statement on the ethics of transplantation.
BMA negotiated extra duty allowances for hospital junior staff.
Government published Green Paper on the Administrative Structure of the Health and Personal Social Services in Northern Ireland.
Joint Consultants Committee met in Belfast.

1970 Government published second English Green Paper on administrative reorganisation of NHS.
Special representative meeting on GMC retention fee.
BMA published report *Health Services Financing.*
Privy Council introduced GMC annual retention fee.
Special representative meeting on Todd Report, second Green Paper, and General Medical Council (6 and 7 May).
Publication of Twelfth Report of Review Body delayed until 4 June. Government refused to implement award in full, and referred report to Prices and Incomes Board. Review Body resigned. BMA imposed sanctions.
General election (18 June). Change of Government.
New Government cancelled reference of Review Body report to Prices and Incomes Board and undertook to re-establish an independent Review Body. BMA withdrew sanctions.
Central Council for Postgraduate Medical Education and Training established.

1971 Brynmor Jones Report on composition of GMC.

BMA published "Memorandum on Association Policy in Relation to Smoking."
Government published "Consultative Document on NHS Reorganisation in England."
Special representative meeting on (*1*) consultative document and (*2*) Industrial Relations Bill.
BMA entered in the Special Register under Industrial Relations Act.

1972 BMA published Chambers Report.
White Paper on NHS reorganisation.
BMA published new model contract for consultants.
Special representative meeting accepted Chambers proposals "in principle."
Government set up committee of inquiry into the GMC, with Dr A W Merrison as chairman.
BMA elected to full membership of Standing Committee of Doctors of the EEC.

1973 United Kingdom entered European Economic Community (1 January).
Annual representative meeting debated proposals for implementing "Chambers in principle," and modified them on the recommendation of the Council.
National Health Service Reorganisation Act passed.
Council dinner attended by Prime Minister (Mr Edward Heath).
Organisation of Petroleum Exporting Countries (OPEC) boosted the world price of oil.

1974 BMA provided presidency and secretariat of Standing Committee of Doctors of the EEC (for three years).
Secretary of State for Social Services (Mrs Barbara Castle) set up the Owen Working Party with the profession to negotiate on (*1*) new consultant contract and (*2*) separation of private practice from NHS hospitals.
Reorganisation of the administrative structure of the National Health Service (1 April).
Report of the Lane Committee on the working of the Abortion Act.
Trade Union and Labour Relations Act 1974

passed. This Act made the BMA a trade union (but it also remained a registered company).
BMA led deputation of health professions to the Prime Minister (Mr Harold Wilson) about NHS financing. They asked for an independent inquiry into financing the service.
Negotiations broke down in Owen Working Party and consultants decided to apply sanctions.

1975 BMA negotiated new "closed-ended" contract for hospital junior staff.
Special representative meeting debated Council's third report on the Chambers proposals, and finally settled a new constitution.
Report of Merrison Committee on the GMC.
Negotiations resumed with Mrs Castle on new consultant contract, and consultants withdrew sanctions.
Special representative meeting on Merrison Report on the GMC.
Publication of consultative document on the separation of private practice from the NHS.
Prime Minister announced appointment of Royal Commission on the National Health Service, but refused to hold up legislation to "phase out" pay-beds. Consultants applied renewed sanctions, together with hospital junior staff who were in dispute about their new contract.
Lord Goodman produced compromise proposals to settle the pay-beds issue.

1976 Goodman proposals approved by consultants, who suspended sanctions.
BMA deputation to Prime Minister (Mr James Callaghan) about impact of Government pay policy on the Professions.
BMA published detailed proposals for new consultant contract.
Health Services Act 1976 passed, enacting the Goodman proposals.

1977 BMA and Royal Colleges published discussion document on ethical responsibilities of doctors in regard to "industrial action."
Special representative meeting debated draft

memorandum of evidence to the Royal Commission on the NHS.

1978 Medical Act 1978 reconstituting the GMC passed.
Government published discussion paper, *Medical Manpower — The Next Twenty Years.*
BMA launched French edition of *You and Your Baby* in Paris, in presence of French Minister of Health.

1979 Report of Royal Commission on the National Health Service.
Review Body's pricing of the new consultant contract led to its rejection by consultants.

1980 Health Services Act 1980 again reorganised administrative structure of the NHS, and reversed the previous Government's policy on private practice.
BMA published *The Handbook of Medical Ethics.*
HRH the Prince of Wales elected President of the Association for 1982-3.

1981 Government found "compelling reasons" for reducing the Review Body's award from 9% to 6%.
Annual representative meeting voted for medical audit organised and administered by the profession.
BMA membership 66 906.

Appendix

Annual Meetings, Chief Officers, et

YEAR	PLACES OF ANNUAL MEETINGS	SESSION	PRESIDENT	CHAIRMAN OF REPRESENTATIVE BODY	CHAIRMAN OF COUNCIL
1932	London	1932-3	The Rt Hon Lord DAWSON of Penn	Dr ERNEST KAYE LE FLEMING	Sir HENRY BRITTEN BRACKENBU
1933	Dublin	1933-4	Professor THOMAS GILLMAN MOORHEAD	Dr ERNEST KAYE LE FLEMING	Sir HENRY BRITTEN BRACKENBU
1934	Bournemouth	1934-5	Dr SYDNEY WATSON SMITH	Mr HENRY SESSIONS SOUTTAR	Dr ERNEST KAYE LE FLEMING
1935	Melbourne (Annual Meeting) London (Annual Representative Meeting)	1935-6	Sir JAMES WILLIAM BARRETT	Mr HENRY SESSIONS SOUTTAR	Dr ERNEST KAYE LE FLEMING
1936	Oxford	1936-7	Sir EDWARD FARQUHAR BUZZARD, Bt	Mr HENRY SESSIONS SOUTTAR	Dr ERNEST KAYE LE FLEMING
1937	Belfast	1937-8	Professor (later Sir) ROBERT JAMES JOHNSTONE	Dr HARRY GUY DAIN	Sir ERNEST KAYE LE FLEMING

EASURER	SECRETARY	EDITOR	GOLD MEDALLISTS
r NATHANIEL BISHOP HARMAN	Dr GEORGE CRANSTON ANDERSON (Medical Secretary) Mr LEYCESTER FERRIS-SCOTT (Financial Secretary)	Dr NORMAN GERALD HORNER	
r NATHANIEL BISHOP HARMAN	Dr GEORGE CRANSTON ANDERSON (Medical Secretary) Mr LEYCESTER FERRIS-SCOTT (Financial Secretary)	Dr NORMAN GERALD HORNER	
r NATHANIEL BISHOP HARMAN	Dr GEORGE CRANSTON ANDERSON (Medical Secretary) Mr LEYCESTER FERRIS-SCOTT (Financial Secretary)	Dr NORMAN GERALD HORNER	
r NATHANIEL BISHOP HARMAN	Dr GEORGE CRANSTON ANDERSON (Medical Secretary) Mr LEYCESTER FERRIS-SCOTT (Financial Secretary)	Dr NORMAN GERALD HORNER	Dr HARRY GUY DAIN
r NATHANIEL BISHOP HARMAN	Dr GEORGE CRANSTON ANDERSON (Medical Secretary) Mr LEYCESTER FERRIS-SCOTT (Financial Secretary)	Dr NORMAN GERALD HORNER	
r NATHANIEL BISHOP HARMAN	Dr GEORGE CRANSTON ANDERSON	Dr NORMAN GERALD HORNER	

YEAR	PLACES OF ANNUAL MEETINGS	SESSION	PRESIDENT	CHAIRMAN OF REPRESENTATIVE BODY	CHAIRMAN OF COUNCIL
1938	Plymouth	1938-9	Dr COLIN DUNROD LINDSAY	Dr HARRY GUY DAIN	Sir ERNEST KAYE LE FLEMING
1939	Aberdeen	1939-40	Dr THOMAS FRASER	Dr HARRY GUY DAIN	Mr HENRY SESSIONS SOUTTAR
1940	London (Annual General Meeting only)	1940-1	Dr THOMAS FRASER	Dr HARRY GUY DAIN	Mr HENRY SESSIONS SOUTTAR
1941	London (Annual General Meeting only)	1941-2	Dr THOMAS FRASER	Dr HARRY GUY DAIN	Mr HENRY SESSIONS SOUTTAR
1942	London	1942-3	Sir HAROLD BECKWITH WHITEHOUSE (died 28 July 1943)	Dr HARRY GUY DAIN	Mr HENRY SESSIONS SOUTTAR
1943	London	1943-4	The Rt Hon Viscount DAWSON of Penn	Dr PETER MACDONALD	Dr HARRY GUY DAIN
1944	London	1944-5	The Rt Hon Viscount DAWSON of Penn (died 7 March 1945)	Dr PETER MACDONALD	Dr HARRY GUY DAIN
1945	London	1945-6	Mr HENRY SESSIONS SOUTTAR	Dr JAMES BLAKELY MILLER	Dr HARRY GUY DAIN
1946	London	1946-7	Sir HUGH LETT, Bt	Dr JAMES BLAKELY MILLER	Dr HARRY GUY DAIN
1947	London	1947-8	Sir HUGH LETT, Bt	Dr JAMES BLAKELY MILLER	Dr HARRY GUY DAIN
1948	Cambridge	1948-9	Sir LIONEL ERNEST HOWARD WHITBY	Dr EDWARD ANDREW GREGG	Dr HARRY GUY DAIN

EASURER	SECRETARY	EDITOR	GOLD MEDALLISTS
NATHANIEL BISHOP HARMAN	Dr GEORGE CRANSTON ANDERSON	Dr NORMAN GERALD HORNER	Dr CHARLES OLIVER HAWTHORNE
JOHN WARDLE BONE	Dr GEORGE CRANSTON ANDERSON	Dr NORMAN GERALD HORNER	
JOHN WARDLE BONE	Dr GEORGE CRANSTON ANDERSON	Dr NORMAN GERALD HORNER	Sir ERNEST KAYE LE FLEMING
JOHN WARDLE BONE	Dr GEORGE CRANSTON ANDERSON	Dr NORMAN GERALD HORNER	
JOHN WARDLE BONE	Dr GEORGE CRANSTON ANDERSON	Dr NORMAN GERALD HORNER	
JOHN WARDLE BONE	Dr GEORGE CRANSTON ANDERSON (died 1 January 1944) Dr CHARLES HILL (appointed 3 March 1944)	Dr NORMAN GERALD HORNER	
JOHN WARDLE BONE	Dr CHARLES HILL	Dr NORMAN GERALD HORNER	
JOHN WARDLE BONE	Dr CHARLES HILL	Dr NORMAN GERALD HORNER	
JOHN WARDLE BONE	Dr CHARLES HILL	Dr NORMAN GERALD HORNER (until December 1946) Dr HUGH ANTHONY CLEGG (from January 1947)	
JOHN WARDLE BONE	Dr CHARLES HILL	Dr HUGH ANTHONY CLEGG	
r ARCHIE MURRELL ACHESON MOORE	Dr CHARLES HILL	Dr HUGH ANTHONY CLEGG	Dr JOHN WARDLE BONE

YEAR	PLACES OF ANNUAL MEETINGS	SESSION	PRESIDENT	CHAIRMAN OF REPRESENTATIVE BODY	CHAIRMAN OF COUNCIL
1949	Harrogate	1949-50	Dr CYRIL WILLIAM CURTIS BAIN	Dr EDWARD ANDREW GREGG (elected Chairman of RB 27 June 1949, and Chairman of Council 29 June 1949) Dr JAMES ALEXANDER BROWN (Acting Chairman of RB from 29 June 1949)	Dr EDWARD ANDREW GREGG
1950	Liverpool (Annual Scientific Meeting) Southport (Annual Representative Meeting)	1950-1	Sir HENRY COHEN	Dr JAMES ALEXANDER BROWN	Dr EDWARD ANDREW GREGG
1951	London	1951-2	Dr ALAN WILLIAM STUART SICHEL	Dr SOLOMON WAND	Dr EDWARD ANDREW GREGG
1952	Dublin	1952-3	Dr PATRICK THEODORE JOSEPH O'FARRELL	Dr SOLOMON WAND	Dr EDWARD ANDREW GREGG
1953	Cardiff	1953-4	Mr JAMES WILLIAM TUDOR THOMAS	Dr SOLOMON WAND	Dr EDWARD ANDREW GREGG
1954	Glasgow	1954-5	Sir JOHN WILLIAM McNEE	Dr IAN DINGWALL GRANT	Dr EDWARD ANDREW GREGG
1955	Toronto (Joint Annual Meeting of British, Canadian, and Ontario Medical Associations) London (Annual Representative Meeting)	1955-6	Dr THOMAS CLARENCE ROUTLEY	Dr IAN DINGWALL GRANT	Dr EDWARD ANDREW GREGG

EASURER	SECRETARY	EDITOR	GOLD MEDALLISTS
ARCHIE MURRELL ACHESON MOORE	Dr CHARLES HILL	Dr HUGH ANTHONY CLEGG	Dr JAMES PETER SPEID JAMIESON
ARCHIE MURRELL ACHESON MOORE	Dr CHARLES HILL (until November 1950) Dr ANGUS MACRAE (from November 1950)	Dr HUGH ANTHONY CLEGG	Dr EDWARD ANDREW GREGG
r ARCHIE MURRELL ACHESON MOORE	Dr ANGUS MACRAE	Dr HUGH ANTHONY CLEGG	
r ARCHIE MURRELL ACHESON MOORE	Dr ANGUS MACRAE	Dr HUGH ANTHONY CLEGG	
r ARCHIE MURRELL ACHESON MOORE	Dr ANGUS MACRAE	Dr HUGH ANTHONY CLEGG	Dr SOLOMON WAND
r LAWRENCE DOUGAL CALLANDER	Dr ANGUS MACRAE	Dr HUGH ANTHONY CLEGG	Sir HENRY SIMPSON NEWLAND
r LAWRENCE DOUGAL CALLANDER	Dr ANGUS MACRAE	Dr HUGH ANTHONY CLEGG	

YEAR	PLACES OF ANNUAL MEETINGS	SESSION	PRESIDENT	CHAIRMAN OF REPRESENTATIVE BODY	CHAIRMAN OF COUNCIL
1956	Brighton	1956-7	Dr ALEXANDER HISLOP HALL	Dr IAN DINGWALL GRANT	Dr SOLOMON WAND
1957	Newcastle-upon-Tyne	1957-8	Mr WELLDON PATRICK TYRONE WATTS	Dr ARTHUR BEAUCHAMP	Dr SOLOMON WAND
1958	Birmingham Southampton (Annual Clinical Meeting)	1958-9	Professor (later Sir) ARTHUR PEREGRINE THOMSON	Dr ARTHUR BEAUCHAMP	Dr SOLOMON WAND
1959	Edinburgh (Joint Annual Meeting of British and Canadian Medical Associations) Norwich (Annual Clinical Meeting)	1959-60	HRH PRINCE PHILIP, Duke of Edinburgh	Dr ARTHUR BEAUCHAMP	Dr SOLOMON WAND
1960	Torquay Middlesbrough (Annual Clinical Meeting)	1960-1	Sir ARTHUR PORRITT	Dr ALFRED TALBOT ROGERS	Dr SOLOMON WAND
1961	Auckland (Annual Meeting and Biennial Conference of New Zealand Branch) Sheffield (Annual Representative Meeting) Canterbury (Annual Clinical Meeting)	1961-2	Sir GEORGE DOUGLAS ROBB	Dr ALFRED TALBOT ROGERS	Dr IAN DINGWALL GRANT (died 17 April 1962) Mr JOHN RAYMOND NICHOLSON LAILEY (from May 1962)
1962	Belfast Newport, Mon. (Annual Clinical Meeting)	1962-3	Mr (later Sir) IAN FRASER	Dr ALFRED TALBOT ROGERS	Mr JOHN RAYMOND NICHOLSON LAILEY

EASURER	SECRETARY	EDITOR	GOLD MEDALLISTS
· LAWRENCE DOUGAL CALLANDER	Dr ANGUS MACRAE	Dr HUGH ANTHONY CLEGG	Sir HENRY HALLETT DALE
· LAWRENCE DOUGAL CALLANDER	Dr ANGUS MACRAE	Dr HUGH ANTHONY CLEGG	Lord ADRIAN
r LAWRENCE DOUGAL CALLANDER	Dr ANGUS MACRAE (until 12 November 1958) Dr DEREK PAUL STEVENSON (from 13 November 1958)	Dr HUGH ANTHONY CLEGG	
r LAWRENCE DOUGAL CALLANDER	Dr DEREK PAUL STEVENSON	Dr HUGH ANTHONY CLEGG	
r LAWRENCE DOUGAL CALLANDER	Dr DEREK PAUL STEVENSON	Dr HUGH ANTHONY CLEGG	
r LAWRENCE DOUGAL CALLANDER	Dr DEREK PAUL STEVENSON	Dr HUGH ANTHONY CLEGG	Mr LAWRENCE DOUGAL CALLANDER Dr IAN DINGWALL GRANT (posthumous)
r LAWRENCE DOUGAL CALLANDER	Dr DEREK PAUL STEVENSON	Dr HUGH ANTHONY CLEGG	

YEAR	PLACES OF ANNUAL MEETINGS	SESSION	PRESIDENT	CHAIRMAN OF REPRESENTATIVE BODY	CHAIRMAN OF COUNCIL
1963	Oxford Stoke-on-Trent (Annual Clinical Meeting)	1963-4	Sir GEORGE WHITE PICKERING	Dr RONALD GEORGE GIBSON	Mr JOHN RAYMOND NICHOLSO[N] LAILEY
1964	Manchester Northampton (Annual Clinical Meeting)	1964-5	Dr ERIC ARTHUR GERRARD	Dr RONALD GEORGE GIBSON	Mr JOHN RAYMOND NICHOLSO[N] LAILEY
1965	Swansea Dundee (Annual Clinical Meeting)	1965-6	Sir CLEMENT PRICE THOMAS	Dr RONALD GEORGE GIBSON	Mr JOHN RAYMOND NICHOLSO[N] LAILEY
1966	Karachi (Joint Annual Meeting of British and Pakistan Medical Associations) Exeter (Annual Representative Meeting) Worcester (Annual Clinical Meeting)	1966-7	Professor HAMID ALI KHAN	Dr ALFRED NORMAN MATHIAS	Dr RONALD GEORGE GIBSON
1967	Bristol Londonderry (Annual Clinical Meeting)	1967-8	Mr ROBERT VICTOR COOKE	Dr ALFRED NORMAN MATHIAS	Dr RONALD GEORGE GIBSON
1968	Sydney (Joint Annual Meeting of British and Australian Medical Associations) Eastbourne (Annual Representative Meeting) Cheltenham (Annual Clinical Meeting)	1968-9	Sir CLARENCE OSCAR FERRERO RIEGER	Dr ALFRED NORMAN MATHIAS	Dr RONALD GEORGE GIBSON

EASURER	SECRETARY	EDITOR	GOLD MEDALLISTS
SOLOMON WAND	Dr DEREK PAUL STEVENSON	Dr HUGH ANTHONY CLEGG	Sir ARTHUR PORRITT, Bt Lord FLOREY
SOLOMON WAND	Dr DEREK PAUL STEVENSON	Dr HUGH ANTHONY CLEGG	
SOLOMON WAND	Dr DEREK PAUL STEVENSON	Dr HUGH ANTHONY CLEGG (until 31 December 1965) Dr MARTIN WARE (from 1 January 1966)	Dr HUGH ANTHONY CLEGG
SOLOMON WAND	Dr DEREK PAUL STEVENSON	Dr MARTIN WARE	Lord COHEN of Birkenhead
r SOLOMON WAND	Dr DEREK PAUL STEVENSON	Dr MARTIN WARE	
r SOLOMON WAND	Dr DEREK PAUL STEVENSON	Dr MARTIN WARE	

YEAR	PLACES OF ANNUAL MEETINGS	SESSION	PRESIDENT	CHAIRMAN OF REPRESENTATIVE BODY	CHAIRMAN OF COUNCIL
1969	Aberdeen Malta (Annual Clinical Meeting)	1969-70	Sir JAMES WILLIAM HOWIE	Dr ARTHUR McDOUGALL MAIDEN	Dr RONALD GEORGE GIBSON
1970	Harrogate Bath (Annual Clinical Meeting)	1970-1	Sir JOHN RICHARDSON, Bt	Dr ARTHUR McDOUGALL MAIDEN	Dr RONALD GEORGE GIBSON
1971	Leicester Aberystwyth (Annual Clinical Meeting)	1971-2	Sir JOHN PEEL	Dr ARTHUR McDOUGALL MAIDEN	Mr WALPOLE SINCLAIR LEWIN
1972	Southampton Cyprus (Annual Clinical Meeting) Inverness (Annual Postgraduate Meeting)	1972-3	Sir THOMAS HOLMES SELLORS	Dr JOHN SIMPSON NOBLE	Mr WALPOLE SINCLAIR LEWIN
1973	Vancouver (Joint Annual Meeting of British and Canadian Medical Associations) Folkestone (Annual Representative Meeting) Coventry (Annual Clinical Meeting) Guernsey (Annual Postgraduate Meeting)	1973-4	Dr PETER JOHN BANKS	Dr JOHN SIMPSON NOBLE	Mr WALPOLE SINCLAIR LEWIN
1974	Hull Jamaica (Annual Clinical Meeting) Isle of Man (Annual Postgraduate Meeting)	1974-5	Sir RONALD ERNEST TUNBRIDGE	Dr JOHN SIMPSON NOBLE	Mr WALPOLE SINCLAIR LEWIN

TREASURER	SECRETARY	EDITOR	GOLD MEDALLISTS
Dr SOLOMON WAND	Dr DEREK PAUL STEVENSON	Dr MARTIN WARE	Dr RONALD GEORGE GIBSON
Dr SOLOMON WAND	Dr DEREK PAUL STEVENSON	Dr MARTIN WARE	
Dr SOLOMON WAND	Dr DEREK PAUL STEVENSON	Dr MARTIN WARE	
Dr JACK ELIUS MILLER	Dr DEREK PAUL STEVENSON	Dr MARTIN WARE	
Dr JACK ELIUS MILLER	Dr DEREK PAUL STEVENSON	Dr MARTIN WARE	
Dr JACK ELIUS MILLER	Dr DEREK PAUL STEVENSON	Dr MARTIN WARE	Dr JAMES CLARK CAMERON

YEAR	PLACES OF ANNUAL MEETINGS	SESSION	PRESIDENT	CHAIRMAN OF REPRESENTATIVE BODY	CHAIRMAN OF COUNCIL
1975	Leeds Aarhus (Annual Clinical Meeting with Danish Medical Association)	1975-6	Sir JOHN ARTHUR STALL-WORTHY	Dr ALEXANDER AITKEN CLARK	Mr WALPOLE SINCLAIR LEWIN
1976	Dublin (Conjoint Annual Meeting of British, Canadian and Irish Medical Associations) London (Annual Representative Meeting) Exeter (Annual Clinical Meeting)	1976-7	Mr BARRY O'DONNELL	Dr ALEXANDER AITKEN CLARK	Dr JAMES CLAR CAMERON
1977	Glasgow Leiden (Annual Clinical Meeting with Royal Netherlands Medical Association)	1977-8	Sir WILLIAM FERGUSON ANDERSON	Dr ALEXANDER AITKEN CLARK	Dr JAMES CLAR CAMERON
1978	Cardiff Ipswich (Annual Scientific Meeting) Gibraltar (Annual Clinical Meeting)	1978-9	Professor WILLIAM LINFORD LLEWELYN REES	Dr EDWARD BRIAN LEWIS	Dr JAMES CLAR CAMERON
1979	Liverpool Nottingham (Annual Scientific Meeting) Hong Kong (Annual Clinical Meeting)	1979-80	Dame ALICE JOSEPHINE MARY TAYLOR BARNES	Dr EDWARD BRIAN LEWIS	Mr ANTHONY HERBERT GRABHAM
1980	Newcastle-upon-Tyne	1980-1	Sir JOHN NICHOLAS WALTON	Dr EDWARD BRIAN LEWIS	Mr ANTHONY HERBERT GRABHAM

TREASURER	SECRETARY	EDITOR	GOLD MEDALLISTS
Dr JACK ELIUS MILLER	Dr DEREK PAUL STEVENSON	Dr STEPHEN PENFORD LOCK	Dr DEREK PAUL STEVENSON
Dr JACK ELIUS MILLER	Dr ELSTON GREY-TURNER	Dr STEPHEN PENFORD LOCK	
Dr JACK ELIUS MILLER	Dr ELSTON GREY-TURNER	Dr STEPHEN PENFORD LOCK	Dr DENIS PARSONS BURKITT Sir JOHN CHARNLEY
Dr JACK ELIUS MILLER	Dr ELSTON GREY-TURNER	Dr STEPHEN PENFORD LOCK	Mr WALPOLE SINCLAIR LEWIN
Dr JACK ELIUS MILLER	Dr ELSTON GREY-TURNER (until 31 December 1979) Dr JOHN DAVID JAYNE HAVARD (from 1 January 1980)	Dr STEPHEN PENFORD LOCK	Sir THOMAS HOLMES SELLORS Lord HUNT of Fawley
Dr JACK ELIUS MILLER	Dr JOHN DAVID JAYNE HAVARD	Dr STEPHEN PENFORD LOCK	Sir JOHN ARTHUR STALLWORTHY

YEAR	PLACES OF ANNUAL MEETINGS	SESSION	PRESIDENT	CHAIRMAN OF REPRESENTATIVE BODY	CHAIRMAN OF COUNCIL
1981	Brighton San Diego (Annual Clinical Meeting with San Diego County Medical Society)	1981-2	Sir JOHN NICHOLAS WALTON	Dr JOHN HENRY MARKS	Mr ANTHONY HERBERT GRABHAM

ꞮREASURER	SECRETARY	EDITOR	GOLD MEDALLISTS
ꞏ ROBERT ANTHONY KEABLE-ELLIOTT	Dr JOHN DAVID JAYNE HAVARD	Dr STEPHEN PENFORD LOCK	

Index

ACCESSION NUMBER
10240
REFERENCE NUMBER
WZ23